Updates in Clinical Dermatology

Updates in Clinical Dermatology aims to promote the rapid and efficient transfer of medical research into clinical practice. It is published in four volumes per year. Covering new developments and innovations in all fields of clinical dermatology, it provides the clinician with a review and summary of recent research and its implications for clinical practice. Each volume is focused on a clinically relevant topic and explains how research results impact diagnostics, treatment options and procedures as well as patient management. The reader-friendly volumes are highly structured with core messages, summaries, tables, diagrams and illustrations and are written by internationally well-known experts in the field. A volume editor supervises the authors in his/her field of expertise in order to ensure that each volume provides cutting-edge information most relevant and useful for clinical dermatologists. Contributions to the series are peer reviewed by an editorial board.

Peter J. Panagotacos • Howard Maibach
Editors

Hair Loss

Advances and Treatments

Editors
Peter J. Panagotacos
University of California San Francisco
San Francisco, CA, USA

Howard Maibach
University of California, San Francisco
San Francisco, CA, USA

ISSN 2523-8884 ISSN 2523-8892 (electronic)
Updates in Clinical Dermatology
ISBN 978-3-031-74313-9 ISBN 978-3-031-74314-6 (eBook)
https://doi.org/10.1007/978-3-031-74314-6

This Springer imprint is published by the registered company Springer Nature Switzerland AG
The registered company address is: Gewerbestrasse 11, 6330 Cham, Switzerland

Preface

When Dr. Howard Maibach, a senior editor of this series "Updates in Dermatology", asked me to write a volume on hair covering what might be new to the subject in the past few decades, I immediately responded in the affirmative. Dermatology became my choice of specialty after having completed a rotation at UCSF Dermatology Clinic during my internship because of Dr. Maibach as a role model. He also steered me to a residency program at Charity Hospital in New Orleans which was well suited for my clinical interests. It was there that Dr. James Burks became a mentor in hair transplantation. In 1980, Dr. Maibach asked me if I would give a lecture at an international meeting in his place. Again, I consented, but only if I could give the lecture on hair transplantation rather than Mycosis Fungoides. That led to over 40 years of lecturing at international meetings and the publication of a book on hair loss meant for patients. My subspecialty in medical and surgical hair restoration, therefore, is in large part due to his guidance early in my career.

In deciding what should be included in this volume, I wanted to include what was new in the diagnosis and treatment of general medical dermatology as well as for androgenetic alopecia. The treatment of the most common form of alopecia, androgenetic alopecia, is covered in Chap. 2 by Dr. Marc Avram and the surgical treatment in Chap. 3 by Dr. Konstantinos Anastassakis. Frontal fibrosing alopecia needed to be covered as it is a new entity that first appeared only a few decades ago. Trichoscopy also needed to be included as it is a new technique for diagnosis in dermatology. Low level laser light therapy became a popular treatment for androgenetic alopecia in the past two decades and is covered in Chaps. 4 and 5.

The next most common form of alopecia we see is alopecia areata which is covered in Chap. 6 with a discussion of JAK inhibitors, PRP and exosomes. To conclude the subject matter covered, I included a chapter on what research is being done today in hair genetics and lastly a chapter on what we may see in the near future in hair cloning.

As editor of this book, I have not attempted to have my biases in treatment affect the other contributors' viewpoints. For example, I do not prescribe low-dose oral Minoxidil because I do not believe the risk vs benefit ratio warrants it. I also do not use most of the popular nutraceuticals which are popular today. These are individual preferences of relatively new treatments, and the reader should be aware of the therapies that are currently being used by hair restoration specialists.

I wrote the introductory chapter of this book on the history of hair loss treatments, a subject I thought I was well versed. However, in doing the research on what's new in the field, I discovered something new about what was old and overlooked. In 1941, Dr. Rattner wrote an excellent article "Ordinary Baldness", in the Archives of Dermatology and Syphilology. In this article, he mentions Dr. Okuda as having done transplants in the 1930s, who only recently has been acknowledged in most publications. He also mentions Dr. Tauber as having "good results from full thickness grafts from the back and sides for the head". It took many months of requesting reprints of the article published by Dr. Tauber before I finally found a librarian in New York City who was able to send me a copy. In the British Medical Journal of Ceylon, Dr. Tauber in describing his method of a rotation flap from the temporal-occipital area to the frontal scalp states "… the flap method is the first and real treatment of choice in alopecia praematura gen. Incipiens" (now known as androgenetic alopecia). This was news to me, and when I read further I found he had given lectures on the subject in Cairo in 1937. So, I'm hoping others in the field will start to recognize Dr. Tauber as the father of hair restoration surgery.

As I finish writing this book, I am closing my 50-year private practice in San Francisco. It is with mixed feelings that I leave the active practice of seeing patients and giving lectures, and I hope I have made a positive contribution in a field I enjoyed so much.

The editor welcomes suggestions for the next edition.

San Francisco, CA, USA Peter J. Panagotacos

Contents

The History of Hair Loss Treatments

1

Peter J. Panagotacos

The History of Medical Hair Loss Treatments

Since the beginning of recorded history, men and women have searched out cures for hair loss. The oldest known prescription is 5000 years old and was for hair loss. Written in the Ebers Papyrus, about 1500 BC, is a prescription for Queen Ses, mother of the Egyptian King Teta, 2000 years earlier. It is not known whether she had Androgenetic Alopecia or Alopecia Areata. There are several prescriptions for hair loss in the Papyrus. The one for Queen Ses was a mixture of "Toes-of-a dog, refuse-of-dates (and) hoof-of-an-ass" (Fig. 1.1) [1, 2].

The Ebers Papyrus is the oldest complete medical text ever found, and it is devoted to treatments for various skin diseases and cosmetic conditions. It includes the oldest known written prescription for treating baldness: a mixture of iron oxide, red lead, onions, alabaster, honey, and fat from a variety of animals, including snakes, crocodiles, hippopotamuses, and lions. The mixture was to be swallowed after first reciting a magical invocation to the Sun God.

Another cure for baldness from the Ebers Papyrus involved swallowing the following "mixture of iron, red lead, onions, alabaster, and honey" while reciting the invocation below:

> "O Shining one, thou who hoverest above!
> O Xare! O Disk of the Sun!
> O Protector of the Divine Neb-Apt!"[3, 4]

Later in the Ebers Papyrus, there are remedies suggested for Alopecia Areata. It was known as "bite hair loss." In 30 CE, Celsus described Alopecia Areata presenting as scalp alopecia in spots, or the "windings of a snake" and suggested treatment with caustic compounds and scarification" [5].

Wigs and hairpieces of various sorts were popular among upper-class Assyrians, Sumerians, Cretans, Carthaginians, and Persians in the Fertile Crescent area of the Middle East." Both sexes seem to have often worn large wigs, as in ancient Egypt" [6].

Wigs were popular among Egyptian royalty at this time as well, and a number of elaborate and well-preserved hairpieces have been found in tombs by archaeologists. Many Egyptian wigs were ornate creations constructed of linen fiber as well as human hair, while others made of metal were more helmet-like. As an example of the importance hair played in certain cultures, certain Egyptian royalty also used "facial hair wigs," specifically fake beards, to signify power. Both male and female royalty wore fake beards [7].

Hippocrates, about 400 BC, described Alopecia Areata and coined the term alopecia

P. J. Panagotacos (✉)
University of California San Francisco,
San Francisco, CA, USA

P. J. Panagotacos, H. Maibach (eds.), *Hair Loss*, Updates in Clinical Dermatology,
https://doi.org/10.1007/978-3-031-74314-6_1

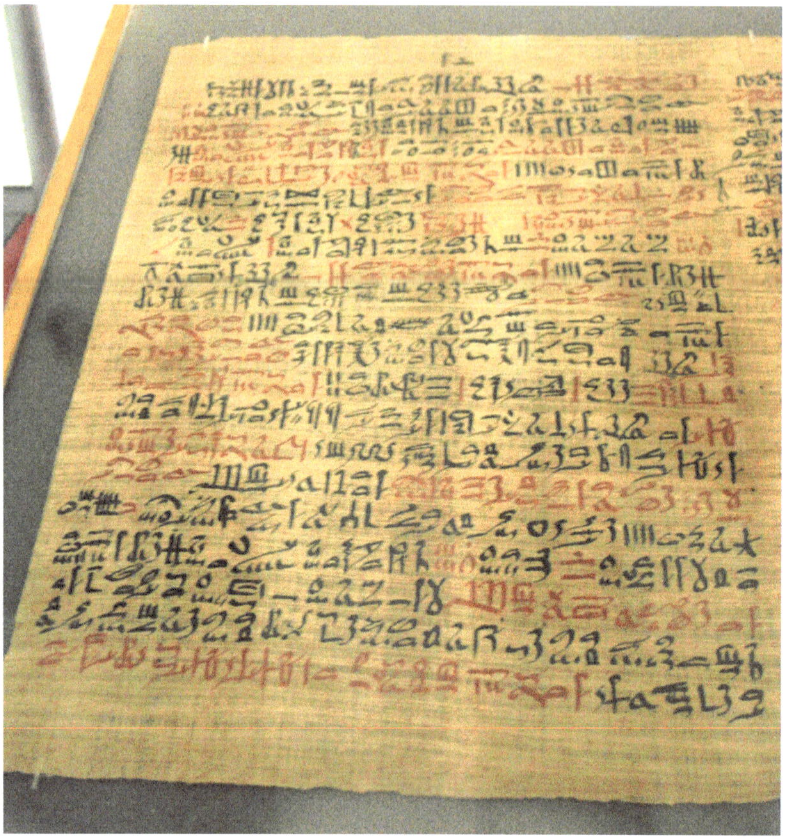

Fig. 1.1 Ebers Papyrus (2023, March 16). In *Wikipedia*

(from the Greek for fox). The term most likely derives from a reference to a mange causing spotty hair loss in foxes [8]. Hippocrates has been depicted in busts and drawings as being very bald. There has been some question as to whether Hippocrates was in fact as bald as depicted in most drawings and busts done of him over the past 2000 years because there were none done while he was alive which remain intact. Most authors assume he was very bald, and the term "Hippocratic baldness" used for centuries not only refers to inherited baldness but to his personal extensive baldness with only a rim of hair in the periphery (Fig. 1.2).

A conventionalized image in a Roman "portrait" bust (nineteenth-century engraving).

We know he prescribed topical treatments such as a mixture of opium, horseradish, pigeon droppings, beetroot, and various spices that were applied to the head. Hippocrates eventually lost it to the extent that today we refer to advanced male pattern baldness as "Hippocratic baldness" [9, 10].

In his collection of astute observations called the "Aphorisms of Hippocrates," he noted that Persian Army eunuchs guarding the king's harem never experienced hair loss. In Aphorism XXVIII, he states: "Eunuchs are not affected by gout, nor do they become bald" [11]. We now know that it is true that castration before or shortly after puberty reduces testosterone and Dihydrotestosterone (DHT) levels in the blood to such a degree that genetic hair loss is prevented [12, 13].

In ancient Rome, hair continued to be a symbol of power and virility. This presented a problem for Julius Caesar, whose hairline was receding even as his empire was expanding. He developed some cosmetic solutions to his hair loss problem. First, he began growing it long in the back and combing it straight forward over his bald spot. Sort of a "comb forward" instead of a "comb-over". This didn't seem to work all that well, perhaps because hair gel would not be invented for another 2000 years [14]. According to Suetonius, Cesar was awarded the Civic

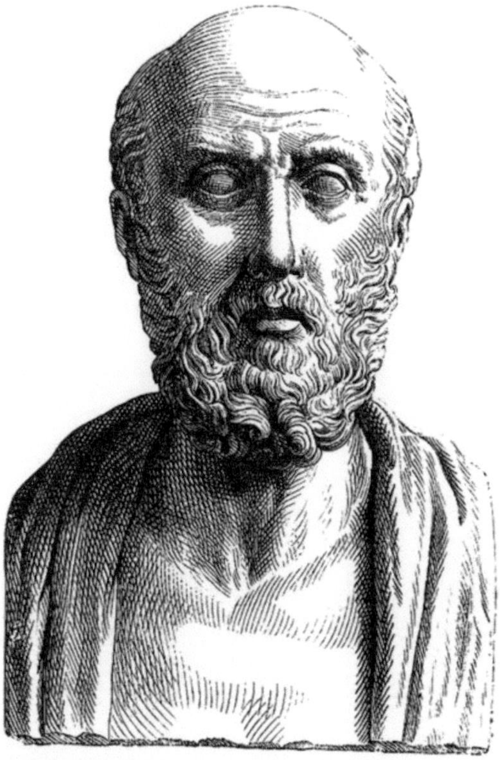

Fig. 1.2 Hippocrates. In *Wikipedia*. https://en.wikipedia.org/wiki/Hippocrates

Crown, a laurel wreath, for his service in the Siege of Mytilene in 81 BC. For the sake of his vanity, he convinced the Roman Senate to allow him to wear it during his role as emperor to hide his baldness [15].

In 1624, King Louis XIII of France began wearing a full wig to camouflage his thinning hair, which began at age 23. Soon, other members of the court followed his example, regardless of their own hair condition. Wigs became symbols of power. The height, length, and bulk of wigs increased with each decade, and giant powdered wigs became the fashion in all French courts [16].

In 1660, King Charles II in England was restored to the throne after his exile in Versailles, where he had been exposed to the French wig craze. The English were not to be outdone by the French. Within a short time, more elaborate giant powdered wigs were worn in English courts than had ever appeared in France [17]. Upper-class American colonists picked up the wig fashion, and by the late eighteenth century, most wealthy people wore false hair to signify their elevated class. However, the American War of Independence and the subsequent French Revolution caused the look of royalty and elevated class distinction to fall out of favor, and wigs pretty much disappeared from the scene [18].

The nineteenth century was the heyday of the "snake oil" salesmen, and for the next 100 years, bottles of hair loss cures with names like "Mrs. Allen's World Hair Restorer," "Ayers Hair Vigour," "East India Oil Hair Restoration," "Skookum Root Hair Growth," "Westphall Auxiliator," "Imperial Hair Regenerator" and the ever popular "Barry's Tricopherous" were sold to hopeful buyers seeking a cure for their hair loss from "modern medicine."

A hundred years later, "snake oil" cures for hair loss continue to be marketed, except now they're sold by beauty salons and barber shops, by mail, cable television, over the Internet, and with great success to listeners of talk radio programs. Barry's Tricopherous, which was founded in 1801, is still being sold in the US as well as Central America. A bottle I obtained from a pharmacy in Honduras in 1970 states on the label, "Guarantees to Restore the Hair to Bald Heads and to Make it Grow Thick, Long and Soft.". The bottle contains alcohol, water, and coloring. For sale on Amazon, the claim is now a "hair dressing for men, women, and children. Instead of using water'. "Tricopherous was produced by Barry's of New York, and although the recipe changed over time, in 1893 it consisted of 97% alcohol, about 1.5% castor oil, 1% tincture of Spanish fly" (Figs. 1.3, 1.4, and 1.5) [19].

During the Victorian era in England in the 1850s, a popular hair loss treatment was cold Indian tea applied to the scalp, followed by a vigorous rubbing of the balding area with fresh lemon juice. This hair loss treatment would probably be better to sip on a hot day than apply to the scalp. It didn't grow hair. The English may have borrowed this remedy from their time in India [20].

The wearing of hats by nearly all men in urban areas around this time was blamed for causing hair loss. From the mid-1800s to the mid-1900s,

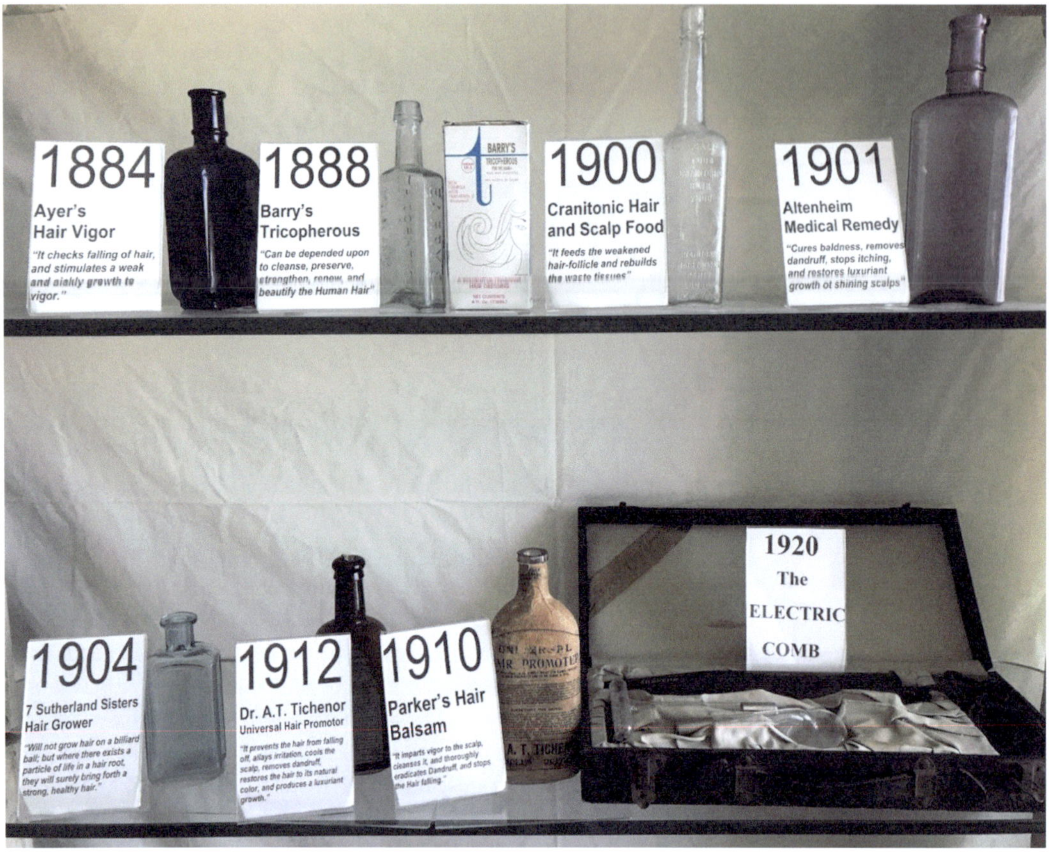
1884
Ayer's
Hair Vigor
"It checks falling of hair, and stimulates a weak
1888
Barry's
Tricopherous
"Can be depended upon to cleanse, preserve,
beautify the Human Hair"
BARRY'S
1900
Cranitonic Hair
and Scalp Food
"It feeds the weakened hair-follicle and rebuilds
1901
Altenheim
Medical Remedy
"Cures baldness, removes dandruff, stops itching, and restores luxuriant growth of shining scalps"
1920
The
ELECTRIC
COMB
1904
7 Sutherland Sisters
Hair Grower
1912
Dr. A.T. Tichenor
Universal Hair Promotor
1910
Parker's Hair
Balsam

Fig. 1.3 Panagotacos personal collection shown at the 2006 ISHRS annual meeting in San Diego [79]

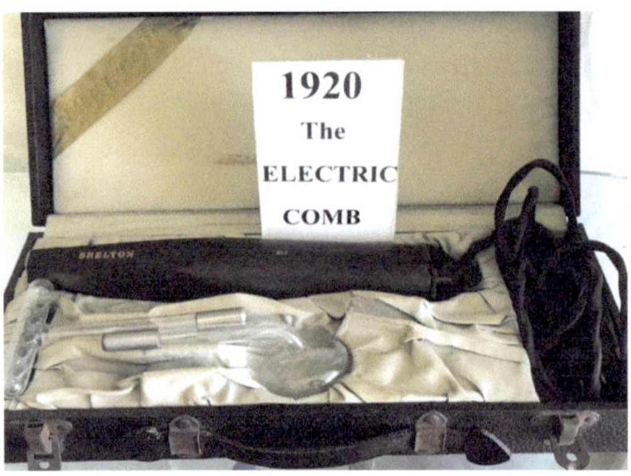

Fig. 1.4 1920 Shelton Electric Comb (author's private collection) delivers an electric shock to the skin and hair

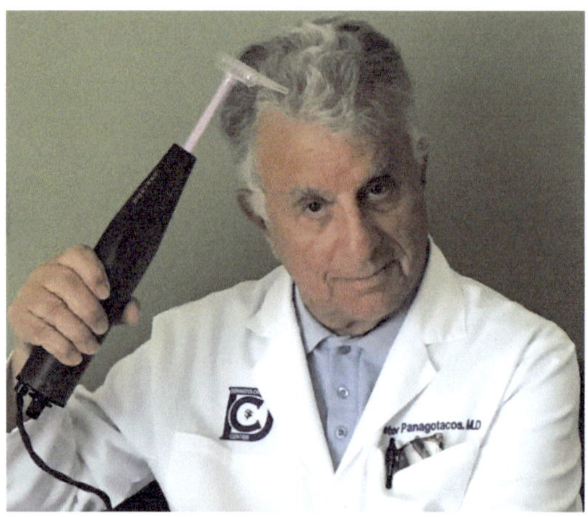

Fig. 1.5 1920 Shelton Electric Comb (author's private collection) delivers an electric shock to the skin and hair

it was thought the hat constricted blood vessels, leading to baldness [21]. Anti-hat advocates urged men to let their hair follicles "breathe" and to allow their scalps to enjoy the benefits of "sun baths" and "air baths." No one seemed to notice the countless men who wore hats who did not lose their hair [22].

The industrial age brought new inventions to the marketplace, solving a countless number of life's little problems. In St. Louis, the Evans Vacuum Cap Company marketed a suction device in 1905 that: "…exercises the scalp and helps to circulate stagnant blood, feeding the shrunken hair roots, and causing the hair to grow…".

This theory stayed alive for decades. Twenty years later, it was published in the Lancet [23] and mentioned by Rattner in his January 1941 article in the Archives of Derm&Syph.: "In 1936 there was described a new method of treatment using the principle of vacuum pressure. No mention was made of the time required to produce the results or of the permanency of the effect, and there were no illustrative photographs. The method, however, was immediately exploited. Vacuum pressure machines quickly found their way into many barber shops" (Fig. 1.6) [22].

In his book Hair Culture, published in 1922, health advocate Bernarr MacFadden wrote: "There is more quackery rampant in connection with hair and scalp care—both by the medical profession and by drug and lotion manufacturers—than there is in any other specialty ever devised for the exploitation of ailing humans". He then went on to say that most hair loss is caused by a lack of physical vigor and unhygienic scalp conditions. He prescribed scalp massage, hair pulling, and vigorous brushing of the scalp [23].

In 1925, the Allied Merke Institute in New York City began selling the Thermocap Treatment device, claiming to stimulate circulation, cleanse clogged-up pores, and nourish dormant hair bulbs with heat and blue light from a special actinic quartz ray bulb. The quartz ray treatment took only 15 min a day. Along with the Thermocap device, the complete Treatment included the Merke Tonic, Merke Dandruff Treatment, and Merke Shampoo Cream.

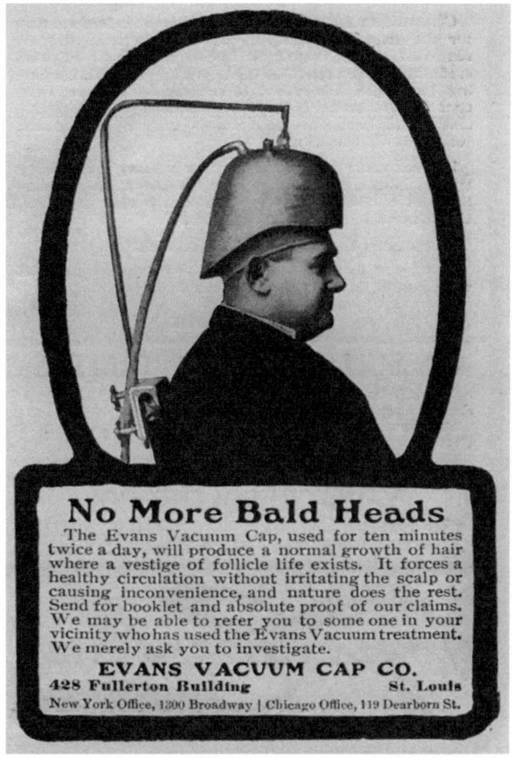

Fig. 1.6 Scientific American, March 24, 1906, p. 261

In 1936, in Cincinnati, the Crosley Radio Corporation diversified a bit from radios, and offered an electric scalp vacuum device claimed to be a "Therapeutic Method for Hair Growth" and called it the X-ER-VAC. It was available for home, local clinic, barbershop, and beauty shop use (Fig. 1.7).

James Hamilton was a Yale anatomist who, while visiting the Kansas State Asylum for the Education of Idiotic and Imbecile Youth in 1942, noted a bald twin visiting his brother who had a full head of hair. It was a common practice in Kansas from 1913–1950s to castrate male patients to keep them docile. Hamilton proved baldness was related to the length of time the subject was exposed to testosterone.

He went on to study identical twins, some of whom were castrated early in life in a 1969 study to prove the concept of the need for an inherited pattern plus testosterone to express the pattern of loss [12].

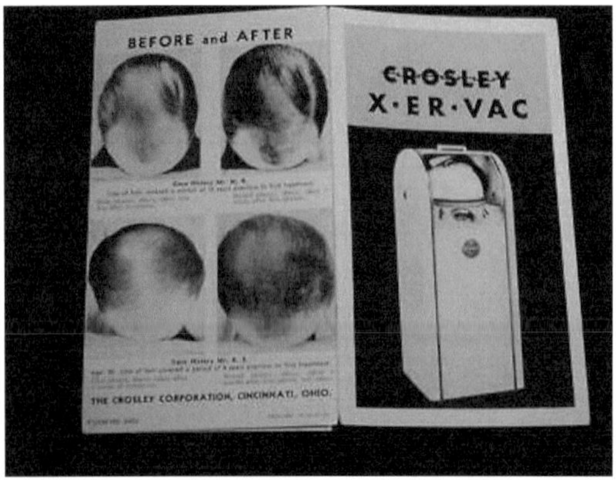

Fig. 1.7 Crosley X-er-Vac photo of a 1937 advertising brochure- a device that advertised an ability to grow hair through Vacuum and Pressure and stimulation of the scalp (author's private collection)

Whereas Hippocrates knew baldness was due to being hot-blooded and castration worked to prevent this, he assumed the hot blood burned the hair roots, it was James Hamilton who proved it was Testosterone in the blood, which was the hormone that was the actual culprit.

Finally, we have the two medications that have actually been proven to the FDA to work,

- Minoxidil-approved in 1988 to stimulate hair
- Finasteride-approved in 1998 to prevent baldness

Minoxidil

Minoxidil, a medication taken in pill form (Loniten) for treating severe high blood pressure, also caused hypertrichosis, in 24% of patients [24]. Clinical trials were established to prove to the U.S. Food and Drug Administration the safety and effectiveness of this promising hair loss treatment medication, but it would be years before the manufacturer could advertise it as a treatment for hair loss. The oral medication was found to cause tachycardia and hypotension in a number of patients and hypertrichosis in many. Sobota commented it "causes minimal pharmacologic **effects** except in the cardiovascular system. The drug does produce hirsutism in humans, an annoying **side effect**, especially in women" [25]. In a review article in 1981 "Ninety-one episodes of pericardial disease have been reported in 1,869 experimental subjects (4.8%). Pericardial tamponade occurred in 21, with eight associated deaths. There are no specific patient characteristics that predict the likelihood of effusion. Since the reaction is both idiosyncratic and potentially fatal, it seems appropriate to continue to limit the use of minoxidil" [26]. The same year, another review article with only 47 patients came to the conclusion the medication was safe [27]. Yet 7 years later, in 1998, Rogaine came on the market as a 2% minoxidil solution with a much safer profile [28, 29].

Combination therapies using topical Minoxidil plus additives have been used for decades. In 1979, I began grinding up Loniten tablets to make a 2% minoxidil solution, dissolving them in a 60 ml bottle of solvent, Nerutorgena Vehicle N, used by dermatologists at that time to make topical minocycline or clindamycin solution for acne. It was composed of mainly alcohol plus propylene glycol. Nia Terazakis began adding tretinoin to a minoxidil solution in the mid-1980s and finding a synergistic action with better growth than with minoxidil alone; results were published in 1986 [30].

Over the past four decades, I began adding tretinoin in small concentrations to either 2% or 5% minoxidil and then an anti-androgen mix that I learned from Dr. Orentreich, which included Beta-dihydroprogesterone 0.05% + Prequenolone 0.1% + progesterone 0.5%. Spironolactone (or more recently, Canrenone, a stronger but less smelly analog) was also added. I also added Betamethasone Valerate, which helped in prevention of scarring of the fine hairs as they went into their final life cycles. When Finasteride and Dutasteride became available in 1992 and 2002, respectively, they too were added. The minoxidil was the stimulant for weak hairs to grow better, whereas the other compounds prevented aging of the hair follicles by blocking the messenger of death, DHT, from getting to the androgen receptor sites on the hair shafts.

Microneedling and topical minoxidil by themselves have been shown to stimulate hair growth, but in combination, the effect was greater, as reported in a review article of 466 patients [31].

Finasteride

A study in the 1970s of a familial group in the Dominican Republic with an enzyme deficiency of 5 alpha-reductase type II proved it was the enzyme that made DiHydroTestosterone- DHT, necessary for the development of male genitalia in utero. The boys in this family never developed prostate cancer, nor did they go bald [32]. Not long after, Merck did a study for the FDA using Finasteride to block the enzyme and came out with 5 mg Finasteride (Proscar) to treat BPH in 1992 and 1 mg Finasteride (Propecia) in 1998 to prevent male pattern baldness [33, 34]. At the American Academy of Dermatology annual meeting in New Orleans in March 2000, the author of this chapter gave a lecture on Hair Restoration and the advantages of using 1 mg Finasteride to prevent ongoing baldness when doing hair transplantation using, as an example, identical twins who had surgery done in the previous 3 years. One of the identical twins had his first hair transplant procedure in 1996, and in 1997 began taking 1 mg Finasteride (before Propecia was released). Two years later, in early 2000, the second twin had a hair transplant procedure. In comparing the photographs of both, it was obvious the first twin had regrowth of hair with a smaller bald spot, and the second twin's bald spot was significantly larger than it was 3 years earlier [35], When asked by Merck, they declined to be part of an advertising campaign as part of an identical twin study using finasteride. As this was the first identical twin study of Finasteride and AGA I think James Hamilton would have been envious that he did not have access to the use of Finasteride when doing his twin studies (Fig. 1.8) [36].

The ability of finasteride to stop baldness in 85% of patients changed the hair transplantation field tremendously as we could transplant into a balding area feeling fairly comfortable that the area would not keep enlarging. An example of a patient who continued to bald beyond what was expected and ran out of scalp donor hair is described near the end of this chapter.

Low Level Laser Light therapy to stimulate hair growth began to have a lot of media coverage in the early 2000s. There was little proof it worked until a study showing it may actually stimulate growth [35]. In 2009, Dr. Hamblin gave a lecture at the ISHRS meeting in Amsterdam, which explained the mechanism of action of LLLTx. Shortly thereafter, the author was sent a prototype of the LaserCap, the original full coverage Low Level Laser device, it proved to be a positive addition in the treatment of androgenetic alopecia, increasing the density on average about 25%, which was equivalent to the effect of 5% minoxidil lotion [37].

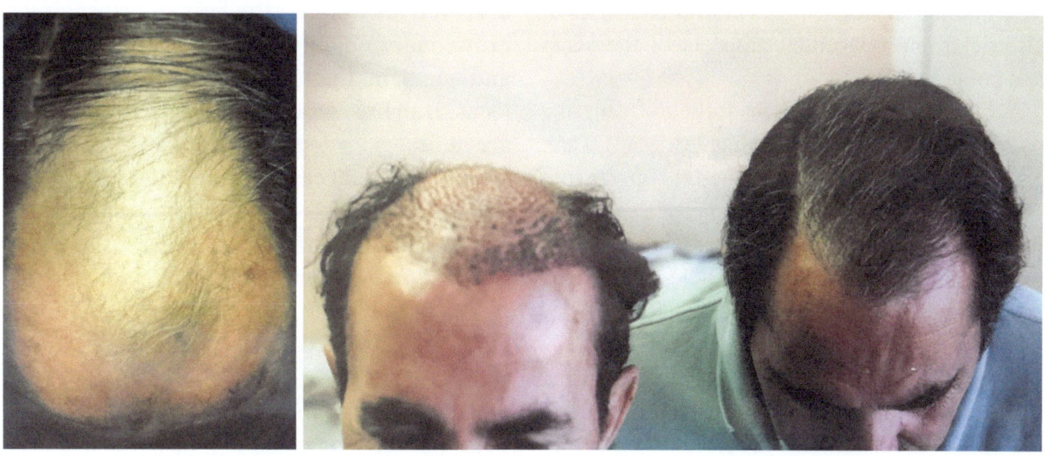

Fig. 1.8 Photo 1. Photo taken by the author in 1996 before any surgeries- both twins had the same degree of baldness. Photo 1 Jan 2000 Identical twin on left 1 week after 2000 grafts in 1999. Twin on right after 1600 grafts in 1996 and oral finasteride 1 mg daily 1997–2000—Hair Restoration lecture: Am Acad of Derm annual meeting New Orleans 2000

In a personal conversation with Dr. Michael Rabin, inventor of the LaserCap, at the ISHRS meeting in Panama in October 2022, he said there was new evidence showing increasing the use of the 30 min 220 diode cap from every other day to daily—at the same time each day- leaving a 24 h refractory period worked better than the initial studie [38]. Wearing the cap shortly after applying a minoxidil lotion seemed to act synergistically with the minoxidil. In the 10 months since changing to this new protocol, I have seen even more growth in my patients.

The History of Surgical Hair Loss Treatments

Hair transplantation experiments from one animal to another were done by Johann Dieffenbach, a plastic surgeon in East Prussia, in 1822 to show that hairs could grow when transplanted from one species to another [39].

In Japan, an ophthalmologist with an interest in hair, Dr. Shoji Okuda, published in the October issue of the Japanese Journal of Dermatology and Urology his method for using hair transplant grafts to replace hair lost from the scalp, eyebrow, mustache, and pubic hair areas. This was the first published account of the modern hair transplantation technique, Okuda, writing these five papers in 1939, claimed to have successfully used homografts for 10 years in over 200 cases of cicatricial and congenital alopecia of the scalp and pubic hair loss.

Dr. Okuda removed hair follicles from the back of his patient's heads using 2.0, 2.5, 3.0 and 3.5 mm punches and transplanted the grafts into new locations 0.5 mm smaller to give the look of having more hair on the face. He found the 1 mm punch transected too many follicles. His work went largely unnoticed in the West because of World War II [40, 41].

Most dermatologists were unaware of the work done by Okuda, however, Rattner, in his article in the Archives of Dermatology and Syphilology, January 1941, states, "Okuda obtained good cosmetic results from tiny homotransplants, and Tauber in the Ceylon Branch of the British Medical Journal, recently claimed good results from full thickness grafts of hair-bearing areas from the sides and back of the head.", which gives Okuda full credit for being the first to do successful hair transplants. This was printed in the Archives of Dermatology in 1941, a journal that almost all dermatologists would have read at that time [22].)The information about Okuda has been assumed to have been lost in Japan because of the war. He also mentions Tauber, who had good results transplanting flaps from the back and sides of the head to correct male pattern baldness a full decade before Dr. Norman Orentreich used 4 mm punch grafts.

There were other surgeons who were using flap grafting to correct scarring and traumatic wounds in the late nineteenth century and early twentieth century, but it was Dr. H. Tauber who was the originator of surgical hair restoration as a correction of Androgenetic Alopecia was known then "asalopecia praematura gen. incipiens". His theory as to the cause of Androgenetic Alopecia was incorrect as he assumed it had to do with overactive sebaceous glands. There were others who used grafts to correct alopecia areata and cicatricial alopecia before Tauber. He was the first to do it to correct AGA. He wrote, **"In the course of my plastic operations according to Passot's method, which consists of transplanting hair bearing cutis from the lateral and posterior scalp to denuded frontal areas, I observed always that the hair so transplanted grows more quickly, is of a far better quality and pigment than when it is in its original locus. Hairloss, seborrhea, skin-irritations etc. are at first retarded and afterwards stopped. I treated about 50 cases on these lines and I was and am convinced that the *flap-method is the first and real treatment of choice in alopecia praematura gen. incipiens*"** [42].

Dr. Tauber wrote this in an article in 1939 of 50 cases he reported in a lecture in 1937 in Cairo (Fig. 1.9).

This was nearly 10 years before Dr. Orentreich wrote his paper on donor dominance and at least 16 years before the description of the Juri Flap [43]. This flap became popular in the 1970s, but the only advantage to the Juri Flap (TPO flap-

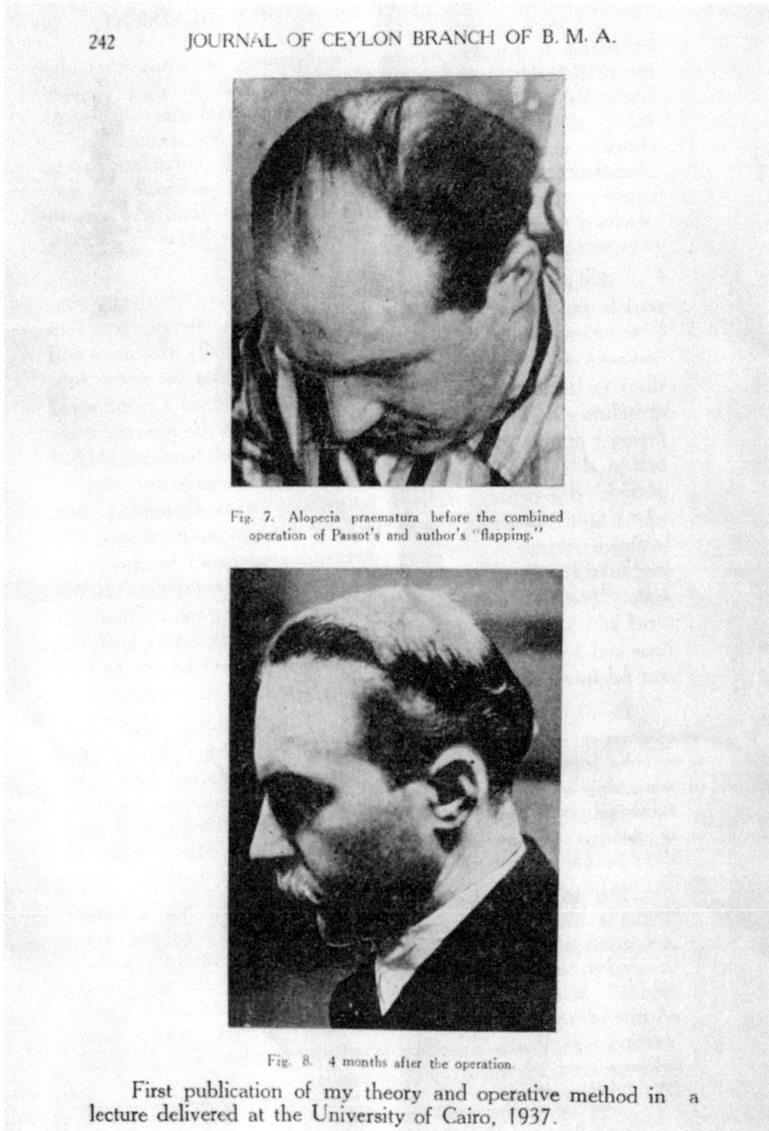
242 JOURNAL OF CEYLON BRANCH OF B. M. A.

Fig. 7. Alopecia praematura before the combined operation of Passot's and author's "flapping."

Fig. 8. 4 months after the operation.

First publication of my theory and operative method in a lecture delivered at the University of Cairo, 1937.

Fig. 1.9 Tauber, H.: Alopecia Praematura and its surgical treatment, J. Ceylon Br. Brit. M. A. 1939, 36, p. 242

Temporal-Parietal-Occipital Flap) was the patient had thick hair growing in the front of his head immediately after the procedure (Fig. 1.10) [44]. This would have taken a year to accomplish with four sessions using the standard 4 mm plug-grafts used. The disadvantage of the procedure was that the patient had excessively dense hair growing in the frontal scalp and a large linear scar in the donor area.

Many patients found this procedure preferable to living with the hair plug—tufted doll's hair look- for months to years. It was only after Follicular Unit Grafting became possible did both the Orentreich 4 mm plug and the TPO—"Tauber Flap"(aka Juri Flap)- become obsolete.

Dr. Tamura, in 1942, pioneered single hair transplants, taking them from the scalp to the pubic area in Japanese women with congenital atrichia [45].

Another observation made by Rattner in 1941 was the cause of baldness was related to glands, which included the gonads. "The striking fact that hippocratic baldness does not occur in women, children or eunuchs points directly to an endo-

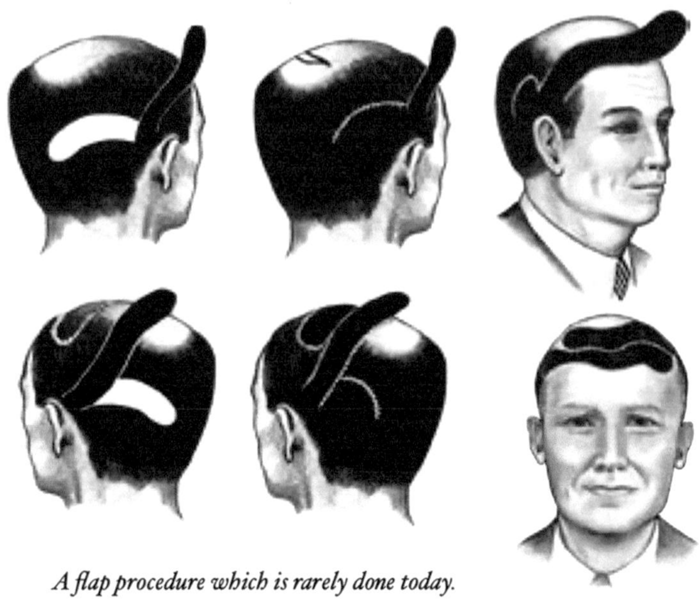

Fig. 1.10 TPO flap—a dense new hairline immediately after the procedure- as described by Tauber and Juri. Illustration by Dr. Alice Do–*Hair Loss Answers*, Panagotacos, P. Elite Books 2005, p. 99

crine factor in its production. The factor is probably in the nature, of a lack of balance of the glands, and the glands which seem most important in the control of hair growth are the adrenals, the gonads, the thyroid and the pituitary" [22]. Okuda's observation precedes, by 20 years, Hamilton's excellent study on twins [36]. Dr. Norman Orentreich was doing a study on vitiligo in 1952. His study involved transferring patches of skin from one part of a patient's body to another. It was noted that a skin graft taken from a hair-bearing area, when placed in a non-hair-bearing area, continued to grow hair at the new site. Soon after making this observation, Dr. Orentreich placed ten punch grafts bearing hair on the front part of the scalp of a patient with severe frontal hair loss. The grafts continued to grow hair in the new location. Dr. Orentreich reported the successful results of the first hair transplant procedure performed in the United States in a paper submitted to the Archives of Dermatology. The reviewers of that journal said the reported results "were not possible" and rejected the paper [46].

Dr. Orentreich was finally able in 1959 to publish his "donor dominance" theory in the New York Academy of Sciences Journal, popularizing and refining the full-size graft hair transplantation technique. The basis of his theory was that 4 mm plugs of hair follicles taken from the back of the scalp would grow when moved to the front or top of the scalp because those hair follicles were genetically programmed to keep growing hair. It was the particular hair follicles that mattered, not the location on the head. This was termed the "Donor Dominance Theory". This concept became the foundation for the entire field of hair restoration surgery. For the next 20 years, full-size grafts were the standard technique for hair transplants. In 1960, Dr. Orentreich is credited for being the first to use the term Androgenetic Alopecia in an article titled "Pathogenesis of alopecia" (Fig. 1.11) [47].

In the 1960s, despite scientific evidence that genetics was the cause of pattern hair loss, other theories continued to be presented by people whose hair loss solution happened to cure the particular theorized cause. Scalp tightness, for example, was advanced as the reason for hair loss, and surgical procedures to "loosen the scalp" with incisions were performed.

Since the 1920s, skin tumors and injured areas of the scalp were removed surgically using a procedure called a "scalp reduction" or, more accurately, "alopecia reduction". In this procedure, the damaged tissue was cut out, and the edges.

of the surgical wound were carefully sewn back together in a manner that left only a very

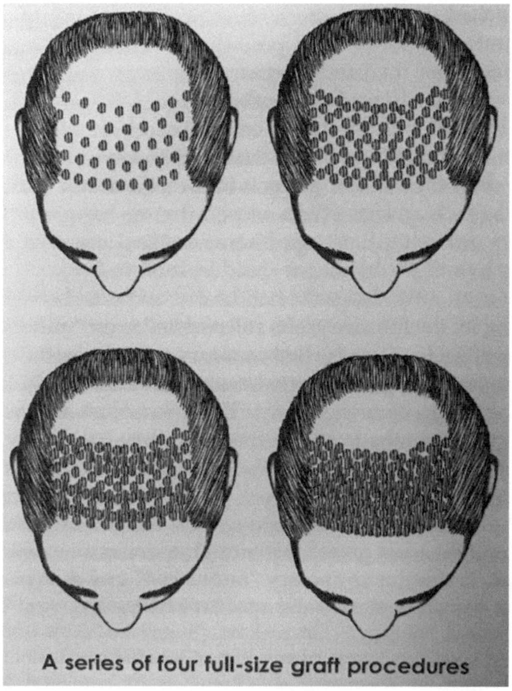

Fig. 1.11 4 mm grafts would be placed in 3.5 mm recipient holes every 3 months, filling in ¼ of the area each time—the procedure would be repeated every 6 weeks to 3 months—taking 6 months to a year to complete and another 4 months for the hair to grow out. This delay is what made the TPO flap the method of choice for men who wanted hair "immediately." Using a checkerboard as an example, the first session would fill in the red squares in every other row, the next session would be the black squares in every other row—etc. Illustration by Dr. Alice Do *Hair Loss Answers*, Panagotacos, P. Elite Books 2005, p. 99

small scar. In 1976, two sets of brothers began what would be called scalp reduction surgery for baldness. The Blanchard brothers [48] published their paper shortly before doctors Martin Unger and Walter Unger published theirs [49]. The article described a method of removing healthy, but hairless, scalp tissue from a patient to simultaneously lift up the fringe of permanently growing hair along the sides and back of the head while making the bald area needing transplants smaller. The article was rejected as "representing nothing new." However, alopecia reductions (bald scalp reductions) were soon regularly performed along with full-size graft hair transplant procedures, because they allowed for increased hair density with full-size graft procedures.

In 1977, at the same time that real advances were being made to remove bald scalp and then transplant into the remaining bald area, new bogus techniques were suggested. One such example was" Bilateral ligature of the superficial temporal arteries and of the posterior auricular arteries is proposed as a treatment for seborrheic alopecia," to cause hypoxia to cure seborrheic alopecia and to decrease DHT to the hairs to prevent baldness in 1300 cases over a 6 year period [50]. The same year, inversion boots were being sold to help increase the blood flow to the scalp to promote hair growth. There are no scientific papers written on inversion therapy; however, the internet confirms the use of inversion as a method to grow hair.

> "Standardized scalp massage is a way to transmit mechanical stress to human dermal papilla cells in subcutaneous tissue. Hair thickness was shown to increase with standardized scalp massage" [51]

During my residency, I was able to visit Dr. Orentreich in his office in New York in 1971. It helped motivate me to spend the next 50 years specializing in hair loss restoration. In 1973, Dr. Orentreich compared research "in baldness to the five years before Neil Armstrong took his giant step for mankind". Others looked upon the treatment of hair loss as a frivolous endeavor for men of medicine. Dr. William Montagna (President of the Society for Investigative Dermatology—1969–1970) considered it an unnecessary endeavor and is quoted as saying, "Baldness is a natural condition, not a disease. If you don't like being bald, get yourself a hairpiece. There's no real problem" [52]. Dr. Orentreich was prescient in predicting the advances in the field, not only did hair transplantation evolve to single hair grafting, but we found a topical medication that promoted hair growth (Rogaine) and then a pill (Propecia) that could block DHT formation and prevent baldness. This was the holy grail of hair restoration. And all this has taken place in only 1% of the 5000 year history of hair loss treatments.

In the 1980s, full-sized 4 mm grafts were then quartered into mini grafts to give a more natural appearance. "The frontal hairline is the most important and difficult part of hair reconstruction. A technique is presented that uses "micrografts" to correct a frontal hairline that looks less than natural, a condition often seen after punch hair grafting (or strip grafting or scalp flaps). With these "micrografts," it is possible to produce a natural-looking, soft frontal hairline" [53], Dr. Emanuel Marritt makes a breakthrough in transplantation by taking one and two hair grafts from the sides of a 4 mm graft and using them to insert into the frontal hairline [54].

In 1984, the United States Food and Drug Administration (FDA) banned synthetic fiber implants, a type of surgical hair restoration procedure where thousands of strands of fibers were implanted in the scalp to simulate the look of real hair. Although the fibers were similar to surgical sutures used by doctors to stitch up wounds, within a short period of time, they would cause bumps, inflammation, infection, scars, and even more hair loss [55].

It was Headinton in 1984 who first described follicular units in a paper on the microscopic anatomy of the scalp [56].

In the late 1980s, Dr. Bobby Limmer, a dermatologist and hair restoration surgeon practicing in Texas, had his surgical team use stereo microscopes rather than less powerful magnifying glasses while preparing micrografts. The more powerful magnification helps his team to preserve naturally occurring clusters of hair follicles in the donor tissue. This advance in dissecting out the hair follicles and leaving behind unwanted skin and fat, produced follicular units of one, two, and three hair grafts. In 1991, Dr. Limmer published an article in Hair Transplant Forum International describing what would become known as follicular unit micrografting and then again in 1994 in The Journal of Dermatologic Surgery and Oncology [57, 58]. Dr. Limmer is considered the father of modern Follicular Unit Grafting.

Hair cloning, "culturing stem cells from the patient's hair follicle", stem cell transplants, hair multiplication and scalp impregnation therapy are all terms for harvesting hair stem cells for the purpose of transplanting an endless supply of new hairs. In the 1990s, stem cells were found in the hair bulge, and attempts to cut a hair in half in the middle of the bulge was proposed in 1993 to produce two hairs. This resulted in two hairs that did not grow well if they survived [59].

In 1997, at the International Society for Hair Restoration annual meeting in Barcelona, I gave a lecture on the need to have caution when assessing the degree a patient may continue to go bald. I presented a case of a 35 year old man who, in 1976, told me his family only had frontal baldness. Over the next 2 years, he underwent eight hair transplants using 4 mm grafts of 30 to 70 grafts per session. The result was very good and lasted for 8 years when he continued to go bald behind and around the transplanted frontal forelock. From 1986 to 1993, he underwent six scalp reduction surgeries to remove the balding areas. Having exhausted the scalp donor hair the patient asked me to use his body hair.

This was at a time when 1 mm FUE grafting had not been perfected, nor did we have Finasteride to stop the process. In 1993, I did a strip excision of suprapubic hair and transplanted 200 grafts of two-haired follicular unit grafts. This was the first patient to have any body hair, in this case, it was pubic hair transplanted to the scalp [60].

My final 35 mm slide in this 1997 presentation stated (Fig. 1.12):

This was the opposite of what Dr. Tamura had done in 1943. Nine months later, a member of the ISHRS who was in the audience at the lecture in 1997 published an article in the ISHRS International FORUM titled "Pubic Hair as Donor Area in Hair Transplantation"- without giving a citation as to where he learned that it was possible [61]. A lecture at a medical conference making new material public qualifies as a publication by most definitions of the word [62]. That material is also covered by copyright law if it was given from written material and or recorded [63]. My lectures at the 1997 ISHRS meeting in Barcelona and subsequent lecture in 2000 at the American Academy of Dermatology meeting in New Orleans meet these qualifications, and claims by others to have been the first to transplant from the body to the scalp are in violation of standard ethical conduct.

The patient I presented as the first to have beard and body hair transplanted to his head, had three facelift surgeries in 1995, 1996, 1997. The tissue that would have been discarded from the beard area to do these procedures was saved in cold saline. Follicular unit grafts were dissected out and transplanted the following day to his scalp. I was able to harvest a total of 1824 beard single-hair follicular unit grafts, which were placed between previously grafted hairs. This was the reverse of what Dr. Okuda had done 60 years earlier and was the first case of body hair to scalp for male pattern baldness.

The patient was later presented as one of three patients I presented at the live patient presentation at the 1999 International Society for Hair Restoration Surgery annual meeting held in San Francisco (Fig. 1.13).

First case of Pubic Hair transplantation to scalp 1993, Beard hair transplantation to scalp 1993–1995. First presented at ISHRS Barcelona 1997 lecture & Live Patient presentation at ISHRS 1999 San Francisco (Figs. 1.14 and 1.15).

In Fig. 1.14, Patient #2 Shows the evolution of full-sized 4 mm grafts done in 1980 to obtain a full head of hair and the serial alopecia reductions which allowed a Type VII Norwood baldness patient to achieve a full head of hair. His final procedure in 1997 was a FUT follicular unit grafting in between the larger grafts, making his frontal hairline more aesthetically pleasing.

Paitent #3-The third patient also was an example of a scalp reduction using Y→T closure with follicular unit grafting in front 1976–1998. Photos taken by author.

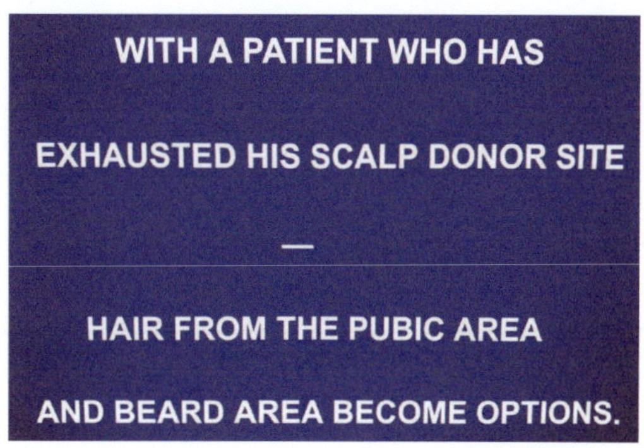

Fig. 1.12 Lecture at 1997 ISHRS annual meeting-actual 35 mm slide from the presentation

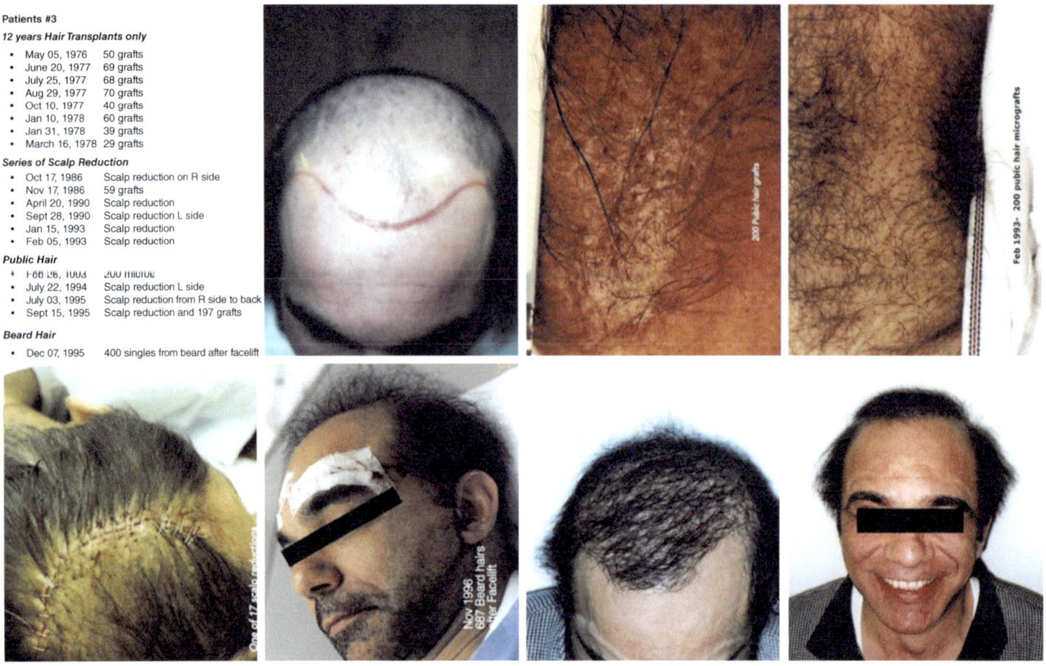

Fig. 1.13 Patient #1—1976–1997 photos take by author

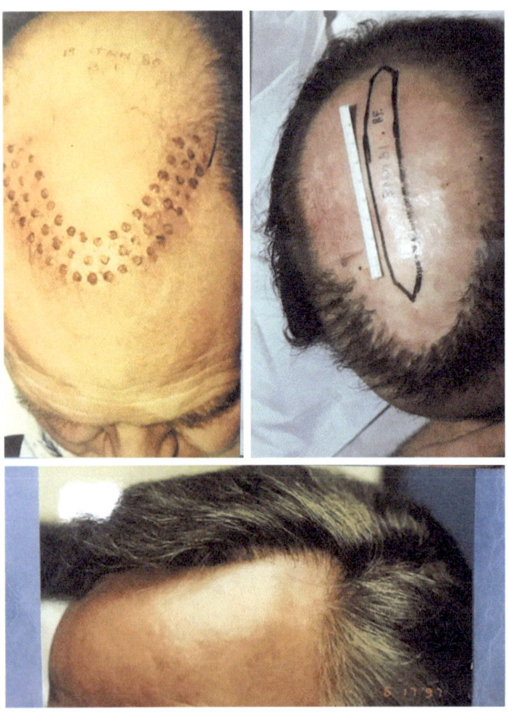

Fig. 1.14 1980–1999 photos taken by author

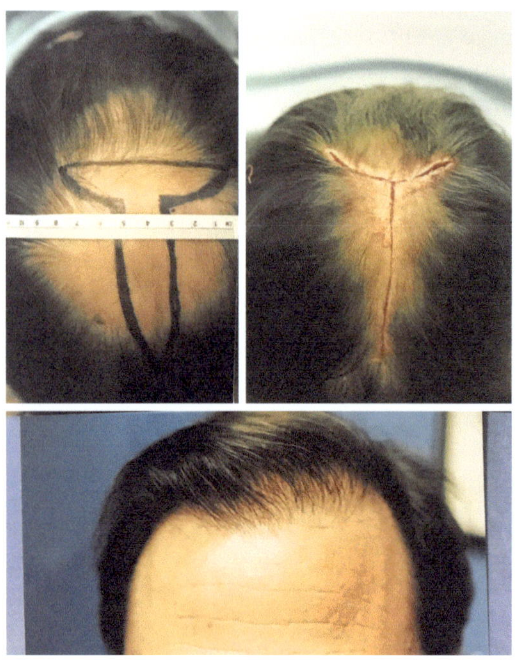

Fig. 1.15 1976–1998

Finasteride: The Medical Treatment Holy Grail

In 1992, Finasteride 5 mg was approved for treating BPH. In 1998, Finasteride 1 mg became the second prescription medication approved by the FDA as a hair loss treatment. In blocking 5 alpha reductase Type II, it lowers DHT by 66% (while raising Testosterone 10%). From 1993–1998, the author treated nearly 500 patients with 1 mg Finasteride made as capsules from the existing 5 mg pill approved for the prostate. In 1998, it is sold in pill form under the brand name Propecia. This medication now makes it possible for men in the early stages of hair loss to keep the hair they have, and even gain back some hair that was recently lost. Eighty-five percent of men stop losing their hair while taking Propecia [64]. In 2002, Dutasteride was approved for treating the prostate, and because it can block both 5 alpha reductase I & II it can lower the DHT 90%, which is extremely valuable for blocking the balding process in men who have inherited more extensive balding patterns [65]. It has also proved to be the drug of choice, in my opinion, in treating post-menopausal women with AGA [66, 67].

With over 50 years of specializing in both medical and surgical hair restoration, I feel quite fortunate to have personally witnessed the advent of Scalp Reductions, Minigrafts, Follicular Unit Grafting (both FUT and FUE), and the discovery of medical treatments which work to stimulate hair growth (minoxidil and LLLTx) as well as prevent AGA (Finasteride and Dutasteride). These treatments have proven to work, and they all were developed in the last 50 years of the 5000 year history of hair loss treatments. The advances in harvesting FUE follicular grafts over the past 20 years have led to a debate over whether sharp punches are better than blunt punches, whether motorized hand pieces that oscillate prevent transection, and whether suction at the time of cutting the skin helps extract healthier grafts (Neograft). All of these have led to continuing improvement in the technique, and with Artificial Intelligence, we now have a robot that has been proven to be more accurate in harvesting FUE grafts than most surgeons who do it manually. In August 2018, the incorporation of an additional laser on the head of the ARTASiX hair transplant robot made it accurate enough so that less than 5% of the grafts were lost to transection, which equaled the ability of most hair transplant surgeons. I purchased the first one off the assembly line in August 2018. The computer operator has to understand that donor areas should not be over-harvested and must be attuned to the patient's well-being. The artistic ability to place the grafts by the robot has not yet equaled what an experienced hair restoration surgeon can do in establishing a natural hairline. Yet, artificial intelligence automation may be the future of hair transplantation if it learns how to implant a natural hairline (Fig. 1.16).

I would like to close this chapter with a note as to the importance of treating hair loss. The question "Why treat hair loss?" seems to be a ridiculous question to many today, but not too long ago, it was seriously asked by many doctors of those who were in the hair restoration field. It would seem self-evident that the loss of hair causes psychological distress in many men and women, yet the literature is resplendent with studies citing the adverse impact of hair loss each time as if it were a new discovery. Many studies have been done showing bald men look

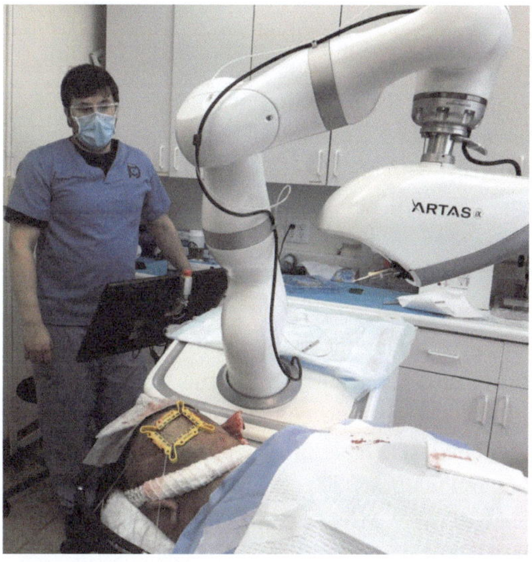

Fig. 1.16 ARTASiX: needs a computer operator, Christopher Panagotacos with ARTASiX

less attractive and 5–10 years older than those with hair. Whether the studies were done with newer digital manipulation of photos or older techniques, the results were the same [22, 68–70]. In 1988 Dr. Albert Kligman wrote: "We already know that **balding men** are viewed as **less attractive**. This could have far-reaching consequences for self-esteem, confidence, ambitiousness, and for success in general" [71]. "In his study of **women** undergoing treatment for primary breast cancer, Freedman found that some **women refused chemotherapy because** of the risk of developing **hair loss**" [72]. Perhaps because the new treatment using JAK inhibitors both orally and topically has generated interest into why we treat this benign disease, the literature again is being flooded with studies to prove the condition is not benign and causes psychological distress [73–76].

In 1993, when I first posted my website www.HairDoc.com as an educational tool for patients, I predicted we would eventually have a topical method of replacing the balding gene using mRNA. I am not a specialist in that field, yet it seemed plausible then as it does to me now. In 1995, it was suggested by Robert Hoffman that we would be able to treat baldness by gene therapy [77]. Research continues to be done in this field [78]. Raquel Cuevas Díaz Durán, Ph.D., the author of the chapter on "Research in hair genetics", explained to me in an email some of the reasons why this has not been accomplished yet. "Regarding the induction of "hairy genes", there are definitely amazing scientific advances like antisense oligonucleotides (ASO) and CRISPR that can silence genes and modify genetic sequences. However, we still don't know exactly which cell subpopulation would have to be modified, when to perform the modification, what DNA loci to modify, and how to keep the modification. I think science has some work to do still identifying specific cell types that become dysregulated. There is also a dysregulation in cell communications. The problem can be the influence of other cells (e.g., immune cells), so if we transplant dermal papilla cells successfully, we can't be sure that the other cells or the extracellular environment will also end up dysregulating them. We still have a lot to understand from the human hair follicles at the molecular level."

I have been waiting patiently for decades for the final success of this process from hair multiplication experts and may have to wait yet another decade.

References

1. Ebers G, Stern L. Papyros Ebers das hermetische Buch über die Arzneimittel der alten Ägypter in hieratischer Schrift. Hrsg. mit Inhaltsangabe und Einl. vers. von Georg Ebers. Mit hieroglyphisch-lateinischem Glossar von Ludwig. Stern. Mit Unterstützung d. Königl. Sächsischen Cultusministeriums. Englmann, Leipzig; 1875.
2. Ali F, Finlayson A. Pharaonic trichology: the Ebers Papyrus. JAMA Dermatol. 2013;149(8):920.
3. Pusey W. The history of dermatology. Springfield, IL: CC Thomas; 1933.
4. Castiglioni A. A history of medicine. New York: Alfred Knopf; 1958.
5. Broadley D, McElwee K. A "hair-raising" history of alopecia areata. Exp Dermatol. 2020;29(3):208–10.
6. https://www.britannica.com/topic/dress-clothing/Mesopotamia.
7. Banka N, Bunagan MJ, Dubrule Y, Shapiro J. Wigs and hairpieces: Evaluating dermatologic issues. Dermatol Ther. 2012;25:260–6.
8. Gollnick H, Orfanos C. Hair and hair diseases. Berlin: Springer; 1990.
9. Trüeb R, Lee W. Male alopecia. Springer; 2014.
10. Homan PG. Baldness: a brief history of treatments, from antiquity to the present. Pharm Hist. 2019;49(1):24–5.
11. Coar T. The Aphorisms of Hippocrates with a translation into Latin and English. A.J Valpy; 1822.
12. Hamilton JB. Male hormone stimulation is prerequisite and an incitant in common baldness. Am J Anat. 1942;71(3):451–80.
13. Price VH. Testosterone metabolism in the skin: a review of its function in androgenetic alopecia, acne vulgaris, and idiopathic hirsutism including recent studies with antiandrogens. Arch Dermatol. 1975;111(11):1496–502.
14. Shareef S, Maranda EL, Shareef F, Augustynowicz A, Tongdee E, Jimenez JJ. Patterns from the past—laurel wreaths and comb-overs. JAMA Dermatol. 2016;152(9):1020.
15. Paterson J. Caesar the man. A companion to Julius Caesar. 2009;10:126–40.
16. DeGalan AM. Lead white or dead white? Dangerous beauty practices of eighteenth-century England. Bull Detroit Inst Arts. 2002;76(12):38–49.
17. Cheesbrough MJ. Wigs. Br Med J. 1989;299(6713):1455–6.

18. Smith MD, editor. The World of the American Revolution [2 volumes]: A Daily Life Encyclopedia [2 volumes]. Bloomsbury Publishing; 2015. p. 261–3.
19. Albert MR. Nineteenth-century patent medicines for the skin and hair. J Am Acad Dermatol. 2000;43(3):519–26.
20. Anand M, Hutheesing K. Book of Indian beauty. Charles E. Tuttle; 1981.
21. Subscriber A. Hats and baldness. Buffalo Med J Mon Rev Med Surg Sci. 1853;8(12):739–40.
22. Rattner H. Ordinary baldness: President's address. Arch Dermatol Syphilol. 1941;44(2):208–9.
23. Macfadden B. Hair culture: rational methods for growing the hair and for developing its strength and beauty. Applewood Books; 2000.
24. Jackson EA, Cardoni AA, Smith GH. Minoxidil (Loniten®, Upjohn). Drug Intell Clin Pharm. 1980;14(7–8):477–82.
25. Sobota JT, Martin WB, Carlson RG, Feenstra ES. Minoxidil: right atrial cardiac pathology in animals and in man. Circulation. 1980;62(2):376–87.
26. Reichgott MJ. Minoxidil and pericardial effusion: an idiosyncratic reaction. Clin Pharmacol Ther. 1981;30(1):64–70.
27. Joekes AM, Thompson FD. Clinical use of Minoxidil (Loniten). J R Soc Med. 1981;74(4):278–82.
28. Rietschel RL, Duncan SH. Safety and efficacy of topical minoxidil in the management of androgenetic alopecia. J Am Acad Dermatol. 1987;16(3):677–85.
29. Zins GR. The history of the development of minoxidil. Clin Dermatol. 1988;6(4):132–47.
30. Bazzano GS, Terezakis N, Galen W. Topical tretinoin for hair growth promotion. J Am Acad Dermatol. 1986;15(4):880–93.
31. Abdi P, Awad C, Anthony MR, et al. Efficacy and safety of combinational therapy using topical minoxidil and microneedling for the treatment of androgenetic alopecia: a systematic review and meta-analysis. Arch Dermatol Res. 2003;315:2775–85.
32. Imperato-McGinley J, Gautier T, Peterson RE, Shackleton C. The prevalence of 5α-reductase deficiency in children with ambiguous genitalia in the Dominican Republic. J Urol. 1986;136(4):867–73.
33. Sudduth SL, Koronkowski MJ. Finasteride: the first 5α-reductase inhibitor. Pharmacotherapy. 1993;13(4):309–29.
34. Shapiro J, Price VH. Hair regrowth: therapeutic agents. Dermatol Clin. 1998;16(2):341–56.
35. Panagotacos P. Lecture—"Hair Restoration" lecture including use of 1m Finasteride. American Academy of Dermatology Annual Meeting New Orleans; 2000.
36. Hamilton J. Effect of castration in adolescent and young adult males upon further changes in the proportions of bare and hairy scalp. J Clin Endocrinol Metabol. 1960;20(10):1309–18.
37. Avram M, Rogers N. The use of low-level light for hair growth: part I. J Cosm Laser Ther. 2009;11(2):110–7.
38. Liu K-H, Liu D, Chen Y-T, Chin S-Y. Comparative effectiveness of low-level laser therapy for adult androgenic alopecia: a system review and meta-analysis of randomized controlled trials. Lasers Med Sci. 2019;34(6):1063–9.
39. Dieffenbach J. Nonnulla de regeneratione et transplantatione. Dissertatio inaguralis. 1822.
40. Okuda S, Jpn J. Dermatol Urol. 1939;46:537–87.
41. Jimenez F, Shiell RC. The Okuda papers: an extraordinary–but unfortunately unrecognized–piece of work that could have changed the history of hair transplantation. Exp Dermatol. 2015;24(3):185–6.
42. Tauber H. Alopecia praematura and its surgical treatment. J Ceylon Br Brit M A. 1939;36:237.
43. Juri JO. Use of parieto-occipital flaps in the surgical treatment of baldness. Plast Reconstr Surg. 1975;55(4):456–60.
44. Kabaker SS. Juri flap procedure for the treatment of baldness: two-year experience. Arch Otolaryngol. 1979;105(9):509–14.
45. Tamura H. Pubic hair transplantation. Jpn J Dermatol. 1943;53:76.
46. Orentreich N. Autografts in alopecias and other selected dermatological conditions. Ann N Y Acad Sci. 1959;83(3):463–79.
47. Orentreich N. Pathogenesis of alopecia. J Soc Cosm Chemists. 1960;11:479–82.
48. Blanchard G, Blanchard B. Obliteration of alopecia by hairlifting: a new concept and technique. J Natl Med Assoc. 1977;69:639–41.
49. Unger MG, Unger WP. Management of alopecia of the scalp by a combination of excisions and transplantations. J Dermatol Surg Oncol. 1978;4:670–2.
50. Marechal RE. New treatment for seborrheic alopecia: the ligature of the arteries of the scalp. J Natl Med Assoc. 1977;69(10):709–11.
51. Koyama T, Kobayashi K, Hama T, Murakami K, Ogawa R. Standardized scalp massage results in increased hair thickness by inducing stretching forces to dermal papilla cells in the subcutaneous tissue. Eplasty. 2016;16:e8.
52. Solomon J. Sprout, Damned Root! Sciences. 1973;13(7):13–7.
53. Nordström REA. "Micrografts" for improvement of the frontal hairline after hair transplantation. Aesth Plast Surg. 1981;5:97–101.
54. Marritt E. Single-hair transplantation for hairline refinement: a practical solution. J Dermatol Surg Oncol. 1984;10(12):962–6.
55. Medical Device Bans. FDA. Content current as of: April 6, 2020. https://www.fda.gov/medical-devices/medical-device-safety/medical-device-bans.
56. Headington JT. Transverse microscopic anatomy of the human scalp: a basis for a morphometric approach to disorders of the hair follicle. Arch Dermatol. 1984;120(4):449–56.
57. Limmer BL. ISHRS Forum. 1991;2(2):8–9.
58. Limmer BL. Elliptical donor stereoscopically assisted micrografting as an approach to further refinement in hair transplantation. J Dermatol Surg Oncol. 1994;20(12):789–93.
59. Kim JC. Paper presented at the International Society of Hair Restoration annual meeting, Dallas, 1993.

60. Panagotacos P. Lecture- pubic and beard hair as alternative sources when scalp donor runs out. Barcelona: ISHRS; 1997.
61. Minotakis C, Giotis C. Pubic hair as donor area in hair transplantation. Hair Transplant Forum Int. 1998;8(4):25.
62. https://www.merriam-webster.com/dictionary/publish.
63. Harding DE. Copyright in lectures, sermons, and speeches. Copyright L. Symp. 1964;14:270.
64. Sawaya ME. Novel agents for the treatment of alopecia. Semin Cutaneous Med Surg. 1998;17(4):276–83.
65. Arif T, Dorjay K, Adil M, Sami M. Dutasteride in androgenetic alopecia: an update. Curr Clin Pharmacol. 2017;12(1):31–5.
66. Olsen EA, Hordinsky M, Whiting D, Stough D, Hobbs S, Ellis ML, Wilson T, Rittmaster RS, Dutasteride Alopecia Research Team. The importance of dual 5alpha-reductase inhibition in the treatment of male pattern hair loss: results of a randomized placebo-controlled study of dutasteride versus finsteride. J Am Acad Dermatol. 2006;55:1014–23.
67. Camacho F, Tosti A. Tratamiento médico de las alopecias femeninas. Monogr Dermatol. 2005;18:92–117.
68. Wells PA, Willmoth T, Russell RJ. Does fortune favour the bald? Psychological correlates of hair loss in males. Br J Psychol. 1995;86(3):337–44.
69. Ricciardelli R. Masculinity, consumerism, and appearance: a look at men's hair. Can Rev Soc. 2011;48(2):181–201.
70. Cash TF. The psychological effects of androgenetic alopecia in men. J Am Acad Dermatol. 1992;26(6):926–31.
71. Kligman AM, Freeman B. History of baldness from magic to medicine. Clin Dermatol. 1988;6(4):83–8.
72. Yeager CE, Olsen EA. Treatment of chemotherapy-induced alopecia. Dermatol Ther. 2011;24(4):432–42.
73. Caro SR. Understanding the profound impact of alopecia areata on patients. Am J Nurs. 2023;123(3):11.
74. Saraswat N, Shankar P, Chopra A, Kumar S, Mitra D, Agarwal R. Impact of psychosocial profile on alopecia areata in pediatric patients: a case control study from a tertiary care hospital in Eastern Uttar Pradesh. Indian J Dermatol. 2020;65(3):183.
75. Villasante Fricke AC, Miteva M. Epidemiology and burden of alopecia areata: a systematic review. Clin Cosmet Investig Dermatol. 2015;24:397–403.
76. Dillon KA. A comprehensive literature review of JAK inhibitors in treatment of alopecia areata. Clin Cosmet Investig Dermatol. 2021;25:691–714.
77. Li L, Hoffman RM. The feasibility of targeted selective gene therapy of the hair follicle. Nat Med. 1995;1(7):705–6.
78. Cooley J. Follicular cell implantation: an update on "hair follicle cloning". Facial Plastic Surg Clin. 2004;12(2):219–24.
79. Panagotacos P. Bogus hair remedy collection. As presented at The International Society of Hair Restoration Surgery, San Diego; 2006.

Hair Loss: Advances and Treatments

2

Marc Avram

Introduction

Hair is one of the few physical attributes we have that we can readily control-its length, color and style. The *involuntary* gradual loss of hair *does* change our physical appearance over time. Hair frames our face and the loss of hair changes our appearance. There are a variety of causes and medical and surgical solutions to treat hair loss. This chapter will be limited to the widely used medical therapies to treat male and female pattern hair loss. Fortunately, we live in an era with safe, effective treatments for both women and men. All can dramatically restore lost hair, partially restore lost hair, prevent further hair loss or not work at all. As with other medical conditions combination therapy and monotherapy can be effective. It is important to let patients know 6–9 months are required to judge the efficacy of any therapy.

As a transplant surgeon, patients will often present for surgery reporting medical therapy failed. On questioning patients often report stopping their medical therapy after 2–3 months secondary to not seeing positive results. It is vital to educate patients that multiple months are necessary to judge efficacy and *all* medical therapy; and if successful they must be continued indefinitely to maintain their efficacy. Two to three months is simply not long enough to judge their efficacy.

Currently, topical, oral and non medical options are available as treatment options. The consultation is the opportunity to review in detail the advantages and disadvantages of each treatment option. Each patient will choose the treatment option they feel most comfortable using regularly. We often supplement the consultation with written materials for the patient to review. If they are not sure which therapy or combination to choose we encourage them to research and call us with any more questions. Understanding the risk benefit and side effects before beginning the treatment increases the chances of long term compliance and success.

Minoxidil Topical and Oral Minoxidil Mechanism of Action

Minoxidil, a vasodilator, was initially developed as an antihypertensive agent. Its ability to stimulate hair growth was discovered serendipitously [1]. Although the exact mechanism of action remains unclear, several key processes have been identified. Minoxidil shortens the telogen phase (resting phase) of the hair cycle and prolongs the anagen phase (active growth phase) [2]. It achieves this by stimulating dermal papilla cells, leading to increased hair follicle size [3]. Additionally, min-

M. Avram (✉)
Private Practice, New York, NY, USA

Clinical Professor of Dermatology, Weill Cornell Medical Center/New York Presbyterian Hospital, New York, NY, USA
e-mail: MAvram@dravram.com

P. J. Panagotacos, H. Maibach (eds.), *Hair Loss*, Updates in Clinical Dermatology,
https://doi.org/10.1007/978-3-031-74314-6_2

oxidil enhances microcirculation around hair follicles, promoting nutrient delivery and hair growth [4]. Furthermore, it reduces the negative effects of dihydrotestosterone (DHT) on hair follicles, a key factor in androgenetic alopecia (AGA) [5].

Efficacy

Both topical and oral minoxidil have demonstrated efficacy in treating hair loss (Table 2.1).

Topical minoxidil remains the only approved medication for both male and female pattern hair loss. Oral minoxidil is not FDA approved but recently has become a popular off label modality for treating hair loss.

Topical minoxidil, most commonly available in 2% and 5% concentrations, has been shown to be effective in stimulating hair growth in men and women with AGA [6]. Research suggests that 5% topical minoxidil is slightly more effective than the 2% formulation [7]. However, it may cause more side effects, particularly in women [8].

Oral minoxidil, while less studied, has shown promising results in treating AGA and other types of hair loss, including alopecia areata [9]. The efficacy of oral minoxidil is dose-dependent, with higher doses (1–5 mg daily) providing better results [4]. However, the risk of side effects also increases with higher doses [10].

Side Effects

Topical minoxidil is generally well-tolerated. Common side effects include local irritation, itching, and scaling [11]. For women hirsutism can occur. If minoxidil creates unwanted hair growth on the face it is also growing hair where the patient wants it on their scalp. Stopping the minoxidil will reverse the drug induced hirsutism but will also cause the loss of minoxidil induced hair growth on the scalp. Many women opt to continue the minoxidil and remove unwanted hair on their face via laser or waxing.

Rarely, systemic absorption can lead to dizziness, tachycardia, and fluid retention [12]. Pregnant and nursing women should avoid using minoxidil due to its potential teratogenic effects [13].

Oral minoxidil has a higher risk of side effects including - dizziness, tachycardia, hypertrichosis [14], fluid retention, pericardial effusion, allergic reaction. Since oral minoxidil is an anti hypertensive medication patients primary physician should be aware of and approve its use before the patient begins using it for their hair loss [15]. The optimal dose of oral minoxidil for hair loss has not been established. The majority of women are being treated with doses ranging from .625–1.25 mg and men 1.25 to 2.5 mg.

Platelet Rich Plasma (PRP) for Hair Loss in Men and Women

Platelet Rich Plasma (PRP) therapy is a non-surgical treatment option for hair loss in both men and women. It has gained popularity in recent years as an effective solution for those experiencing male or female pattern hair loss. PRP has been used as a therapeutic option in a variety fields of medicine from orthopedic surgery to dental surgery. It has become a popular treatment option for hair loss since it is a natural treatment option that

Table 2.1 Minoxidil for hair loss

Attribute	Description
Product name	Minoxidil (brand names: Rogaine, Regaine, and others)
Type	Topical medication
Indication	Androgenetic alopecia (pattern hair loss) in men and women
Mechanism of action	Vasodilator, increases blood flow to hair follicles, stimulates hair growth and prolongs growth phase
Concentrations	Men: 5% solution or foam; Women: 2% solution or 5% foam
Application frequency	Once daily (morning or evening)
Onset of action	3–6 months of continuous use for visible results; optimal results after 1 year
Duration of Treatment	Long-term; discontinuation may lead to hair loss reversal

Table 2.2 Side effects of PRP

Common side effects	Rare side effects
• Mild pain or discomfort at the injection site • Temporary shedding of existing hair follicles	• Infection, scarring, dyschromia

if successful can maintain or regrow hair without the need for daily therapy.

Mechanism of Action

PRP therapy involves the use of a patient's own blood plasma enriched with platelets. Platelets are small blood cells that play a crucial role in wound healing and tissue regeneration. They contain numerous growth factors such as platelet-derived growth factor (PDGF), vascular endothelial growth factor (VEGF), and transforming growth factor (TGF), which can stimulate hair follicle regeneration and promote hair growth [15].

When PRP is injected into the scalp, the high concentration of growth factors in the platelets can stimulate dormant hair follicles, increase blood circulation to the hair follicles, and promote the proliferation of dermal papilla cells [16]. This, in turn, can lead to a thicker hair shaft, increased hair density, and overall improved hair growth.

How to Perform PRP Therapy: PRP Therapy Involves Several Steps

Blood Collection: Blood (usually about 20–40 mL) is drawn from the patient's arm. Separation of PRP: The collected blood is then centrifuged an average of 10 min to separate the plasma and platelets from the red and white blood cells. This results in a concentration of platelets in the plasma, hence the name Platelet Rich Plasma.

Injection of PRP: PRP is then injected into the areas of the scalp with thinning hair using a small caliber needle. The injections are usually given at multiple sites, about 1 cm apart, across the area being treated. It is vital to inject the PRP where it will have maximum impact on the hair cycle which in the zone of the deep dermis to superficial subcutaneous tissue.

Side Effects (Table 2.2)

It is important to note that while PRP therapy has shown promising results in various studies, individual responses may vary, and it may not be effective for everyone. Also, PRP therapy is often considered as a part of a multi-modal approach to hair loss treatment, which may include other treatments such as minoxidil, finasteride, low level light therapy or hair transplantation.

Conclusion

PRP therapy is an effective option for hair loss in both men and women [17–19]. It involves the use of the patient's own platelet-rich plasma, which contains growth factors that can stimulate hair follicle regeneration and promote hair growth. Several studies have supported its efficacy in increasing hair density and thickness with minimal side effects. However, individual responses may vary, and it may not be effective for everyone. It is always advisable to consult a healthcare professional or a dermatologist before starting any new treatment for hair loss.

Finasteride

Finasteride is a 5-alpha-reductase inhibitor commonly used for the treatment of male pattern loss. It is available in both oral and topical formulations, with oral finasteride being widely used and well-researched, while topical finasteride is a relatively newer form of treatment.

Mechanism of Action

Male pattern hair loss is characterized by the miniaturization of hair follicles, leading to thinner and shorter hairs. The main androgen responsible for

Table 2.3 Side effects

Side effect	Description
Decreased libido	A reduced interest in sexual activity is the most common side effect
Erectile dysfunction	Difficulty in achieving or maintaining an erection
Ejaculation disorders	This includes decreased volume of ejaculate
Testicular pain	Some men experience discomfort or pain in the testicles
Depression	Some users have reported mood changes, including increased feelings of depression
Gynecomastia	This is the enlargement or swelling of breast tissue in males
Skin rash	Although less common, some men may develop a skin rash

this is dihydrotestosterone (DHT), which is formed from testosterone by the enzyme 5-alpha-reductase. Finasteride works by inhibiting the 5-alpha-reductase enzyme, thereby reducing the conversion of testosterone to DHT [20]. This leads to a decrease in DHT levels in the scalp and serum, which in turn reduces hair follicle miniaturization and promotes hair growth [21].

Clinical Studies Supporting Efficacy: Oral Finasteride

Oral finasteride has been extensively studied and is proven to be effective in the treatment of AGA in men. A landmark study conducted by Kaufman et al. found that after 1 year of treatment with oral finasteride, 86% of men had increased or maintained hair count compared to baseline [22]. Another 5-year study conducted by Leyden et al. found that finasteride not only increased hair count but also improved hair quality and scalp coverage [23]. Moreover, a meta-analysis conducted by Liu et al. concluded that oral finasteride significantly increased hair count and improved patient self-assessment of hair growth.

Oral Finasteride

The most common side effects of oral finasteride are related to sexual function and include decreased libido, erectile dysfunction, and ejaculatory disorders. These side effects occur in a small percentage of men and are usually reversible upon discontinuation of the medication. Other less common side effects include breast tenderness and enlargement, and rash. There have been reports of men complaining of long-term persistent sexual side effects and/or depression called post finasteride syndrome. It is rare. The precise incidence is yet to be determined [24–29] (Table 2.3).

Topical Finasteride

Topical finasteride is generally well-tolerated and has a lower incidence of side effects compared to oral finasteride. This is because topical finasteride has less systemic absorption and therefore lower systemic DHT suppression [23]. The most common side effects of topical finasteride are local skin reactions such as itching, redness, and scaling. Systemic side effects, such as those affecting sexual function, are rare but can occur [30].

Conclusion

Oral finasteride is a well-established and effective treatment for AGA in men, with numerous studies supporting its efficacy in increasing hair count and improving hair quality. However, it is associated with a risk of sexual side effects, which has led to the development of topical finasteride as an alternative treatment option. Topical finasteride has shown promising results in preliminary studies, with a lower incidence of side effects compared to oral finasteride. However, more research is needed to establish its long-term efficacy and safety.

Low-Level Light Therapy for Male and Female Pattern Hair Loss

Low-level light therapy (LLLT), also known as photobiomodulation, is a non-invasive treatment option for androgenic alopecia (AGA), commonly known as male and female pattern hair loss. It involves the use of low-power lasers or light-emitting diodes (LEDs) to deliver red or near-infrared light to the scalp, which is believed to promote hair growth and improve hair density.

Mechanism of Action

The exact mechanism by which LLLT promotes hair growth is not fully understood, but several key processes are believed to be involved. LLLT is thought to increase adenosine triphosphate (ATP) production in the mitochondria of hair follicle cells, leading to increased cell proliferation and hair growth [31]. Additionally, LLLT may increase blood flow to the scalp, promoting nutrient and oxygen delivery to the hair follicles [32]. Furthermore, LLLT is believed to modulate inflammatory cytokines and growth factors, reducing inflammation and promoting hair growth [33].

Studies Supporting Efficacy

Numerous studies have been conducted to assess the efficacy of LLLT in the treatment of AGA in both men and women. A randomized, double-blind, sham device-controlled study conducted by Jimenez et al. found that men who received LLLT treatment for 26 weeks showed a statistically significant increase in hair density compared to those who received sham treatment. Similarly, a study conducted by Lanzafame et al. found that both men and women who received LLLT treatment for 16 weeks showed a statistically significant increase in hair density compared to those who received sham treatment [34]. Additionally, a meta-analysis conducted by Gupta et al. concluded that LLLT is a safe and effective treatment for AGA in both men and women, with a moderate effect size [35, 36].

Side Effects

LLLT is generally well-tolerated and associated with minimal side effects. The most common side effects are mild and transient, such as scalp itching, warmth, or redness. Serious side effects, such as burns or scars, are rare and usually associated with improper use of the device. It is important for patients to use the device according to the manufacturer's instructions and consult a healthcare professional if they experience any unusual symptoms.

Conclusion

Low-level light therapy is a non-invasive, safe, and effective treatment option for androgenic alopecia in both men and women. It works by increasing ATP production, promoting blood flow, and modulating inflammatory cytokines and growth factors. Numerous studies support its efficacy in improving hair density and overall hair health. While mild and transient side effects, such as scalp itching, warmth, or redness, may occur, serious side effects are rare. It is important for patients to use the device according to the manufacturer's instructions and consult a healthcare professional if they experience any unusual symptoms.

References

1. Friedman ES, Friedman PM, Cohen DE, Washenik K. Minoxidil for androgenetic alopecia. Exp Opin Drug Saf. 2002;1(2):195–200.
2. Messenger AG, Rundegren J. Minoxidil: mechanisms of action on hair growth. Br J Dermatol. 2004;150(2):186–94.
3. Uno H, Cappas A, Brigham P. Action of topical minoxidil in the bald stump-tailed macaque. J Am Acad Dermatol. 1987;16(3 Pt 2):657–68.
4. Lachgar S, Charveron M, Gall Y, Bonafe JL. Minoxidil upregulates the expression of vascular endothelial growth factor in human hair dermal papilla cells. Br J Dermatol. 1998;138(3):407–11.
5. Olsen EA, Whiting D, Bergfeld W, et al. A multicenter, randomized, placebo-controlled, double-blind clinical trial of a novel formulation of 5% minoxidil topical foam versus placebo in the treatment of androgenetic alopecia in men. J Am Acad Dermatol. 2007;57(5):767–74.
6. Blume-Peytavi U, Hillmann K, Dietz E, Canfield D, Garcia BN. A randomized, single-blind trial of 5% minoxidil foam once daily versus 2% minoxidil solution twice daily in the treatment of androgenetic

alopecia in women. J Am Acad Dermatol. 2011;65(6):1126–1134.e2.
7. Olsen EA, Dunlap FE, Funicella T, et al. A randomized clinical trial of 5% topical minoxidil versus 2% topical minoxidil and placebo in the treatment of androgenetic alopecia in men. J Am Acad Dermatol. 2002;47(3):377–85.
8. Lucky AW, Piacquadio DJ, Ditre CM, et al. A randomized, placebo-controlled trial of 5% and 2% topical minoxidil solutions in the treatment of female pattern hair loss. J Am Acad Dermatol. 2004;50(4):541–53.
9. Sinclair R, Wewerinke M, Jolley D. Treatment of female pattern hair loss with oral minoxidil. Australas J Dermatol. 2005;46(1):27–30.
10. English RS, Barazesh JM, McClellan JH, Washenik K, Shupack JL. A higher incidence of pericardial effusion in patients taking oral minoxidil for hair loss. J Am Acad Dermatol. 2019;80(2):497–8.
11. Olsen EA, DeLong ER, Weiner MS. Long-term follow-up of men with male pattern baldness treated with topical minoxidil. J Am Acad Dermatol. 1987;16(3 Pt 2):688–95.
12. Price VH. Treatment of hair loss. N Engl J Med. 1999;341(13):964–73.
13. Levy LL, Emer JJ. Female pattern alopecia: current perspectives. Int J Womens Dermatol. 2013;5(3):243–51.
14. Rathnayake D, Sinclair R. Innovative use of spironolactone as an antiandrogen in the treatment of female pattern hair loss. Dermatol Clin. 2010;28(3):611–8.
15. Trink A, Sorbellini E, Bezzola P, et al. A randomized, double-blind, placebo- and active-controlled, half-head study to evaluate the effects of platelet-rich plasma on alopecia areata. Br J Dermatol. 2013;169(3):690–4.
16. Cervelli V, Garcovich S, Bielli A, et al. The effect of autologous activated platelet-rich plasma (AA-PRP) injection on pattern hair loss: clinical and histomorphometric evaluation. Biomed Res Int. 2014;2014:760709.
17. Gentile P, Garcovich S, Bielli A, et al. The effect of platelet-rich plasma in hair regrowth: a randomized placebo-controlled trial. Stem Cells Transl Med. 2015;4(11):1317–23.
18. Alves R, Grimalt R. A randomized placebo-controlled, double-blind, half-head study to assess the efficacy of platelet-rich plasma on the treatment of androgenetic alopecia. Dermatol Surg. 2018;44(4):541–7.
19. Giordano S, Romeo M, Lankinen P. A meta-analysis on evidence of platelet-rich plasma for androgenic alopecia. Int J Trichology. 2017;9(1):1–10.
20. Dallob AL, Sadick NS, Unger W, et al. The effect of finasteride, a 5 alpha-reductase inhibitor, on scalp skin testosterone and dihydrotestosterone concentrations in patients with male pattern baldness. J Clin Endocrinol Metab. 1994;79(3):703–6.
21. Kaufman KD, Olsen EA, Whiting D, et al. Finasteride in the treatment of men with androgenetic alopecia. J Am Acad Dermatol. 1998;39(4 Pt 1):578–89.
22. Kaufman KD, Rotonda J, Shah AK, Meehan AG. Long-term treatment with finasteride 1 mg decreases the likelihood of developing further visible hair loss in men with androgenetic alopecia (male pattern hair loss). Eur J Dermatol. 2008;18(4):400–6.
23. Leyden J, Dunlap F, Miller B, et al. Finasteride in the treatment of men with frontal male pattern hair loss. J Am Acad Dermatol. 1999;40(6 Pt 1):930–7.
24. Liu L, Zhao S, Li F, Li E, Kang R, Luo L, Luo J, Wan S. Effect of 5α-reductase inhibitors on sexual function: a meta-analysis and systematic review of randomized controlled trials. J Sex Med. 2016;13(9):1297–310.
25. Suchonwanit P, Thammarucha S, Leerunyakul K. Minoxidil and its use in hair disorders: a review. Drug Des Dev Ther. 2019;13:2777–86.
26. Caserini M, Radicioni M, Leuratti C, Terragni E, Iorizzo M, Palmieri R. Effects of a novel finasteride 0.25% topical solution on scalp and serum dihydrotestosterone in healthy men with androgenetic alopecia. Int J Clin Pharmacol Ther. 2016;54(1):19–27.
27. Traish AM, Hassani J, Guay AT, Zitzmann M, Hansen ML. Adverse side effects of 5α-reductase inhibitors therapy: persistent diminished libido and erectile dysfunction and depression in a subset of patients. J Sex Med. 2011;8(3):872–84.
28. Mondaini N, Gontero P, Giubilei G, Lombardi G, Cai T, Gavazzi A, Bartoletti R. Finasteride 5 mg and sexual side effects: how many of these are related to a nocebo phenomenon? J Sex Med. 2007;4(6):1708–12.
29. Rahimi-Ardabili B, Pourandarjani R, Habibollahi P, Mualeki A. Finasteride induced depression: a prospective study. BMC Clin Pharmacol. 2006;6:7.
30. Suchonwanit P, Iamsumang W, Rojhirunsakool S. Efficacy of topical combination of 0.25% finasteride and 3% minoxidil versus 3% minoxidil solution in female pattern hair loss: a randomized, double-blind, controlled study. Am J Clin Dermatol. 2019;20(1):147–53.
31. Avci P, Gupta GK, Clark J, Wikonkal N, Hamblin MR. Low-level laser (light) therapy (LLLT) for treatment of hair loss. Lasers Surg Med. 2014;46(2):144–51.
32. Chung H, Dai T, Sharma SK, Huang YY, Carroll JD, Hamblin MR. The nuts and bolts of low-level laser (light) therapy. Ann Biomed Eng. 2012;40(2):516–33.
33. Hou X, Yuan S, Liu D, Hu X. Low-level light therapy of male and female pattern hair loss: a multicenter, randomized, sham device-controlled, double-blind study. Am J Clin Dermatol. 2019;20(2):313–21.
34. Jimenez JJ, Wikramanayake TC, Bergfeld W, et al. Efficacy and safety of a low-level laser device in the treatment of male and female pattern hair loss: a multicenter, randomized, sham device-controlled, double-blind study. Am J Clin Dermatol. 2014;15(2):115–27.
35. Lanzafame RJ, Blanche RR, Chiacchierini RP, Kazmirek ER, Sklar JA. The growth of human scalp hair in females using visible red light laser and LED sources. Lasers Surg Med. 2014;46(8):601–7.
36. Gupta AK, Foley KA. A critical assessment of the evidence for low-level laser therapy in the treatment of hair loss. Dermatol Surg. 2017;43(2):188–97.

3 Hair Transplantation—From the "Ancient" 4 mm Plugs to the Latest Follicular Unit Excision Technique: 8 Decades of Painful Progress

Anastasakis Konstantinos

Introduction

Hair Restoration Surgery (HRS) has weathered a tumultuous history, bearing the weight of a questionable reputation for decades. Dating back to the 1960s, the results of earlier techniques and the misuse of more contemporary approaches have left an indelible mark on countless patients, leading to the stigmatization of HRS within both the medical community and the public perception.

Regrettably, the past of HRS is marked by instances of poor surgical judgment, thoughtlessness, and a steadfast adherence to outdated practices. The repercussions of these mistakes have been profound, with the acquisition of knowledge through experience proving to be a slow and arduous process. However, amid the shadows of controversy, a cadre of ambitious and ethical surgeons has risen to question the entrenched "dogmas" of earlier HRS techniques. These pioneers embarked on experimental journeys aimed at achieving natural results and surmounting surgical challenges. Their dedication to advancing the scientific foundation of HRS led to the dismantling of older, obsolete, and illogical techniques that had plagued the field for decades.

By tracing the evolution of HRS, this work aims to provide a comprehensive understanding of the challenges faced, the mistakes made, and the transformative efforts that have paved the way for a more ethical, scientifically grounded, and patient-centric approach to HRS with the latest surgical technique, Follicular Unit Excision (FUE).

Lessons From the Past

Surgical techniques exhibit ongoing evolution and refinement over time, benefiting from advancements in technical instrumentation and accumulating experience, thereby enhancing their efficacy. HRS, however, has historically been entrenched in scientific dogmatism, impeding the progression of surgical methods. HRS has suffered from prolonged periods of scientific stagnation, resulting in millions of patients bearing the residual effects of unnatural results (Fig. 3.1).

In addition to the archetypal "Punch Graft Technique," alternative approaches such as scalp lifts, scalp reductions, and flaps were prevalent until the early 1990s. These alternatives emerged as responses to the suboptimal outcomes associated with the punch graft technique, providing avenues for exploration. The pivotal departure from punch grafts involved the introduction of the "Strip Excision Technique"or Linear Strip Excision (LSE). This technique entailed extracting a horizontal-ellipsoid strip of scalp skin from the

A. Konstantinos (✉)
Anastasakis Hair Clinic, Athens, Attiki, Greece

P. J. Panagotacos, H. Maibach (eds.), *Hair Loss*, Updates in Clinical Dermatology,
https://doi.org/10.1007/978-3-031-74314-6_3

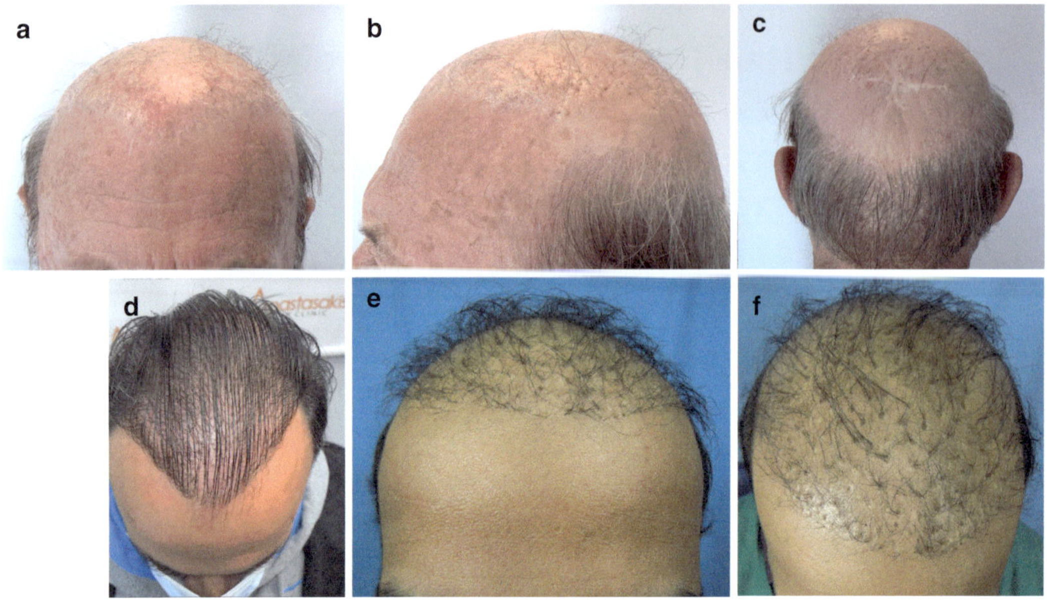

Fig. 3.1 (**a–c**) A typical elderly patient and veteran of HRS, with signs of punch grafts and scars from several scalp reductions, who has been wearing hair prosthesis to cover the terrible results, (**d**) excessively flared, triangular hairline with unnatural multi-FU grafts (minigrafts) that looks artificial, "aggressive", draws attention, (**e, f**) Punch grafts spread on a larger surface gave this horrible appearance. Scar tissue in the perimeter of punch grafts creates pitting (from [1]) [2]

occipital area, followed by the surgical approximation of the wound edges [3]. The extracted strip graft was subsequently dissected into smaller grafts, namely micrografts (partial follicular units) and minigrafts (groups of >1 follicular unit) [4].

LSE swiftly became the new "Gold Standard," marking a transformative period where the success and acceptance of mini/micrografting curtailed the enthusiasm for alopecia reduction, scalp lifts, and 4-mm punch grafting procedures. LSE presented a safe, relatively easy-to-learn technique that yielded results embraced by both patients and surgeons alike (Fig. 3.2) [5].

While it optimized donor area management and improved the thickness and naturalness of HRS results, cosmetic challenges persisted in the recipient area compared to natural hair growth, including tufted hair, pitting, cobblestoning, and "see-through" complications with mini- and micrografts.

In the early 1990s, Dr. Bobby Limmer [6] and Bernstein et al. [7] culminated decades of HRS refinement by embracing the histologic observation by Headington [8]. Headington presented that hairs do not grow singly but rather in natural groups known as Follicular Units (FUs). This seminal insight led to the development of Follicular Unit Transplantation (FUT). The technique prioritized preserving the intact, naturally occurring individual FU during all procedural steps, avoiding fragmentation into smaller units (older micrografts) or fusion into larger ones (older minigrafts) for reasons of economy of size and minimal trauma [7, 9]. Imitating nature by transplanting natural FUs offered numerous cosmetic advantages, marking the pinnacle of HRS evolution concerning graft type, size, naturalness, and recipient area density [10].

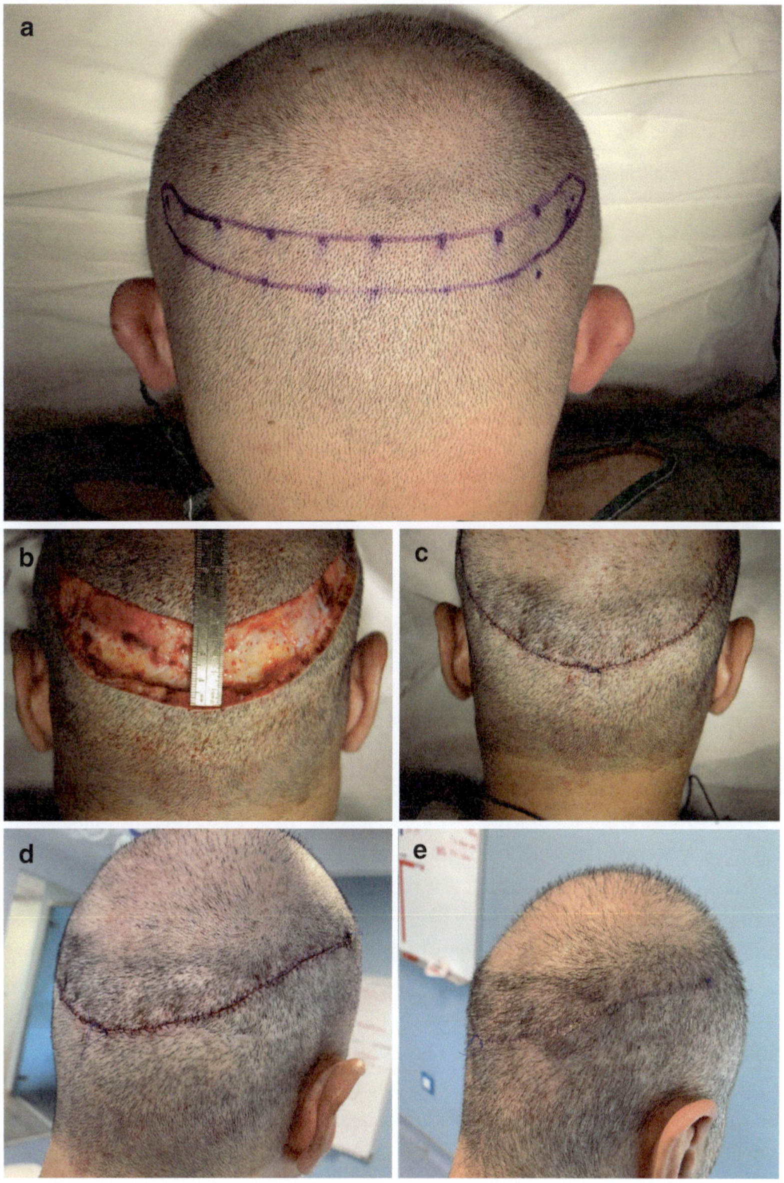

Fig. 3.2 (**a**) The LSE incision must follow the curvature of the skull. (**b**) When a 15-mm wide strip is excised, it will double in width due to elasticity, but (**c**) meticulous, tensionless 2-layer suturing will approximate the edges seamlessly. (**d–e**) Result immediately after wound suturing and at 12 days post-op. Even this imperceptible LSE scar is not acceptable by patients anymore

Great Expectations!

The inherent trajectory of every cosmetic surgical discipline should lead to enhanced cosmesis. With the introduction of Follicular Unit Transplantation (FUT), the recipient area achieved impeccable naturalness, subsequently elevating patient expectations regarding the donor area (Fig. 3.3). In due course, patients began deeming even the slightest Linear Strip Excision (LSE) scar on the posterior scalp as "unacceptable," irrespective of the cosmesis achieved in the recipient area (Fig. 3.2d, e). Particularly among younger LSE patients, frustration arose due to the cosmetic limitation of being unable to adopt very short haircuts on the back and sides of the head. Those with scars from prior LSE procedures or individuals who, unfortunately, developed poor scars due to surgical misjudgment or idiosyncratic reasons faced profound distress regardless of the result on the recipient area.

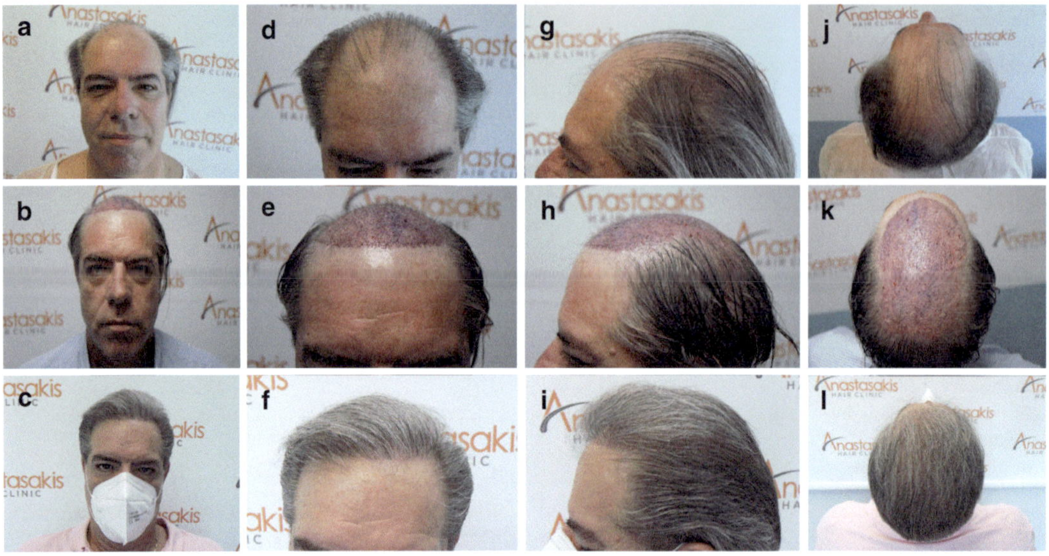

Fig. 3.3 (**a–l**) Result of LSE on Stage VI patient with thick caliber, salt-n-pepper hair, after a megasession with 4000 FUs and overall 11,000 hairs, offering an impressive result!

The quest for graft extraction without the "cosmetic cost"of a linear scar emerged as a new frontier, prompting pioneering surgeons to tackle this challenge. Consequently, the Follicular Unit Extraction (FUE) technique was presented in 2002, involving the use of minuscule circular punches to dissect and extract intact follicular units (FUs) in situ. This innovation sparked an unprecedented race among practitioners to master the FUE technique, propelling the field forward through ongoing refinement of techniques and the invention of new tools. The evolution of FUE became a dynamic force in response to the burgeoning demand for improved cosmesis and the desire to liberate patients from the constraints imposed by linear scars in the donor area.

Evolution/Revolution!

The technique later coined as Follicular Unit Excision (FUE) by Rassman et al. [11] was not entirely novel; similar concepts had been explored in the 1970s and continued to evolve during the initial years of LSE. However, a comprehensive historical examination of the FUE technique lies beyond the scope of this paper. Rassman et al. [11] published their innovated FUE technique (originally named Follicular Unit Extraction) in a peer-reviewed medical journal in 2002, elucidating the procedure's intricacies, advantages, and limitations. They refined the earlier technique of Inaba [12] (1996), rendering it more efficient and applicable to an extensive number of grafts within a reasonable surgical timeframe while preserving high survival rates. [11] Using a manual extraction device, Rassman et al. employed a handle with a custom 1 mm punch connected to it, featuring adjustable depth control (Fig. 3.4).

The punching device was positioned directly over an individual Follicular Unit (FU), and the punch was advanced with a rotating/pushing movement of the fingers and thumb, scoring through the epidermal and dermal layers. The partially mobilized FU was then delicately extracted with forceps (Fig. 3.5). The resulting cylindrical hole, approximately 1 mm in diame-

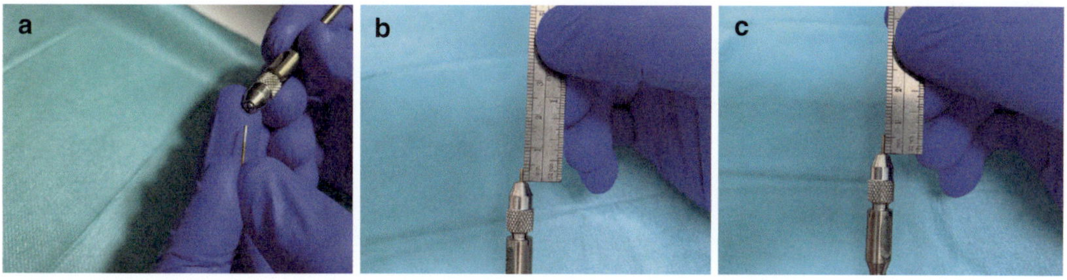

Fig. 3.4 (**a**) A manual extraction device used for FUE similar to the one used by Rassman et al. [11] (**b, c**) The punch is connected to a handle, and the depth can be adjusted according to the length of the FU, anywhere between 2 and 5 mm (From [13], used with permission)

ter, was left open and healed rapidly by secondary intention, yielding an imperceptible circular scar (Fig. 3.6). This innovative technique held the promise of the "holy grail" of HRS: achieving natural and thick results in the recipient area without visible scarring in the donor area. However, this simplistic depiction overlooks the myriad challenges faced by the authors and the numerous complexities encountered by subsequent FUE pioneers in their attempts to replicate and advance the original technique.

The promised merits of FUE motivated physicians worldwide to promptly adopt the novel "FUE procedure". Many prominent HRS surgeons launched aggressive marketing campaigns without prior adequate training and a nuanced understanding of its intricacies. In retrospect, FUE proved to be significantly more challenging than initially perceived, leading many practitioners to generate, for several years, results that Rassman termed a "Follicular Holocaust" rather than achieving superior outcomes compared to LSE [14].

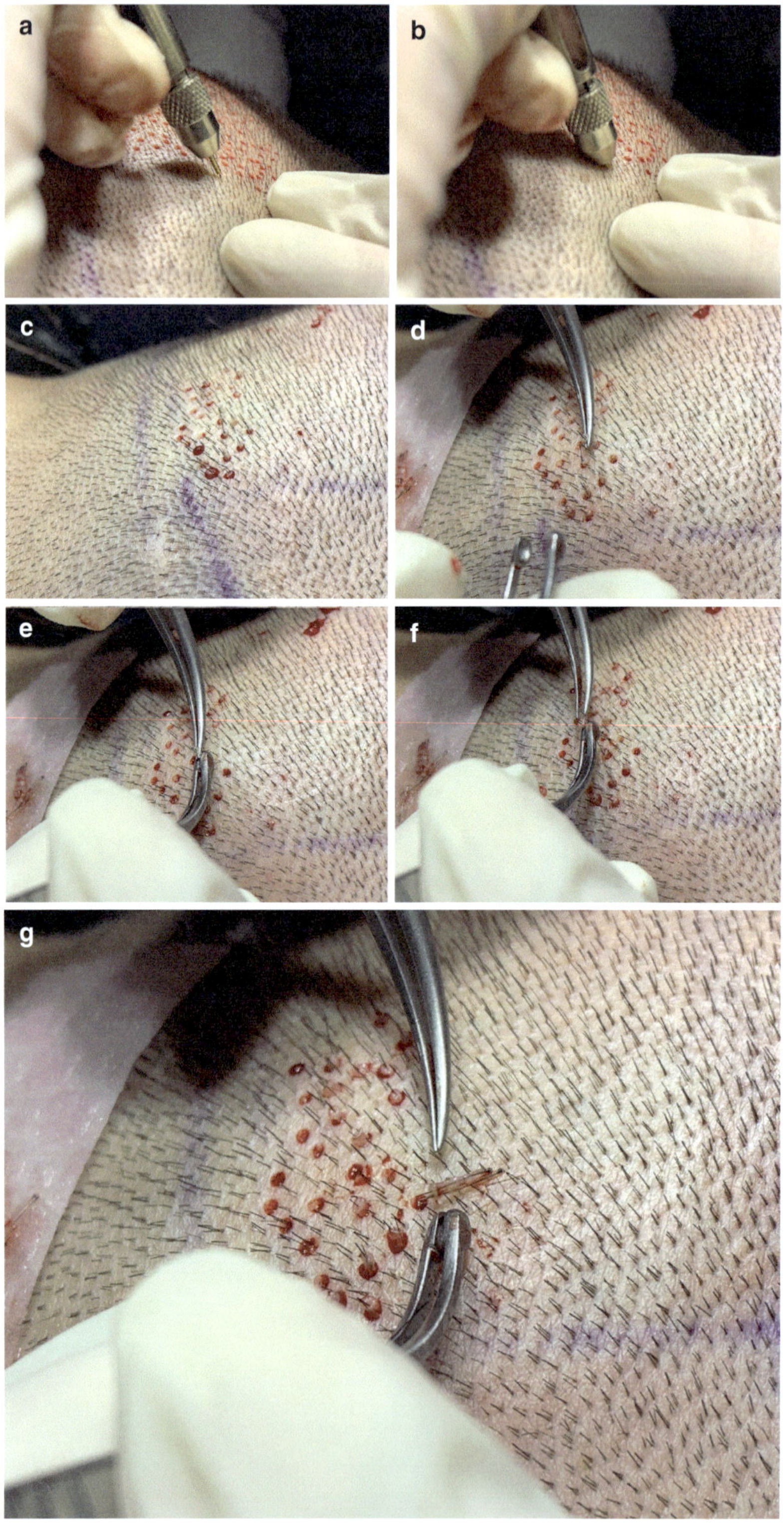

Fig. 3.5 The **sequence of steps** the surgeon must repeat thousands of times during each FUE session is: (**a**) punch alignment, centering, engagement, (**b**) accurate and controlled advancement, (**c**) With proper dissection, a graft usually elevates 0.5–1 mm and (**d**) can be extracted using one or (**e, f**) two forceps. (**g**) Extracted grafts are then collected and stored (From [13], used with permission)

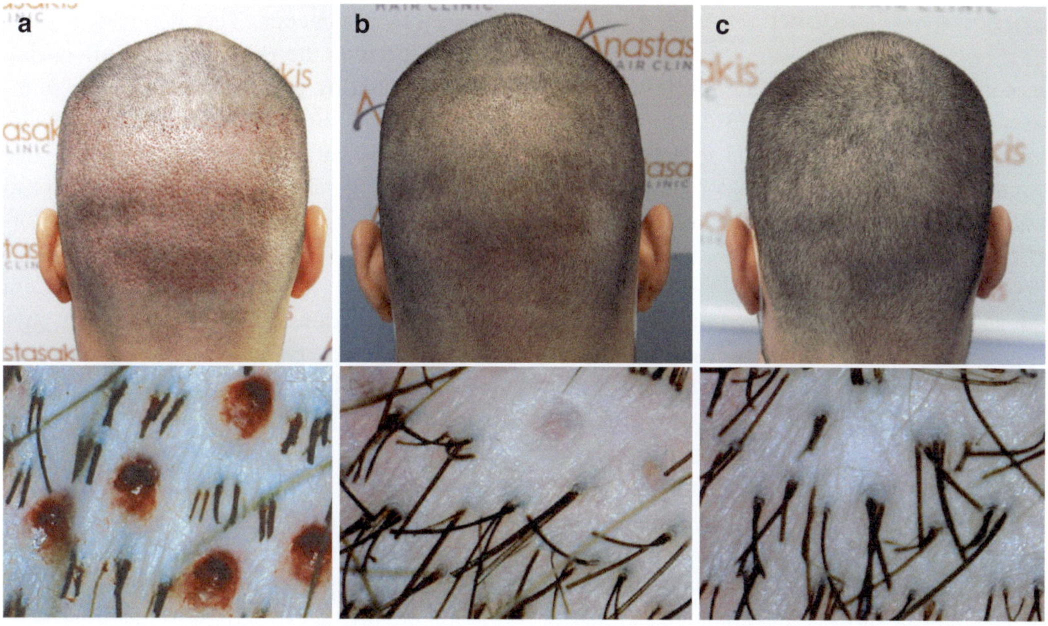

Fig. 3.6 (**a, c**) Global and corresponding macro images of the donor area immediately after FUE harvesting (**a**), at 48 h (**b**), and at 5 days post-surgery (**c**). The incisions are fully healed

Less Scars, More Candidates!

As previously elucidated, FUE emerged as a strategic response to the suboptimal donor scar outcomes associated with the LSE technique. Essentially, FUE represented a reimagination of the archetypal 4 mm punch grafting technique, albeit with the use of tiny punches, 1 mm in diameter or less, instead of 4 mm.

The primary motivation behind employing FUE lies in its ability to circumvent the creation of a visible linear scar, thereby allowing patients the flexibility to wear their hair short. Beyond this fundamental advantage, patients were assured of several side benefits, including markedly reduced post-operative discomfort or pain [15, 16], expedited surgical recovery, minimal disruption to an active professional, personal, or social lifestyle, an increase in scalp donor capacity (enabling safe harvesting from areas superior and more anterior to the ears and the nape of the neck), diminished limitations imposed by scalp laxity, and the prospect of expanding the potential donor area to include body hair [17].

Furthermore, FUE proved to be particularly advantageous for specific patient demographics. (a) Young patients, who are inherently at a higher risk for developing wider scars after LSE [18], can undergo FUE without such concerns. (b) Additionally, individuals with limited areas of alopecia other than androgenetic alopecia [19] (AGA) or those requiring inherently small sessions (e.g., eyebrows, eyelashes, mustache) have found FUE to be an ideal solution. (c) Furthermore, individuals with previous LSE surgeries seeking to camouflage older scars by implanting FUs inside the existing scar without removing it [20], and (d) patients with a history of wide scars or hyper-elastic skin have discovered viable solutions through FUE; (e) Patients with scars from various causes, including dermatologic conditions (scarring alopecias), trauma, or neurosurgical procedures [21], can also benefit from FUE.

The versatility of FUE not only addresses the aesthetic concerns of patients but also extends its applicability to diverse clinical scenarios, making it a valuable and multifaceted tool in the realm of HRS.

Spread and Conquer!

In contrast to LSE, harvesting grafts with FUE does not involve the creation of a linear incision; instead, it entails the creation of thousands of circular incisions. These incisions rapidly contract and heal, resulting in inconspicuous tiny circular scars that are difficult to discern, even upon close inspection. It is acknowledged that the punctuate FUE scars pose minimal practical concern and are aesthetically less conspicuous than a linear scar for the majority of patients.

However, to dispel a common misconception influenced by enthusiasm and deceptive advertising, it is crucial to recognize that FUE is not a scarless technique but rather a scar-spreading technique. Notably, scar tissue produced during even an ideally executed FUE session is several times larger in surface area compared to that of an average, uncomplicated LSE session with the same number of grafts extracted.

Remarkably, over the course of the two decades of FUE evolution, a noteworthy shift in focus has occurred among both HRS surgeons and patients, redirecting attention from the recipient area to the donor area. With the advent of the FUE technique, emphasis has been placed on the incisional aspect to minimize transection rates and enhance extraction speed. Consequently, there is a prevalent preoccupation with the details of punches, devices, and the postoperative appearance of the donor area, inadvertently diverting attention from the primary motivation that brought the patient to seek treatment initially: the desire for thick and naturally growing hair in areas affected by baldness. The evolving landscape of FUE has prompted a shift in priorities, necessitating a balanced perspective that encompasses both the donor and recipient areas to optimize outcomes and align patient expectations with the true goals of HRS.

The Game-Changer

The advent of a technique that promised minimal scar visibility, reduced pain, and broader eligibility resonated beautifully with both patients and neophyte surgeons. This heralded a paradigm shift within the HRS industry, influencing public demand by positioning itself as a minimally invasive surgical option. This shift not only altered patient expectations but also imposed new demands on service providers to meet the evolving requirements of this transformative process.

In the first decade of the FUE era (2002–2012), extensive discourse among physicians, ancillary personnel, the public, and various media platforms on the internet ensued, evaluating the comparative value of FUE versus LSE harvesting. Regrettably, numerous claims of the “superiority” of newer techniques were often driven more by marketing agendas and self-promotion than by rigorous scientific evaluation. [11] Despite this, a compelling motivation among doctors to promptly integrate FUE into their repertoire emerged as patient demand increased [11].

In contrast to other medical and surgical technologies, where major corporations are typically involved in research, development, education, and dissemination, the field of FUE experienced a distinct lack of such evolution. Physicians found themselves grappling with solutions to the challenges posed by FUE failures independently, with the responsibility falling squarely on their shoulders and those of their patients. Over time, practitioners managed to address these challenges, but not without incurring substantial costs along the way. The trajectory of FUE integration into clinical practice highlighted both the promise and challenges associated with pioneering techniques in the ever-evolving landscape of HRS.

Getting It Right

The rationale behind FUE involves employing a circular punch to excise a tissue column comprising an intact FU along with all layers of the skin. This process entails releasing the fold of arrectores and severing the adherence of surrounding dermal collagen, followed by a gentle yet firm extraction of the graft (Fig. 3.5). In the context of the preceding sentence, "intact" is the key term; the surgeon must exert every effort to prevent any trauma to the harvested hair follicles, with transection or amputation representing the most severe forms of injury.

The extremely delicate nature of the FU renders it susceptible to various forms of harm during the harvesting process, giving rise to a multitude of challenges inherent in extracting individual FUs with tiny punches while avoiding follicular transection or amputation. [11] In summary, the successful extraction of FUE grafts involves specific universal steps: targeting, incision/scoring, extraction, and collection. Apart from the preparatory stage, the surgeon is tasked with the meticulous extraction of each graft intact, repeating this sequence thousands of times during each FUE session. While patients may easily express a powerful preference for FUE over LSE, it is crucial to acknowledge that FUE harvesting is a tedious procedure that takes a toll on the surgeon's patience, energy levels, and enthusiasm.

Tough as They Come!

The challenges encountered in FUE harvesting proved to be more formidable than initially perceived. Unlike LSE, FUE surgery does not necessitate general surgical skills or proficiency in tissue approximation and suturing, eliminating a genuine barrier to entry that previously existed for HRS Surgeons. This new lower barrier, stemming from a perceived diminished need for surgical skills and the absence of multiple surgical staff trained in laborious microscopic dissection, led to an explosion of neophyte providers globally. The initial perception of FUE as a less invasive and "easier" procedure overshadowed the stark reality of the protracted learning curve required for proficient FUE donor harvesting [22]. Nearly two decades since the first publication on FUE, the dedicated efforts of numerous surgeons have contributed to substantial enhancements in FUE techniques and technologies, consequently elevating the overall quality of service, albeit more recently. Presently, it is widely acknowledged that successful FUE donor harvesting demands crucial technical, surgical, and artistic prerequisites with zero tolerance for error.

First, Do No Harm!

In the context of FUE harvesting, preserving the FU in its intact anatomy presents a formidable challenge. The primary obstacle in FUE lies in the blind introduction of the punch, which precludes visualization of the FU bulbs or the arrector muscle. Natural FUs, housing 1–4 hairs, exhibit the narrowest surface cross-section, and their inherent tendency to splay apart in random, unpredictable directions and angles in deeper layers poses a risk of transection by the diving punch (Fig. 3.7) [23]. Additionally, maintaining precise punch orientation to the follicular angle proves exceedingly challenging, and even minimal deviations during the push and twist movement will result in the transection of one or more bulbs.

An equally crucial challenge in FUE donor harvesting pertains to the variability of the donor area. The viscoelastic properties of the skin, resembling the biomechanical characteristics of solids and the viscous properties of fluids, contribute to the unpredictability of donor harvesting. The skin's soft tissue, composed of layers with distinct modulus and elastoplastic properties [22], interacts with the punch, subjecting it to various opposing forces such as friction, torque, tangential force, axial force, and oscillating force. These forces can lead to subluxation, overheating, or other forms of injury to the FU, as detailed elsewhere [24]. Patient-to-patient variations in the epidermis, dermal-epidermal junction, and subcutaneous tissue further compound the challenges in donor harvesting and achieving minimal follicular transection rates. [22]

Given the nuanced variations in technique among experts and patients, the fine details of proper FUE donor harvesting are elaborated upon elsewhere [2], while the fundamental principles are discussed herein. [2, 13]

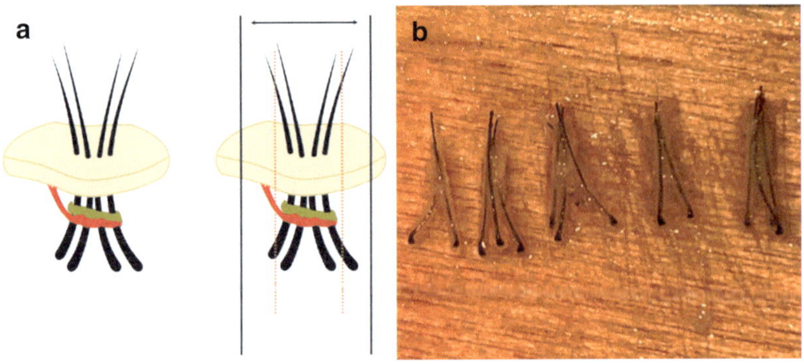

Fig. 3.7 (**a**) Follicles show varying degrees of splay as they extend deeper. Orange dotted lines show how a punch width determined by follicular grouping at the skin surface would damage the two outer follicles. Black lines show how a larger punch would preserve the unit, albeit at the expense of a much larger surface wound. (**b**) FUs with 2 and 3 hairs harvested from a patient with wavy hair showing various degrees of natural splaying. (From [13], used with permission)

Driving Forces of Change

The collaborative endeavors of a handful of surgeons have substantially enhanced the techniques, technologies, and tools associated with FUE, resulting in a noteworthy improvement in service quality and results since 2002. Presently, employing various available FUE approaches, practically all patients can undergo successful harvesting [25], marking a significant achievement. Nevertheless, this progress has been a protracted and challenging journey for both surgeons and patients, who encountered failures as practitioners learned to adapt their techniques incrementally, one step and one patient at a time.

Over time, a shift occurred as most surgeons transitioned from manual handles to motorized devices. While this transition led to a manifold increase in graft harvesting rates, surgeons recognized the need for enhanced control and dexterity compared to manual punching. FUE device manufacturers, designed various automated devices to expedite the process and reduce transection rates, broadly categorized into rotating and oscillating groups. The most popular include the S.AF.E. System (Surgically Advanced Follicular Extraction) [25, 26], Powered Cole Isolation Device (PCID), WAW (Devroye Instruments, Brussels, Belgium), and Mamba device (Trivellini Tech). In the case of oscillating devices, the punch does not rotate in one direction but rather oscillates back and forth, mimicking the manual punch. Concerning the rotating device, the punch rotates in one direction and the operator can control the speed and torque. Newer devices incorporate programmable controls for rotation, oscillation, vibration, or their combination to facilitate and enhance the FUE dissection process [27]. Some devices, such as (NeoGraft Solutions, Dallas, TX) and SmartGraft (Vision Medical, Glen Mills, PA), include suction for graft extraction but may pose a risk of reduced graft survival due to desiccation injury from constant airflow [28].

Regarding punch selection, two distinct schools of thought emerged during FUE evolution, focusing on blunt and sharp dissection approaches. Jim Harris MD introduced the blunt punch, termed the “S.A.F.E. technique” [26], while the alternative approach employs a sharp punch with a “stop” to limit penetration depth. [24] This school advocates that sharp punches minimize friction and thrust force that could damage follicles. However, the choice between sharp and blunt punches does not resolve the dilemma, as various physical and technical factors influence punch-cutting dynamics, tissue distortion, and graft injury. These factors include punch shape, diameter, tip shape, edge sharpness, location and diameter of dissecting edge, punch wall thickness, and punch metal type. Consequently, a diverse array of incisional techniques has emerged, employing sharp, serrated, non-serrated, dull, hybrid, trumpet punches, and other designs (Fig. 3.8). Details on punch design categories, engineering, punch incision geometry, and metallurgy fall beyond the scope of this chapter and can be sourced elsewhere. [24, 26, 29]

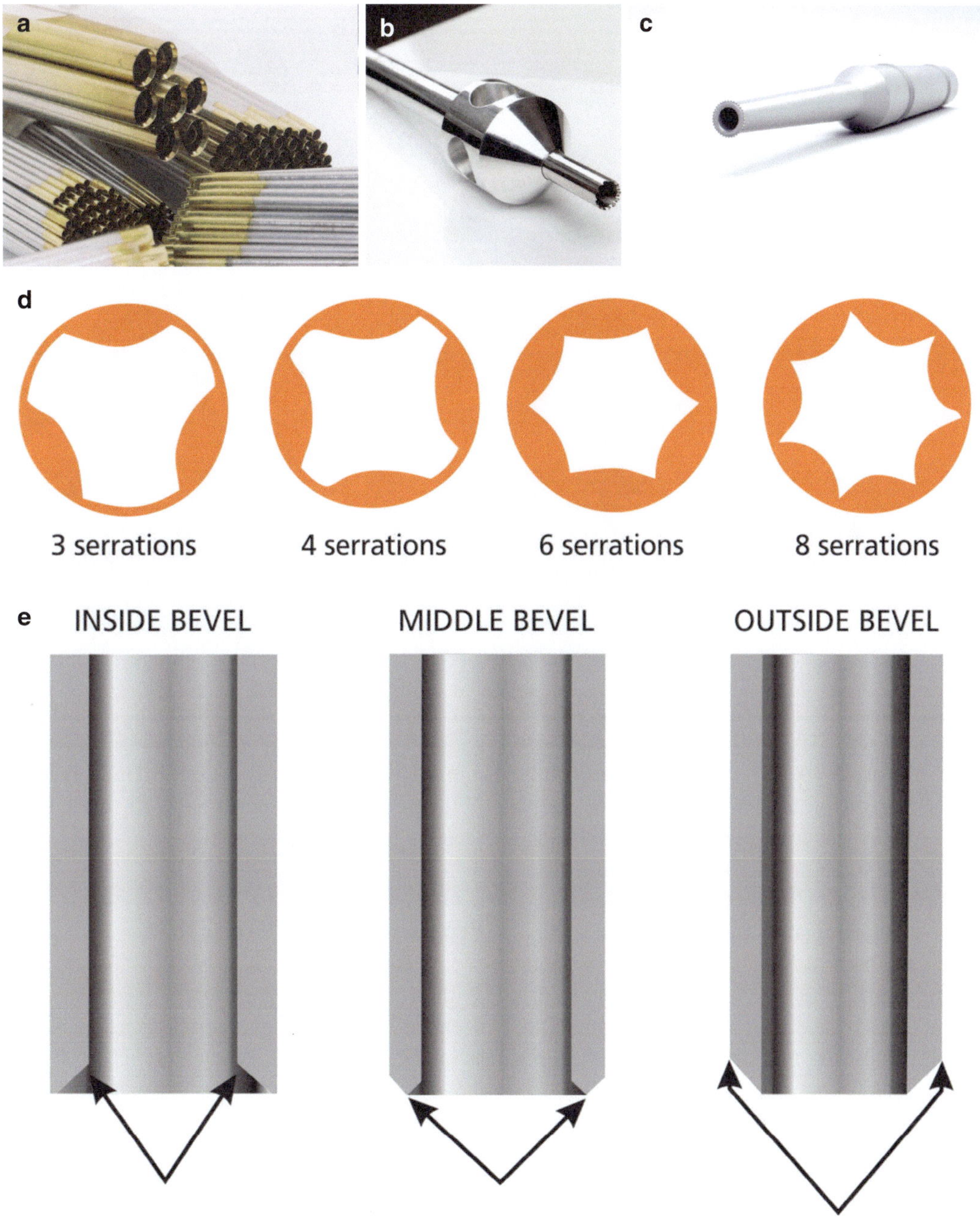

Fig. 3.8 Punch cutting edge styles: (**a**) titanium tip sharp punches, (**b**) a serrated punch, and (**c**) a flared punch. (**d**) The serrated punch cutting edge shows multiple cutting edges and different designs. (**e**) The sharp punch shows the different locations of the cutting edge: inside, middle, or outside. (From [13], used with permission)

Minimally Invasive But With a Thousand Cuts

Walter Unger [30] astutely noted in response to the original FUE publication [11] that FUE entails a substantial increase in the total length of incisions compared to conventional LSE harvesting. For instance, extracting 2000 FUs using an FUE punch with a diameter $D = 1$ mm, would result in a wound length (perimeter) totaling 6280 mm, equivalent to CFUE $\approx$ 6.3 m. In contrast, employing LSE harvesting from an average

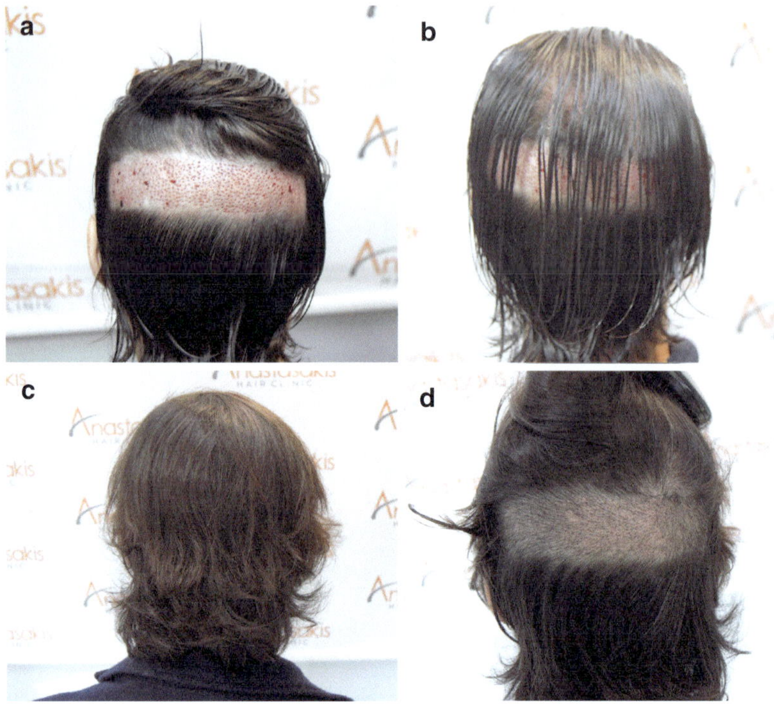

Fig. 3.9 (**a–d**) Patient with a partial, microstrip, shave who needed 600 FUs for a hairline touch-up. The top hair fully covers the shaved area, even with wet hair. Notice that FUs are not harvested too densely and the technique should be used only on patients with an excellent donor area. Notice that on day 5 the trimmed "window" is completely covered by top hair, when hair is dry. (From [13], used with permission)

donor area (80 FUs/cm^2) would yield a wound length of Cstrip = 400 mm = 0.43 m. Consequently, FUE's nearly 15-fold increase in incision length challenges its characterization as minimally invasive, as was often proclaimed in the initial years. Each FUE incision's scar surface, considering a 1-mm diameter punch and a perfectly vertical entry, calculates to E_{FUE} = 1570 mm^2, equivalent to a scar surface of 4 × 4 cm. In comparison, a typical 2 mm wide scar from the 180-mm LSE wound equals 360 mm^2, representing five times less scarring for the same number of grafts.

The diameter of the punch is not even the most determining factor in wound ceation in FUE. Notably, introducing the punch at an angle of 30° results in a 100% increase in the trauma caused by the punch (Fig. 3.9) [31]. Despite the remarkable results of LSE harvesting combined with a trichophytic closure in terms of minimal scarring, this benefit is generally observed from the doctor's perspective. Conversely, from the patient's standpoint, FUE is perceived as a more minimally invasive and patient-friendly method [32], even though it leads to 5–10 times more scarring than LSE!

Pros and Cons of FUE

With a cumulative experience exceeding two decades since 2002, the comprehension of the advantages and disadvantages of FUE for both the patient and surgeon has become extensive. The ensuing "objective pros and cons" of FUE presuppose excellent technical skills of the physician, suitable tools, and superb artistic perception (Table 3.1). It is crucial to acknowledge that inadequately performed FUE by an untrained, or unauthorized provider, will incur significant drawbacks such as diminished graft survival, depletion of donor area reserves, and the risk of overharvesting.

Table 3.1 An objective comparison of LSE versus FUE donor harvesting methods when both are performed "lege artis"

	Linear strip excision	Follicular unit excision
Naturalness of the result	Yes, usually better density/coverage per session	Yes, can offer higher number of hairs/cm^2
Fatigue of patient-surgeon	Less tiring	Especially exhausting for both patient and surgeon
Shaving of donor area	Not needed	Needed most of the times
Healing time: donor area	On average 2 weeks until stitches are removed and fully healed at 12 months	Fully in 5–7 days, but can be reharvested at 4–6 months
Period for complete healing of the recipient area	About 10–14 days	About 10–14 days
Duration of discomfort in the donor area	Between 2 days to a few weeks	Typically, 1 day, but it can last for weeks if the area is overharvested
Amount of time after which the patient may return to work	2–3 days	Usually, the next day
Exercise restriction	3–4 weeks for light exercise, 12–16 weeks for heavy weightlifting	1 weeks for weight training, 2–3 weeks for contact sports
Wearing short hairstyle in the donor area	Rarely possible	100% possible
Time until the next session	10–12 months for the donor area to recover	Next day: different donor region 4–6 months: reharvesting the same region
Postoperative donor area discomfort	Mild to moderate	Minimal
Nerve damage, numbness, permanent pain	Rare	No
Visible scarring with short hair	May occur	Very rare
Reaction to sutures	Rare, especially absorbable ones	Never
Percent of time the doctor operates on the patient	10–30%	80–90%
Type of grafts	Trimmed to the precise shape and size desired by the surgeon	Grafts are extracted from the donor area and often thin and lacking in supportive tissue
Graft placement	Equally good with forceps or implanters	Implanters are preferred
Quality of grafts	Excellent and predictable, "customized" graft quality	Can be considerably lower depending on tools, technique, and patient variability
Transection rate	1–2% with an experienced surgeon and surgical team	Depends on the training and skill of the surgeon
		Approx. 1–5% in expert hands; can be >70% in inexperienced hands
Stitches/staples required	Yes	No
Tissue cutting/excising	Significantly lower cutting and scarring surfaces, but the linear scar may be noticeable	Several times more cutting and scarring surfaces, but spread out and less conspicuous
Excessive bleeding during or after the procedure	Rare	No
Experience and skill of the surgeon	Most often very high	It can range from highly experienced surgeons to inexperienced novices or even non-medical operators
Permanence of harvested grafts	Excellent, all grafts are harvested from the "safest" donor area	Only 25–30% of grafts are harvested from the "safest" donor area

(continued)

Table 3.1 (continued)

	Linear strip excision	Follicular unit excision
Possibility of megasessions (>3000 grafts)	Yes, even up to 5000 FUs for expert teams	Not advisable in 1 day
Type of hair where technique can be applied	All	Not recommended for kinky, coily, curly, or white hair
Suitability for female candidates	Preferred technique	Rarely due to the requirement to trim the entire donor area
Camouflage of older donor area scars	Challenging as a fresh scar is formed	Brilliant, one can even implant body hair grafts within the scar
Number of grafts that can be harvested over a lifetime	More grafts can be extracted in a lifetime before evident thinning of the donor area	Less grafts can be extracted before evident thinning of the donor area
Cost per graft	Lower	Higher
Cost of instrumentation	High initial investment only for microscopes	Higher, especially with motorized devices, and expensive disposable punches
Cost of the surgical team	High	Minimal

Positives for the Surgeon

The following arguments are valid as long as surgery is performed by an experienced and ethical surgeon.

- The surgeon can ensure heightened patient satisfaction with the appearance of the donor area compared to LSE.
- FUE cases requiring 1500–2000 FUs in 1 day can be efficiently completed by an experienced surgeon alone assisted by 1 or 2 assistants, eliminating the need for the large assisting staff of LSE.
- FUE does not necessitate general surgical or LSE harvesting and suturing skills; however, it still demands artistic, diagnostic, and technical skills that require years of development.
- FUE is suitable for a wide range of candidates, including those previously deemed inoperable due to reduced laxity after multiple previous HRS procedures.
- Most importantly, the surgeon can selectively harvest grafts, achieving a higher number of hairs/cm^2 for improved coverage while avoiding excessive grafting FUs/cm^2, promoting better survival and a fuller look with lower and safer recipient area densities.
- Due to the small incision size, serious complications such as scalp necrosis are extremely rare, particularly in experienced hands [33].
- The cost of equipment can be minimized, especially when opting for a manual punch over motorized systems.
- FUE is excellent in repairing the results of older techniques [34], such as LSE surgery, punch grafts, flaps, etc. FUE offers a genuine solution without exchanging an old scar for a potentially thinner one, as seen in other types of scar repair [35].
- FUE can be uniquely effective in camouflaging any type of scalp scar caused by burns, scarring alopecias, trauma, or neurosurgical procedures [21] without having to remove the previous scar, just by implanting FUE grafts inside the scar surface.
- With minimal equipment and staff requirements, the surgeon can easily travel and operate in different locations or countries, significantly expanding the customer base.
- FUE procedures garner highly favorable responses from patients, who perceive them as less invasive compared to LSE, considering FUE a “newer” technique, and often opt in for surgery with minimal consultation.
- FUE can be combined in the same session with LSE and/or BHT in cases requiring the highest number of grafts, a scenario not feasible with FUE or LSE alone under “no tension” donor closure [36]. The Combo Technique (TCT) involves creatively combining harvesting techniques to maximize the number of safely extracted grafts in one session and

expand the lifetime hair donor capacity. TCT is invaluable in a large percentage of cases, in both virgin and non-virgin donor areas. It allows the advantages of both major harvesting techniques to be brought together and helps patients reach their cosmetic goals sooner and safer than with either technique alone. The indications, details, and merits of TCT, as well as a comprehensive decision algorithm for proper TCT, are presented elsewhere [37].

Positives for the Patient

- If FUE is executed "lege artis", the patient can maintain a very short hairstyle even after extensive harvesting and several FUE sessions.
- Post-operative discomfort is minimal; post-surgical painkillers are rarely required.
- Surgical recovery is rapid, with incisions typically healing in just 3–5 days. This leads to minimal downtime and easily concealable wounds.
- Patients with active lifestyles face no significant exercise restrictions, allowing them to resume standard simple activities even on the next day and heavy training in a week.
- Scalp laxity limitations and issues arising from multiple previous donor area scars of any source are practically nonexistent.
- Complications related to nerve and vessel injuries are exceedingly rare, although reports of widespread anagen effluvium in the donor area [22] exist when harvesting is extremely extensive or inappropriate tools are used.
- Patients with advanced AGA may undergo two or three consecutive FUE sessions on consecutive days to cover their cosmetic goals sooner.
- Technician/assistant involvement in FUE can be kept to a minimum.
- FUs from various body areas, such as the beard, chest, abdomen, back, hands, legs, and genitals, can be successfully transplanted. (see Body Hair Transplant)

Negatives for the Surgeon

- FUE necessitates the acquisition of an entirely new skill-set by the surgeon: precise, skillful, strategic FUE harvesting.
- The success of FUE relies significantly on accuracy and speed, both of which evolve with time, focused practice, and experience. The required timeframe is measured in years, not months.
- While prior surgical experience is not mandatory for FUE, the learning curve is notably protracted.
- FUE harvesting demands considerable time and requires more of the physician's time compared to LSE harvesting [38].
- The repetitive nature of FUE harvesting makes it a tedious procedure, impacting the surgeon's patience, energy levels, and enthusiasm over thousands of repetitions per case.
- Prolonged FUE sessions can lead to eye strain and fatigue, chronically wearing down the surgeon.
- Extended FUE sessions may contribute to back and neck problems for the surgeon, potentially progressing to chronic conditions. Attention to ergonomics and positioning is crucial to prevent long-term injuries.
- Surgical time encompasses strategic graft selection by the surgeon to ensure judicious harvesting without over-harvesting any specific area.
- Mastery of different FUE techniques and proficiency in using various devices and/or punches are necessary for customizing each procedure to the individual patient.
- Reharvesting an area again with FUE is exponentially more challenging than extracting grafts from a virgin donor area. Since most patients will need multiple FUE sessions, this occurrence is more of a standard than an exception.
- Excessive FUE harvesting (overharvesting) leads to diffuse donor area thinning, resembling scalp disease. Overharvesting is cosmetically more problematic than a wide LSE scar, and is often impossible to camouflage with any hair length.

Negatives for the Patient

- The primary drawback is the reduction of total donor capacity when exclusively utilizing the FUE technique, which limits the number of grafts safely harvested over one session and one's lifetime [39]. Of course, TCT solves this problem
- A notable concern with FUE, in most hands, is the higher follicular transection rate compared to LSE.
- Significant apprehensions revolve around the fragility of the inherently skinnier FUE grafts compared to LSE grafts [40].
- The FUE procedure is prolonged compared to an LSE session, leading to patient fatigue [41].
- Daily graft extraction is limited, necessitating multiple sessions over 2 or 3 days, or 6–12 months after the previous harvest.
- The standard higher cost per graft in FUE, compared to LSE harvesting, is attributed to the tiring nature of the procedure, requiring substantial experience and specialization, primarily performed by the surgeon.
- Complete shaving of the entire donor area to 1–2 mm (total shave) is required in FUE, is associated with social discomfort. However, the rising popularity of long-hair FUE addresses this concern among patients and surgeons.
- Women will not agree to shave the donor area to help the surgeon identify hair follicles and their exit angle when performing FUE.
- Extensive microscopic devascularization injury in the donor area may lead to permanent "thin" areas. This can occur after multiple FUE sessions or a single injudicious harvest.
- African FUs or very curly/coily hair with a powerful "character" beneath the skin carries an increased risk of graft transection in FUE.

Social and Post-Transplant Concerns in FUE

In order to perform FUE harvesting under proper conditions, the entire donor area must be shaved down to 1 mm (total shave) since the surface necessary to offer the same number of grafts is 5–8 times more extensive than with LSE. For most patients, the considerable benefits of FUE more than offset the social problems seen with the shaved donor area, which have to be managed for the first week or so after an FUE procedure.

There is a demographic of HRS candidates who, for professional, social, or personal reasons, are highly self-conscious of their appearance and do not consider that the benefits of FUE will counterbalance the social awkwardness of a fully shaved donor area. Older male patients who typically have no intention to ever buzz-cut their hair might also be included in this group, and therefore, the cosmetic "freedom" that FUE offers is irrelevant to them. Others are reluctant to trim their hair because scars from previous LSE operations will show.

Solutions to bypass these issues have been offered, in which individual FUs are painstakingly harvested throughout the donor area without shaving the surrounding hairs. These include partial-shaving "tunnels" (microstrip shaving) along the back and sides of the head, each 2 to 3 cm wide, leaving the overlying longer hairs to conceal the trimmed hairs (Fig. 3.9) [42]. Another idea is an individual follicular trim isolation technique, first described by Harris, trimming only those hairs that will be extracted [19]. These techniques are very time-consuming, and unless the surgeon is highly experienced, harvested areas may be left with significant thinning. These techniques risk creating a so-called "zebra effect" or "flag-sign" scarring due to horizontal rows of the scalp that are thinned out from FU harvesting,

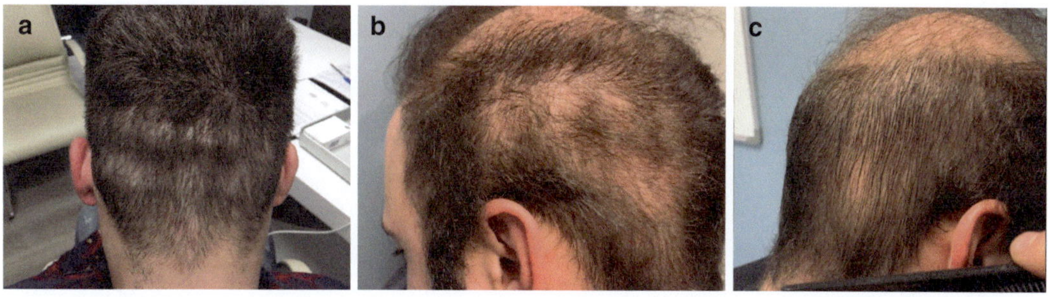

Fig. 3.10 (**a**) Partial-shaving done wrong, creating a "window" effect (flag-sign, zebra-sign), with two centrally thinned areas surrounded by denser hair. This can only be covered by hair longer than 3 cm, (**b**) Partial shaving was done 3 times on the same patient, leaving a severely thin "window" of hair on both sides (**c**), right side of the same patient). If this patient requires more grafts, he can only hope for a very careful performed LSE surgery in the future. (From [13], used with permission)

which is cosmetically worse than a strip scar (Fig. 3.10). Recently, long-hair FUE has been suggested to by-pass all these issues, but a small number of grafts can be extracted safely per day (<800 FUs) [43].

Body-to-Scalp FUE: Heavenly Body or Body Blow?

FUE allowed for the first time to easily harvest body hair follicles and use them in HRS. Body-to-Scalp Hair Transplantation (BHT) involves the harvesting of FUs from areas other than the scalp and their transplantation into the scalp or other hairy areas. Of course, beard and other body donor hair differ in characteristics (maximum length, caliber, color, growth cycles, etc.) from the scalp donor hair since they are typically shorter, single-haired, thinner, and less "shiny" compared to scalp hair. Surprisingly, when these FUs are transplanted to the scalp, they gradually show an ability to reshape their morphology and iteratively converge to the recipient tissue environment by significantly prolonging anagen duration, eventually growing much longer than earlier.

Combining or "mixing" BHT FUs with scalp donor FUs on selected individuals was initially presented as a "miracle solution" that could increase the number of potentially transplantable FUs enormously and expand the candidate pool to cases that were previously deemed inoperable. When the initial enthusiasm was subdued through bitter experience, graft harvesting in BHT proved to be very challenging, having a very long learning curve, with characteristically high follicular transection rates, and often disappointing postoperative graft survival. Especially when non-beard BHT grafts are harvested, the donor area heals slower, and local complications are more frequent than in the scalp.

Notably, only highly trained FUE experts will successfully employ BHT, and not even those may claim that the results on the recipient area are consistent and predictable. Most experts consider BHT as an ultimate, "last resort" solution [44] that should be applied under specific, unique circumstances and for the following indications:

- Cases with extremely unfavorable donor-to-recipient needs ratio. Low donor reserves can be attributed to low donor density, narrow donor fringe, retrograde alopecia, previous surgical or post-traumatic scarring, extensive donor miniaturization, diffuse thinning, and very fine, straight hair. High recipient needs can result from big skull size, advanced AGA, early age of onset, rapid progression of AGA, low-residual hairline, and high hair-to-scalp color contrast. In all these cases, however, the surgeon should first follow established guidelines/protocols on scalp donor area harvesting. The surgeon should not rely on BHT grafts to "save the day" (Fig. 3.11).
- Camouflage of scalp scars, from previous LSE surgery, punch grafts, flaps, burns, or other

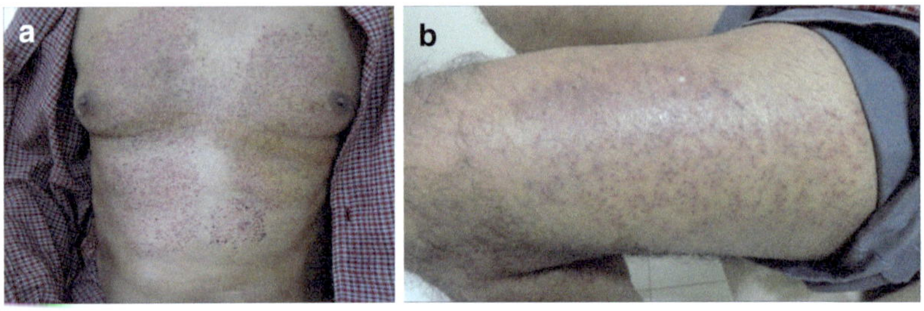

Fig. 3.11 (**a**, **b**) Extensive BHT harvesting of follicles from the chest, upper abdomen, back, arms and thighs, on a 63-year-old male with depleted scalp donor area. Overall, 8900 body FUs were harvested and transplanted in 9 sessions within 18 months. According to the authors, there was a 47% transection rate (From [45])

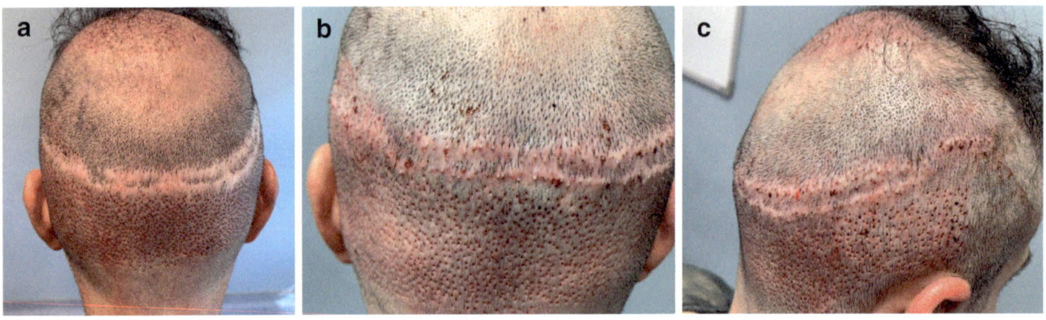

Fig. 3.12 (**a**–**c**) Scar repair of previous FUT surgery using beard grafts, during a combined FUE + BHT session. These thick hairs will offer an efficient scar camouflage, breaking the continuous hairless image of the scar even with shorter hair. The harvested scalp FUs were used exclusively in the recipient areas

injuries for which the patient is unwilling to use "precious" scalp FUs or when the scalp donor area is naturally poor or depleted due to previous surgery (Fig. 3.12) [20, 46].

- Combining or "mixing" beard FUs with scalp donor FUs to improve recipient area density and/or the cosmetic result in individuals with depleted/overharvested scalp donor area [47]. "Combination grafting" of scalp-plus-beard hair not only increases the total number of donor hair but enhances results because of the larger diameter and coverage value of beard hair.
- Lack of adequate donor scalp hair in cicatricial alopecia where scarring is so extensive that there is inadequate scalp donor hair to provide adequate coverage in scarring patches [48].
- Use of thin body hair follicles in areas where hair thickness, growth rate, and length desired are optimal for body hair but not for scalp hair. These include areas where a "thin look" is preferable, such as feathering the hairline [49], use on the temple points, or the reconstruction of eyelashes [50], eyebrows [51], etc.
- To reconstruct small areas of beard in Zones 1–3, which are necessary for secondary sexual male characteristics. In that case, one can recycle beard hair from other, less important beard areas (Fig. 3.13).

Controversial applications of BHT that will not be further analyzed include:

- Increase in coverage/density of recipient area in individuals with high levels of miniaturization in the scalp donor area (such as DUPA patients),
- "Recharging" of donor area after FUE overharvesting. Notably, this is a highly debated approach.

Overall, the experience gathered in BHT has been substantial since the late 2000s. It clearly has a place in modern HRS on many occasions

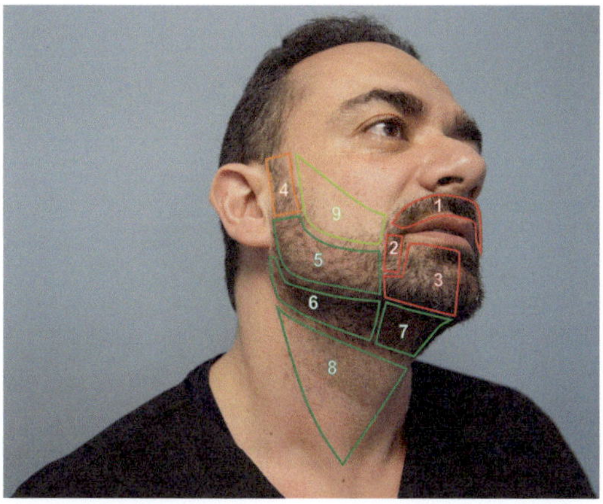

Fig. 3.13 Zones 1, 2, and 3 are "Red Zones", necessary for secondary sexual male characteristics and are strictly avoided during BHT harvesting. Also, these are the first zones to transplant when reconstructing the beard. Zone 4 (sideburns) should be avoided for styling purposes. The most preferred zones are "Green Zones" 5–8, with carotid, submandibular, submental, and mandibular areas being preferred in descending order. Submandibular zone (5) harvesting carries the risk of injuring facial nerve and/or artery, and buccal/zygomatic zone (9) harvesting can result in visible white-spot scarring. However, in zone 9, hairs are usually more scattered and not desirable, regardless of beard style. Thus, removing them can additionally help to create a desirable, more refined beard look. (From [52])

but is performed at an acceptable standard by only very experienced surgeons.

Female Patients and FUE Rarely Make a Match

The principal cosmetic advantage of FUE from the patient's perspective is the freedom to maintain a truly short hairstyle, since there should be no visible signs of surgery even after extensive harvesting and several FUE sessions. However, this inherent benefit of FUE rightfully leaves female HRS candidates unimpressed as very few, if any, will ever cut their hair too short, at least willingly.

Women with any alopecia that is eligible for HRS, most often FPHL or scarring alopecias, will rarely, if ever, agree to entirely shave the donor area to help the surgeon identify hair follicles and their exit angle when performing FUE. This understandable unwillingness to shave the donor area makes FUE megasessions practically impossible for these female patients. Therefore, the size of an FUE session in these women is limited to techniques such as "microstrip shave" or "camouflage-to-go", which will offer a smaller number of FUs compared to a full FUE session. Therefore, LSE surgery is typically preferred in women. However, one should remember that in most women with FPHL, the donor area often presents a high ratio of miniaturized hair follicles. In these cases, the surgical advantage of cherry-picking "healthier" grafts with FUE can be a determining factor in the final result and should be explained to these specific female candidates [53].

The Uncomfortable Controversies of FUE

The promises made by FUE have been alluring to both patients and surgeons from the outset. However, akin to all aspects of life, these promises come with associated costs. To achieve high-quality, intact FUE grafts, minimize transection, and provide reliable results, surgeons must carefully consider several crucial factors inherent to the FUE technique.

Harvesting Rationale and Pattern

The fundamental premise is that donor area FUE scars, typically appearing as hypopigmented, pinpoint atrophic macules/dots, should seamlessly integrate with the remaining hair, resembling an unharvested donor area to escape notice. The surgeon must adhere to specific guidelines [54]:

- Create the smallest scars possible: select punch size, type, and angle of entry meticulously, based on individual patient characteristics.
- Strategically harvest grafts: utilize a zigzag pattern, skipping neighboring FUs to prevent the formation of a visible, linear 2 FU-area void of hair.

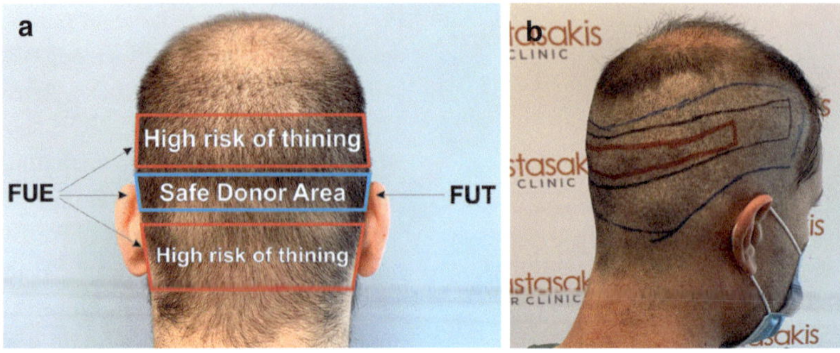

Fig. 3.14 (**a**) The more spread-out protocol of extraction in FUE requires harvesting into "unsafe areas". The long-term consequences of this widespread practice of "FUE-only surgeons" are worrisome; (**b**) The blue line outlines the "extended SDA" used for FUE harvesting; the black line the "safest" SDA used in LSE harvesting; the red line considers the female SDA. The female SDA is much shorter in length and less wide. (From [56])

- Properly space excisions: ensure that remaining hair emerges superior to the excision site, preventing mottling and the risk of local devascularization that could lead to scalp necrosis if accumulated.
- Widely distribute excision sites: implement a uniform distribution to avoid a "window" effect (central thinned area surrounded by denser hair). Overall, the surgeon must homogeneously "thin" the entire donor area to conceal surgical signs. When FUE white dots are uniformly spread, they offer the most aesthetic benefits.

All these considerations necessitate the area of harvesting to be generally five to six times the area of a donor strip for the equivalent number of grafts [55]. This raises the controversy surrounding the concept of "unsafe" Safe Donor Area (SDA) and the risk of "hair graft overharvesting."

Is the Safe Donor Area Safe Enough?

LSE surgeons efficiently extract 100% of their grafts within the established Safe Donor Area (SDA), easily obtaining over 6000 FUs in two or three sessions over the years. In contrast, FUE surgeons aiming for a comparable graft quantity must extend their harvesting beyond the traditional SDA limits, encompassing potential "danger zones" or truly "unsafe zones." These areas, containing hair that may miniaturize over time, pose risks to long-term graft viability (Fig. 3.14). This protocol of artificially expanding the harvesting area and extracting nonpermanent grafts creates a paradox [57]:

- The surgeon is forced to leave behind unharvested thousands of optimal grafts within the true SDA to provide coverage for adjacent FUE white dots.
- Follicles harvested beyond the true SDA limits are prone to future loss due to miniaturization, resulting in a "temporary" hair transplant for a large number of the transplanted grafts (Fig. 3.15) [58]. Moreover, future balding may encroach into the harvested donor zone, leading to visible FUE scars and dissatisfied patients. The surgeon must also avoid creating zones of significantly lower hair density, opting for an "even thinning" of the donor area compared to natural density, even in areas immediately adjacent to the balding margins (Fig. 3.15) [59].
- Despite efforts to preserve density evenly, the risks of future balding encroaching into the harvested donor areas and the potential visibility of donor scarring remain [60].

Overall, FUE surgeons face the challenge of harvesting from unpredictable donor areas that may miniaturize in the future, making it impractical to guarantee the longevity of all harvested FUs in the recipient area throughout the patient's life. Consequently, some renowned FUE surgeons

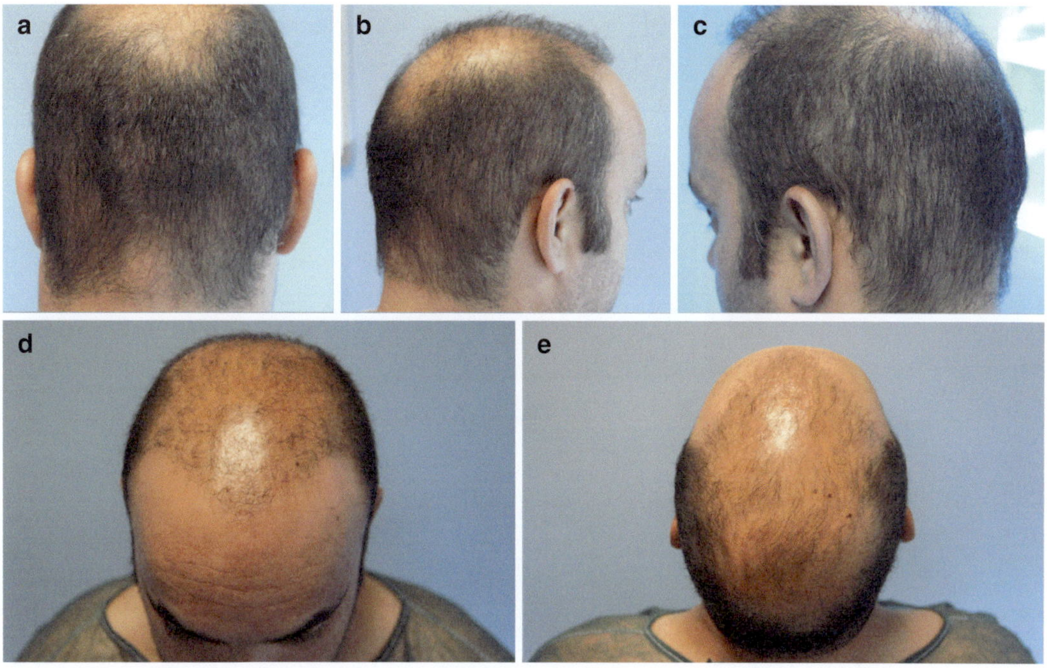

Fig. 3.15 (**a–e**) Moth-eaten, thin donor area after one FUE session, which also resulted in minimal growth. Notice the window effect with the thicker fringe of hair over the harvested area

exclusively accept patients for megasessions under the condition of indefinite oral Finasteride use, banking on its potential to "secure" the donor area. Nonetheless, this approach carries inherent risks, given the uncertainty of medication efficacy over a lifetime.

Is Overharvesting Avoidable?

Evaluating the permissible number of harvested grafts and surgical trauma in FUE before reaching a noticeable decrease in coverage remains an ongoing challenge. No single algorithm comprehensively integrates all the various factors to predict the minimum adequate remaining donor area density following FUE. Therefore, surgical experience and prudent harvesting are paramount.

Unfortunately, the global surge in FUE popularity has led to a massive rise in cases of donor area overharvesting, resulting in severe cosmetic defects ranging from visibly moth-eaten donor areas to near-complete donor alopecia (Fig. 3.16). Overharvesting leads to "donor area depletion," involving not only excessive hair removal but also cumulative scar surface, subclinical vascular damage, and hidden transections causing significant miniaturization of donor hairs and reduced coverage [14]. Notably, diffuse thinning after excessive FUE harvesting poses a greater cosmetic challenge than an LSE scar, resembling a pseudo-syphilitic scalp disease that is impossible to camouflage. Unlike a linear scar that can be hidden by longer hair above the scar, longer hair in the overharvested FUE area may appear overly "thin" and "see-through," more noticeable adjacent to the denser fringe at the balding border. Shorter hair may reduce the "see-through" effect but could expose white dots. Like a poor LSE scar dictating permanently longer donor hair, an overharvested FUE donor area may limit the patient to very short hair or a very specific length to balance transparency and scar visibility. This contradicts the expectation of cosmetic freedom associated with the supposedly "scarless" FUE method, revealing it as an intentional misnomer and fraudulent. To predict FUE harvest limits and prevent overharvesting, some FUE experts pro-

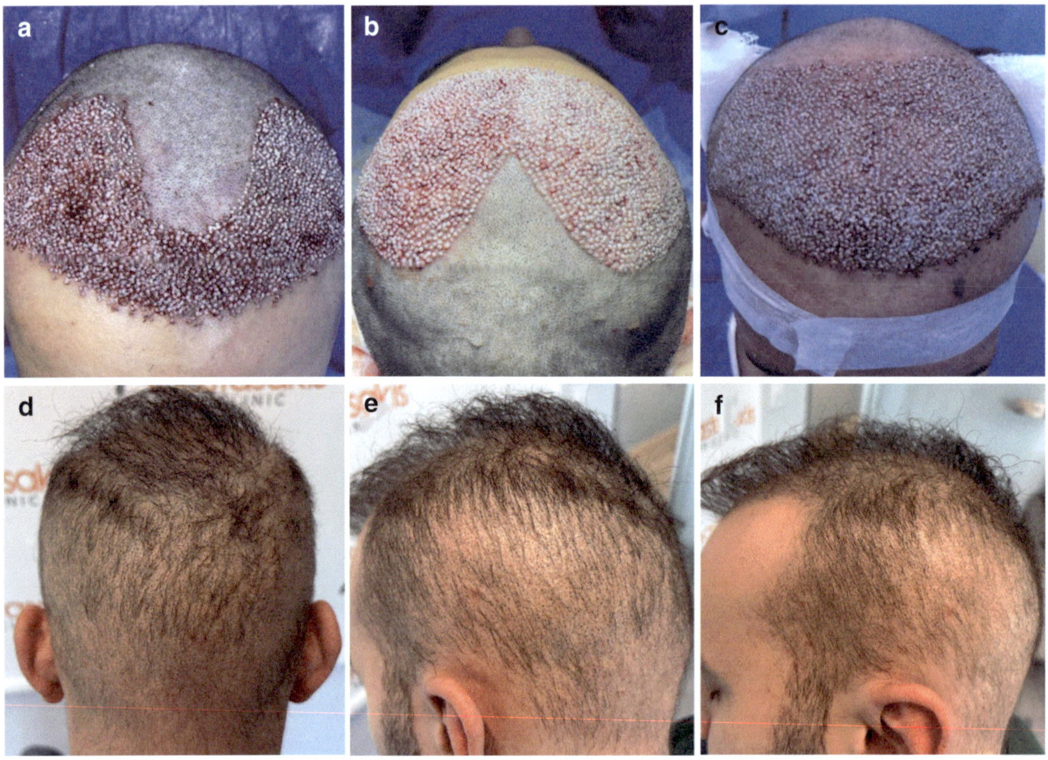

Fig. 3.16 (**a–c**) A typical "black-market" clinic's FUE megasession example with 5000–6000 grafts extracted in 1 day. Note the size of the grafts due to the use of a very large punch, making the area seem denser to the untrained eye. (**d–f**) The results of this practice are detrimental to the donor area. Notice the decimated "pseudo-syphilitic" donor area, which even failed to improve with scalp micropigmentation. (From [61])

pose guidelines based on the initial "Hair Coverage Value" [62] derived from hair shaft diameters and hair count/cm^2. However, no metric or index can substitute for clinical judgment and thoughtful consideration [63].

How Can One Minimize Graft Injuries?

The incidence of injuries to FUE grafts is variable and strongly influenced by the surgeon's skills. Follicular transection stands out as a prevalent form of injury associated with FUE. Minimizing the transection and injury rates primarily relies on the surgeon's expertise, encompassing experience, eyesight, hand-eye coordination, and maneuvering capabilities. Additionally, the details of the technique play a pivotal role, including the FUE extraction devices, punch type, punch size, and harvesting speed. Patient-specific factors, such as prior FUE scarring [64], hair shaft exit angulation [65], skin visco-elastic properties, and other considerations, contribute to the overall transection and injury rates. Ultimately, the operator's proficiency significantly determines the rate of graft transection and injury during FUE procedures, with comprehensive details on the correct technique available in the extensive literature [66].

How Do FUE Grafts Compare to LSE Grafts?

FUE grafts undergo forceful extraction from the surrounding tissue, exhibiting a typically slimmer profile with less perifollicular tissue and minimal fat peribulbar. This characteristic has led to the perception that FUE grafts are compara-

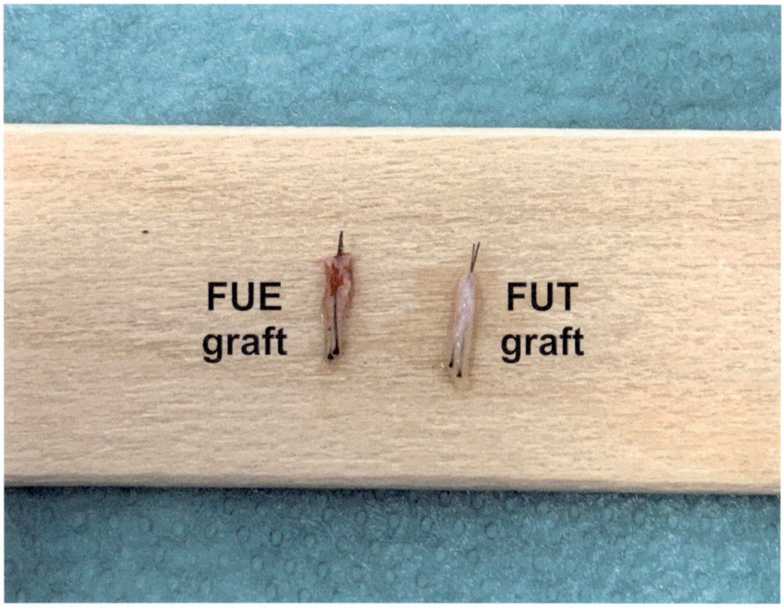

Fig. 3.17 Example of a typical FUE graft (left) vs. an LSE graft (right). One can easily see the pear shape of the microscopically prepared FUSS graft and the partly denuded appearance of the usual FUE graft. Newer devices and punches allegedly address this issue of graft denudation

tively more "fragile" than their LSE counterparts, potentially posing a higher risk of diminished survival rates [39]. The quality of grafts significantly influences the success of FUE procedures, with microscopically slivered and created grafts obtained through LSE regarded as the "gold standard" (Fig. 3.17). However, as experience, refined technique, and appropriate instrumentation come into play, it becomes evident that FUE grafts, under these optimal conditions, do not lag in terms of quality, and their survival rates become comparable to those of LSE grafts.

Are FUE Megasessions Safe?

In recent times, FUE megasessions are being touted as contemporary alternatives to LSE megasessions. Advances in technology, improved punch designs, enhanced training, and accumulated experience, driven in part by greed, ego, and ambition, have enabled surgeons to push the boundaries of FUE megasessions well beyond 1500 FUs in a day. Some have engaged in a competitive "race," attempting heroically extensive FUE megasessions involving several thousand grafts in a single sitting, often overlooking considerations such as transection rates, missed attempts, and ultimate growth outcomes. This narrative introduces a significantly different dimension, sparking controversy regarding the safety of such practices.

Rassman et al. have proposed a mathematical relationship defining a "safe FUE megasession," emphasizing a limit to the number of extracted grafts the human scalp can safely heal. They argue that exceeding this limit poses risks associated with residual donor area trauma. Undeniably, the patterns of FUE donor removal markedly differ from those of a 5000-graft LSE surgery, justifying a lower graft limit for FUE megasessions. As the number of harvested FUs increases and incisions are placed in closer proximity within the confined donor area, there is a potential for irreversible cumulative damage to scalp microvasculature. Unfortunately, documentation on the microvascular risks of FUE megasessions remains scarce. Vascular complications, including (a) focal areas of scalp necrosis and (b) increased donor area miniaturization in the remaining hairs due to hidden transections, are more common than reported. As FUE megasession numbers escalate, injudicious harvesting from the finite donor supply leads to decimated, see-through, moth-eaten, and thin donor areas—a characteristic outcome associated with indiffer-

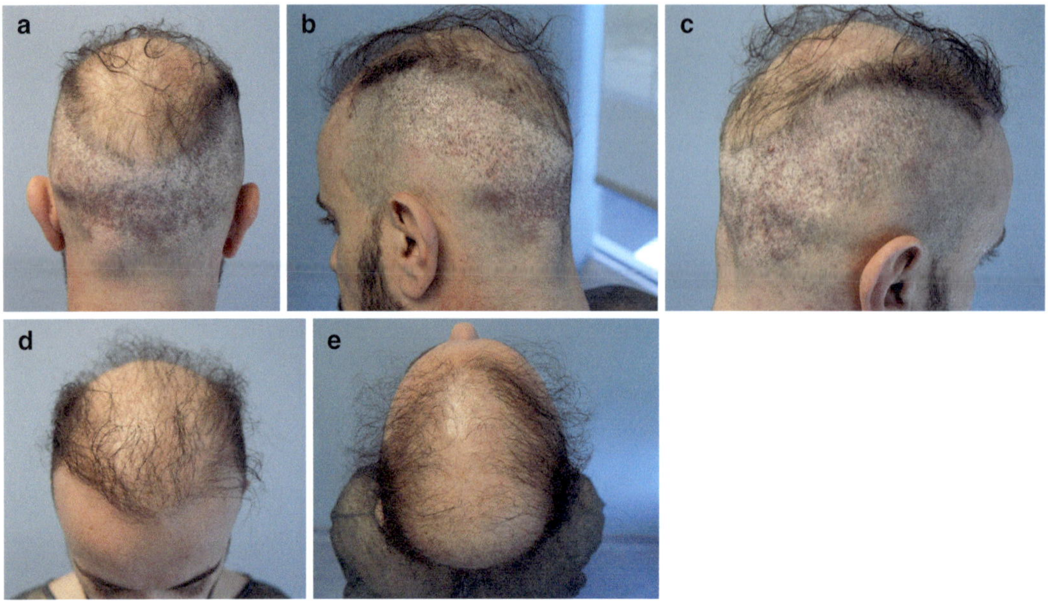

Fig. 3.18 (**a–c**) An unlucky Stage VI patient who was operated on in a "hair mill" clinic that offered "unlimited grafts in one session." The donor area is overharvested, showing dreadful donor scarring, overlapping scars, focal areas of atrichia, subclinical vascular damage, and even hypoesthesia. The result on the recipient area left the patient emotionally devastated. (**d**, **e**) Despite the huge number of transplanted "grafts", probably >6000-7000 of surely transected or severely damaged "grafts", no more than 300-350 hairs have grown overall, a survival rate of <5%

ent operators, often anonymous technicians operating on unsuspecting patients in low-cost FUE destinations (Fig. 3.18).

Interestingly, according to the results of a new member survey conducted by the International Society of Hair Restoration Surgery (ISHRS), 68% of members reported performing an average of one procedure per patient in 2021 to achieve the desired HRS result. This represents a significant improvement, as ISHRS members estimated an average of 3.4 procedures in 2019 and 5 procedures in 2016 were needed per patient to achieve the desired result. This represents a considerable transformation resulting in enhanced results with fewer procedures for male and female patients who benefit from the latest refined HRS techniques, both LSE and FUE [67].

Ethical Considerations of FUE Delegation

The surge in FUE's popularity can be primarily attributed to the aggressive marketing campaigns by FUE device manufacturers and illicit clinics. This heightened patient interest in FUE has resulted in a proliferation of delegating harvesting steps, or the entire procedure, to nonphysicians who bear minimal responsibility for the potential damage inflicted using sub-standard "working models" [68]. Three prevalent models characterize this widespread trend:

The "Turnkey" Model

In the United States and Canada, these illicit clinics operate in a subtle way, using the following paradigm:

- An established plastic surgeon, dermatologist, or other physician purchases a commercially marketable FUE device that can help perform one step of the HRS procedure.
- Instead of performing the procedure themselves, these physicians hire technicians by the day to perform most, if not the entire, procedure-including surgery planning and surgery execution (e.g., graft removal, hairline design, and making scalp incisions to place the grafts). Occasionally, the FUE device manufacturer dispatches technicians to operate it in the doctor's practice.

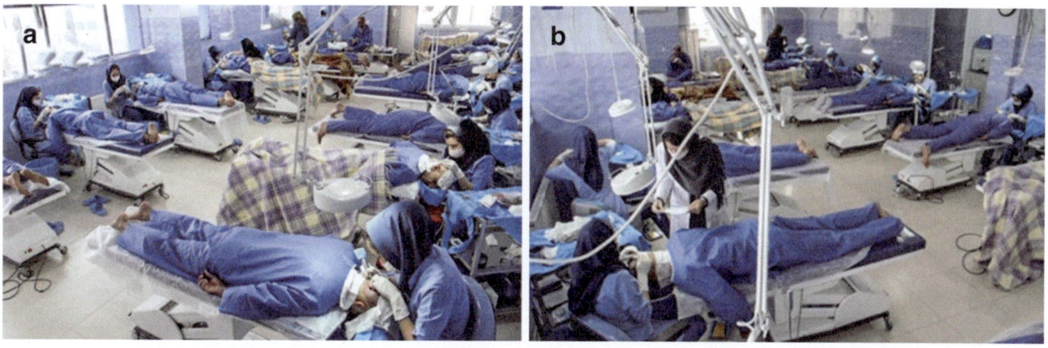

Fig. 3.19 (**a**, **b**) Photographs from a "black market" hair transplantation clinic in a Middle Eastern country. In this picture, more than 14 patients are simultaneously operated by non-medical personnel under unscrupulous hygienic conditions. (photo courtesy of ISHRS, with permission, all rights reserved)

- These doctors, though offering FUE procedures under their name/brand, possess limited or zero knowledge of the HRS procedure. Nevertheless, patients are being led to believe either a doctor will be performing the procedure or assured by a doctor that the technicians are "experts and as good as any doctor in performing hair transplants".
- Automated and robotic devices may align with this "fly-in, fly-out" model involving roving technicians, contributing to the unethical commoditization of FUE.

The "Hair-Farm" Model

This is the prevalent paradigm in heavily promoted FUE destinations globally. Unscrupulous clinics in these destinations lure patients from around the world to travel for HRS procedures using misleading advertising claims, such as "unlimited number of grafts", "all-inclusive packages", very low prices and "guaranteed results". Patients wrongfully assume that the lower cost is attributed to the low labor cost in that country when, in reality, the explanation lies in the most unethical application of "economy of scale": FUE surgical procedures are illegally performed by technicians who do not have medical licenses or surgical training and are reimbursed per "head".

- The FUE promotion appears to endorse technicians/assistants performing the entire FUE procedure under "physician supervision" as a legal façade for local laws,
- One physician, not necessarily a surgeon, allegedly oversees dozens of simultaneous surgeries conducted by technicians in an otherwise legal facility,
- These unlicensed technicians will often harvest on every patient over 6000 "grafts" in one sitting using tiny punches (0.6 mm), resulting in less than 2000 partially transected grafts, along with more than 4000 extracted pieces of scalp skin, all transplanted as "FUE grafts",
- This model typically yields disastrous cosmetic results, depletes the donor area [69], and precludes future procedures due to donor exhaustion, posing severe consequences for patient well-being and significant health risks with little to no recourse for correction (Fig. 3.19).
- Extensive scarring, unnatural hairlines, poor hair growth, wrong hair direction, depleted donor area, and infections are the rule in these clinics, that paradoxically, remain in business for years (Fig. 3.16).

The "In-House" Model

Staff members within an experienced clinic team take on FUE harvesting or the entire procedure without proper training, presenting inherent risks to patient outcomes and safety.

This model seems more benign than the others, yet still it is unethical since service is substandard.

How Did HRS Go So Wrong With FUE?

Modern HRS techniques, especially FUE and BHT, have endorsed a "cosmetic revolution" in HRS and allowed the industry to bounce back from decades of bad results. In modern HRS, hair is transplanted in the same way as it grows, mimicking natural hair growth in terms of numbers and growth patterns. Results of modern "lege artis" FUE are completely natural and indistinguishable from normal hair, and it is not an overstatement to claim that results can change the patient's life.

What seems not to have changed is the "attraction" this field exerts to physicians and businessmen who enter the field for a "quick buck". Combined with the desperate young hair loss patients who will do anything to get their hair back, this field is constantly threatened by both outside and inside "enemies".

Unfortunately, even today, modern HRS techniques alone cannot protect the patient from substandard work or classic surgical mistakes, such as poor surgical judgment and skill, poor artistic perception, operating on a non-suitable candidate, or a patient with unrealistic expectations, as well as delegating HRS to non-medical personnel. Even today, HRS procedures are often advertised as ordinary consumer products; hair loss clinics go into a cut-throat price war, targeting uniformed, naive hair loss patients, whereas HRS procedures performed by non-physicians in "hair-farms" in certain international FUE destinations are probably the most serious problems of modern HRS.

The International Society of Hair Restoration Surgery (ISHRS), a global non-profit medical association and the leading authority on hair loss treatment and restoration with more than 1200 members throughout 70 countries worldwide, has been raising awareness of these issues for years. Their awareness campaign "Fight the F.I.G.H.T.", which stands for Fight the Fraudulent, Illicit & Global Hair Transplants, addresses the alarming problem of unlicensed non-physicians performing HRS worldwide [70].

In an unregulated FUE landscape, the field of HRS is encountering a growing threat to its reputation due to the escalating prevalence of suboptimal outcomes delivered by unlicensed practitioners. These practitioners often operate on unsuitable surgical candidates, make unrealistic promises, engage in overharvesting of donor areas, and create unnatural hairlines [71, 72]. It is tragic to put the beautiful FUE results produced by skilled HRS surgeons side-by-side with the disfiguring results of these "money mills [65].

Dr. Rassman recently issued a cautionary note, suggesting that the role of surgeons in the technical delivery of HRS may diminish in the coming years compared to their traditional involvement in LSE surgery. He anticipates that future FUE teams could comprise as few as two members, utilizing cost-effective implanters and/or robotic devices to offer daily sessions of acceptable quality, albeit with average size (<2000 grafts) [73]. While this perspective paints a somewhat bleak picture, it is not universally accepted, and some maintain a more optimistic outlook for the future of the HRS field [74]. The future is in the hands of ethical physicians who will guide the hair loss patient to the proper treatment strategy that incorporates the correct use of modern HRS techniques.

Conclusion

In transforming the Hair Restoration Surgery (HRS) landscape, Follicular Unit Excision (FUE) has ushered in a new era marked by continual advancements in techniques and tools, enabling dedicated surgeons to consistently achieve excellent outcomes. The aesthetic benefits and heightened patient satisfaction offered by FUE are undeniable. Despite its seemingly straightforward nature, FUE demands a mastery that evolves over years, mandating a unique combination of dexterity, training, dedication, enthusiasm, cognitive clarity, scientific knowledge, and experience. However, the surge in "illicit-market" clinics providing low-cost FUE surgeries, often administered by untrained technicians, poses a serious threat, resulting in cosmetic issues and complications for unsuspecting patients. It is imperative to recognize that FUE is a surgical procedure, and its practice should be confined to licensed physicians extensively trained in the technical and aesthetic facets of HRS. Only when these essential criteria are met can the cosmetic outcomes of FUE rival, and sometimes surpass, those of Linear Strip Excision (LSE), all without the encumbrance of a linear donor scar. Clearly, the adage holds true—properly executed, one can indeed have their cake and eat it too!

Conflict of Interest None declared.

References

1. Anastassakis K. Punch grafts: holes in the head. In: Androgenetic alopecia from A to Z. Cham: Springer; 2023. https://doi.org/10.1007/978-3-031-10613-2_2.
2. Cole JP. An analysis of follicular punches, mechanics, and dynamics in follicular unit extraction. Facial Plast Surg Clin North Am. 2013;21(3):437–47.
3. Pierce HE. The strip graft as a means of hairline replacement. J Natl Med Assoc. 1977;69(7):509–10.
4. Bernstein RM, Rassman WR, et al. Standardizing the classification and description of follicular unit transplantation and mini-micrografting techniques. The American Society for Dermatologic Surgery, Inc. Dermatol Surg. 1998;24(9):957–63.
5. Stough DB 3rd, Mendoza F, Freilich IW. Surgical procedures for the treatment of baldness. Cutis. 1986;37(5):362–5.
6. Limmer BL. Elliptical donor stereoscopically assisted micrografting as an approach to further refinement in hair transplantation. J Dermatol Surg Oncol. 1994;20(12):789–93.
7. Bernstein RM, Rassman WR, Szaniawski W. Follicular transplantation. Int J Aesthet Restor Surg. 1995;3:119–32.
8. Headington JT. Transverse microscopic anatomy of the human scalp. A basis for a morphometric approach to disorders of the hair follicle. Arch Dermatol. 1984;120(4):449–56.
9. Bernstein RM, Rassman WR. The logic of follicular unit transplantation. Dermatol Clin. 1999;17(2):277–95.
10. Bernstein RM, Rassman WR. The aesthetics of follicular transplantation. Dermatol Surg. 1997;23(9):785–99.
11. Rassman WR, Bernstein RM, McClellan R, Jones R, Worton E, Uyttendaele H. Follicular unit extraction: minimally invasive surgery for hair transplantation. Dermatol Surg. 2002;28(8):720–8.
12. Inaba M. Androgenetic alopecia: modern concepts in pathogenesis and treatment. Tokyo: Springer; 1996. p. 238–45.
13. Anastassakis K. Follicular unit excision (FUE). In: Androgenetic alopecia from A to Z. Cham: Springer; 2023. https://doi.org/10.1007/978-3-031-10613-2_10.
14. Rassman WR, Pak J, Kim J. Follicular unit extraction: evolution of a technology. J Transpl Technol Res. 2016;6:158.
15. Kim YS, Na YC, Park JH. Comparison of postoperative pain according to the harvesting method used in hair restorative surgery. Arch Plast Surg. 2019;46(3):241–7.
16. Garg S, Garg AK. Study of ropivacaine block to reduce post-operative pain after strip harvesting, and the relationship of strip width to post-operative pain. Hair Transpl Forum Int. 2019;29(5):186–8.
17. Harris JA. New methodology and instrumentation for follicular unit extraction: lower follicle transection rates and expanded patient candidacy. Dermatol Surg. 2006;32(1):56–61.
18. Habif T. Clinical dermatology. 5th ed. Amsterdam: Elsevier; 2015.
19. Harris JA. Follicular unit extraction. Facial Plast Surg. 2008;24(4):404.
20. Umar S. Use of beard hair as a donor source to camouflage the linear scars of follicular unit hair transplant. J Plast Reconstr Aesthet Surg. 2012;65(9):1279–80.
21. Wu WY, Otberg N, Kang H, Zanet L, Shapiro J. Successful treatment of temporal triangular alopecia by hair restoration surgery using follicular unit transplantation. Dermatol Surg. 2009;35(8):1307–10.
22. Garg AK, Garg S. Donor harvesting: follicular unit excision. J Cutan Aesthet Surg. 2018;11(4):195–201.
23. Bernstein RM, Rassman WR. New instrumentation for 3-step follicular unit extraction. Hair Transpl Forum Int. 2006;16(1):229.
24. Mohebi P, Straga J. Dynamics of FUE. Hair Transpl Forum Int. 2017;27(6):232–6.
25. Lam SM, Williams K. Hair transplant 360: follicular unit extraction (FUE). 1st ed. New Delhi: Jaypee Brothers Medical Publisher; 2016. p. 252.
26. Harris JA. The SAFE system: new instrumentation and methodology to improve follicular unit extraction (FUE). Hair Transpl Forum Int. 2004;14(5):157.
27. Mohebi P, Lorenzo J, Devroye JM, et al. FUE Research Committee Chair's Message: standardization of the terminology used in FUE: part I. Hair Transpl Forum Int. 2013;23(5):165–8.
28. Epstein GK, Epstein J, Nikolic J. Follicular unit excision: current practice and future developments. Facial Plast Surg Clin North Am. 2020;28(2):169–76.
29. True R, et al. A 2019 guide to currently accepted FUE and implanter terminology. Hair Transpl Forum Int. 2019;29(3):98–106.
30. Unger W. Commentary. Dermatol Surg. 2002;28(8):720–8.
31. Zontos G, Rose PT, Nikiforidis G. A mathematical proof of how the outgrowth angle of hair follicles influences the injury to the donor area in FUE harvesting. Dermatol Surg. 2014;40(10):1147–50.
32. Park JH, You SH. Various types of minor trauma to hair follicles during follicular unit extraction for hair transplantation. Plast Reconstr Surg Glob Open. 2017;5(3):e1260.
33. Karacal N, Uralo M, Dindar T, Livao M. Necrosis of the donor site after hair restoration with follicular unit extraction (FUE): a case report. J Plast Reconstr Aesthet Surg. 2012;65(4):87–9.

34. Vogel JE. Hair restoration complications: an approach to the unnatural-appearing hair transplant. Facial Plast Surg. 2008;24(4):453–61.
35. Yoo H, Moh J, Park JU. Treatment of postsurgical scalp scar deformity using follicular unit hair transplantation. Biomed Res Int. 2019;2019:3423657.
36. Crisostomo MR, et al. Untouched strip: a technique to increase the number of follicular units in hair transplants while preserving an untouched area for future surgery. Surg Cosmet Dermatol. 2011;3(4):361–4.
37. Anastassakis K. The combo technique: joined forces. In: Androgenetic alopecia from A to Z. Cham: Springer; 2023. https://doi.org/10.1007/978-3-031-10613-2_30.
38. Mohebi P, Carman T. How I do it: serial extraction–placement FUE technique. Hair Transpl Forum Int. 2016;26(3):104–5.
39. Josephitis D, Shapiro R. A side-by-side study of FUT vs. FUE graft availability in the same patients and its implications on lifetime donor supply and management. Hair Transpl Forum Int. 2019;29(5):177–85.
40. Beehner ML. A comparison of hair growth between follicular-unit grafts trimmed "skinny" vs. "chubby". Dermatol Surg. 1999;25(4):339–40.
41. Ors S, Ozkose M, Ors S. Follicular unit extraction hair transplantation with micromotor: eight year's experience. Aesthet Plast Surg. 2015;39(4):589–96.
42. Park JH. How i do it: direct non-shaven FUE technique. Hair Transpl Forum Int. 2014;24(3):103–10.
43. Boaventura O. Long hair FUE and the donor area preview. Hair Transpl Forum Int. 2016;26(5):200.
44. Saxena K, Savant SS. Body to scalp: evolving trends in body hair transplantation. Indian Dermatol Online J. 2017;8(3):167–75.
45. Mysore V. Body hair transplantation: case report of successful outcome. J Cutan Aesthet Surg. 2013;6(2):113–6.
46. Jones R. Body hair transplant into wide donor scar. Dermatol Surg. 2008;34(6):857.
47. Saxena K, Saxena DK, Savant SS. Successful hair transplant outcome in cicatricial lichen planus of the scalp by combining scalp and beard hair along with platelet rich plasma. J Cutan Aesthet Surg. 2016;9(1):51–5.
48. Poswal A. Body hair transplant: An additional source of donor hair in hair restoration surgery. Indian J Dermatol. 2007;52(2):104–5.
49. Umar S. The transplanted hairline: leg room for improvement. Arch Dermatol. 2012;148(2):239–42.
50. Umar S. Eyelash transplantation using leg hair by follicular unit extraction. Plast Reconstr Surg Glob Open. 2015;3(3):e324.
51. Umar S. Eyebrow transplantation: alternative body sites as a donor source. J Am Acad Dermatol. 2014;71:e140–1.
52. Anastassakis K. Body hair transplantation FUE (BHT FUE). In: Androgenetic alopecia from A to Z. Cham: Springer; 2023. https://doi.org/10.1007/978-3-031-10613-2_11.
53. Anastassakis K. Hair restoration surgery in female patients. In: Androgenetic alopecia from A to Z. Cham: Springer; 2023. https://doi.org/10.1007/978-3-031-10613-2_32.
54. ISHRS Follicular Unit Excision Advancement Committee. FUE clinical practice guidelines. Hair Transpl Forum Int. 2019;29(4):139–50.
55. Bernstein RM. Controversies: FUE and donor depletion: age and the donor zone in FU hair transplants. Hair Transpl Forum Int. 2013;23(3):86–93.
56. Anastassakis K. Overview of safe donor area. In: Androgenetic alopecia from A to Z. Cham: Springer, 2023. https://doi.org/10.1007/978-3-031-10613-2_15.
57. Haber R. FUT fights back. Hair Transpl Forum Int. 2015;25(5):177–87.
58. Knudsen R. Controversies: the temporary hair transplant: a novel idea or making a virtue out of necessity? Hair Transpl Forum Int. 2018;28(2):6.
59. Knudsen R. Notes from the Editor Emeritus: the temporary two-thirds transplant? Hair Transpl Forum Int. 2014;24(5):165.
60. Bernstein RM. Commentary on robotic follicular unit extraction in hair transplantation. Dermatol Surg. 2015;41(2):279.
61. Anastassakis K. Paradigm shift from linear strip to follicular unit excision in hair restoration surgery. Facial Plast Surg. 2024;40(2):129–45. https://doi.org/10.1055/s-0043-1777311.
62. Erdogan K. Coverage value and graft calculation. Presented at the World FUE Institute Meeting; 2015.
63. Keene SA, Rassman WR, Harris JA. Determining safe excision limits in FUE: factors that affect, and a simple way to maintain, aesthetic donor density. Hair Transpl Forum Int. 2018;28(1):1–11.
64. Mohmand MH, Ahmad M. Transection rate at different areas of scalp during follicular unit extraction/excision (FUE). J Cosmet Dermatol. 2019;19(7):1705–8.
65. True R. Notes from the Editor Emeritus, 2014–2016: my journey in the evolution of FUE. Hair Transpl Forum Int. 2019;29(1):7–9.
66. Lam SM, Williams KW. Hair transplant 360, volume 4: follicular unit excision. 2nd ed. New Delhi: Jaypee Brother Medical Publishers; 2021.
67. https://ishrs.org/2022-practice-census/.
68. Knudsen RG. Notes from the Editor Emeritus: ethics and follicular unit extraction. Hair Transpl Forum Int. 2016;26(4):133.
69. Huang YL, Lee MC, Chang SL, Hu S, Chang CS, Lin YF, Cheng CY. Harvested vs estimated follicular units in hair transplantation. J Cosmet Dermatol. 2019;18(3):902–90.
70. https://fightthefight.ishrs.org/.
71. Williams G. Medical and professional ethics: spotlight on surgery by unlicensed practitioners. Hair Transpl Forum Int. 2018;28(5):192–3.
72. Knudsen R. Controversies: what should the ISHRS do about non-physicians performing hair transplantations? Hair Transpl Forum Int. 2012;22(3):83.
73. Rassman WR. The future of hair transplantation. Hair Transpl Forum Int. 2015;25(5):198–9.
74. Keene SA, et al. Response to Dr. Rassman's opinion on the future of hair restoration surgery. Hair Transpl Forum Int. 2015;25(6):264–5.

Photobiomodulation for Alopecia: Mechanisms of Action

4

Michael R. Hamblin

Introduction

Photobiomodulation was discovered in 1967 by Endre Mester working at the Semelweiss University in Hungary [1]. Mester had obtained an example of the newly invented ruby laser, and commenced a series of experiments designed to answer two questions: (a) Can laser irradiation of an experimental tumor transplanted into a mouse or rat produce any cures?; (b) Does repeated laser irradiation of the skin in a mouse or rat cause skin cancer? However Mester's ruby laser did not have sufficient power to produce cures in an experimental tumor, and repeated irradiation did not cause any cases of skin cancer [2]. Nevertheless these experiments did produce highly interesting and useful results [3]. Mester found that incisions that had been made to transplant the tumors healed more rapidly in the laser-treated animals than in controls [4], and moreover the hair grew back faster in the shaved regions of the skin when treated with the ruby laser [5]. Mester named this phenomenon "laser biostimulation" and it later became known as "low-level laser therapy" (LLLT) [1]. Recently an international consensus agreed on the use of the term "photobiomodulation, PBM" to replace LLLT [6] for three reasons. Firstly, there was no agreement on what the term "low" actually meant. Secondly the growing realization that non-coherent light sources such as light-emitting diodes (LEDs), could perform as well as lasers [7], meant that including the term "laser" was no longer appropriate. Thirdly, the realization that many of the applications involved inhibition of biological processes, rather than the more usual stimulation, meant that the term "modulation" was more appropriate.

Although the early studies in the PBM field mainly used red light (600–700 nm), it was subsequently found that near-infrared (NIR) light (760–1000+ nm) was equally (if not more) effective [8]. Light in the low 700 nm wavelength spectrum does not appear to be particularly effective for PBM applications [9, 10]. This double peak in the action spectrum (~660 and ~850 nm) reflects the absorption spectrum of cytochrome c oxidase (CCO), unit IV in the mitochondrial respiratory chain [11]. Together with studies showing the effects of light on isolated mitochondria, these observations led to the most widely-held hypothesis that PBM stimulates respiration

This chapter is an updated version of a previous paper "Photobiomodulation for the management of alopecia: mechanisms of action, patient selection and perspectives.
Hamblin MR. *Clin Cosmet Investig Dermatol.* 2019;12:669–78. https://doi.org/10.2147/CCID.S184979". Since this paper is open access no permissions are necessary for the reprinted material.

M. R. Hamblin (✉)
Laser Research Centre, Faculty of Health Science, University of Johannesburg, Doornfontein, South Africa

P. J. Panagotacos, H. Maibach (eds.), *Hair Loss*, Updates in Clinical Dermatology, https://doi.org/10.1007/978-3-031-74314-6_4

in mitochondria, increasing electron transport, oxygen consumption, and ATP synthesis [12]. One as yet unconfirmed hypothesis suggests that this may be due to photodissociation of inhibitory nitric oxide from the heme and copper centers contained within CCO [13].

For a number of years the main uses of PBM were in the areas of wound healing, or reducing pain and inflammation in musculoskeletal disorders [14, 15]. However starting at the beginning of the twenty-first century, PBM was actively investigated as a treatment for different forms of hair loss [16–21].

Hair loss or alopecia affects the majority of the population at some time over their lifespan, and those afflicted are increasingly demanding some type of treatment. A healthy head of hair has great social significance for humans. Healthy hair indicates health, youth and vigor. Male pattern baldness is taken to be a sign of age and loss of vigor, and is often concealed or alternatively the entire head may be shaved. There is enormous demand for drugs and other treatments that can slow down or reverse hair loss; this has led to the creation of a multibillion-dollar industry [22]. In the USA > \$3.5 billion is spent every year on treating hair loss [23]. It has been stated that "mental disorders such as anxiety, depression, social phobia, posttraumatic stress disorder, and suicidal thoughts are increased among alopecia patients" [24].

The hair follicle (HF) is a complex mini-organ embedded in the skin and is composed of the papilla, matrix, root sheath and bulge [25]. There are between 250,000 and 500,000 individual HFs on the human scalp. Hair grows in cycles during which it moves sequentially from one phase to another (Fig. 4.1). In normal HFs the anagen growth phase can last between 2–6 years. This is followed by a short catagen involution-phase, which lasts 1–2 weeks, and then by a telogen resting-phase lasting 5–6 weeks. The old hairs are then shed, the anagen phase begins over again, and a new hair is produced. Normally, up to 90% of the HFs are in anagen phase, while 10–14% are in telogen and 1–2% in catagen [26].

The most important cells in the HF are those in the dermal papilla (DP). These cells produce signals to control sequential cycling of the follicular epithelium [27]. It is thought that epithelial stem cells, which reside in the bulge area of the HF, can respond to the signals from the DP [14]. These stem cells give rise to progenitor cells, which then become transiently amplifying cells that migrate downward into the deep dermis. These cells differentiate into matrix cells that actually produce the hair shaft, and the sheath. Several growth factor families are involved in HF cycling, namely fibroblast growth factor, EGF, hepatocyte growth factor, IGF-I, and TGF-β [27]. Signal transducer and activator of transcription 3 (stat3) is the most important transcription factor involved in spontaneous HF cycling [28]. There is also another stat3-independent pathway involving PKC, which is also involved in HF cycling, and can be triggered after hair plucking.

A series of signaling pathways are involved in each step of primary hair development and differentiation. These pathways have been elucidated in various mechanistic studies of embryogenesis [29]. Wingless type (Wnt) signaling is crucial for the initiation of HF development [30]. Wnt-protein is a ligand that binds to a cell-surface receptor, a 'Frizzled' family member, which then transduces the signal to the intracellular protein 'Dishevelled' (Dsh). Dsh causes the accumulation of β-catenin in the cytoplasm (by protecting it from degradation) and its eventual translocation into the nucleus where it can act as a transcriptional co-activator of transcription factors that belong to the TCF/LEF family (T-cell factor/lymphoid enhancer factor). 'Sonic hedgehog' (Shh) signaling plays an important role in both embryonic and adult HF development. Shh binds to and inhibits the extracellular domain 'Patched,' allowing the intracellular domain 'Smoothened' to accumulate and inhibit the proteolytic cleavage of the Gli (glioma-associated oncogene) family of zinc-finger transcription factors [31].

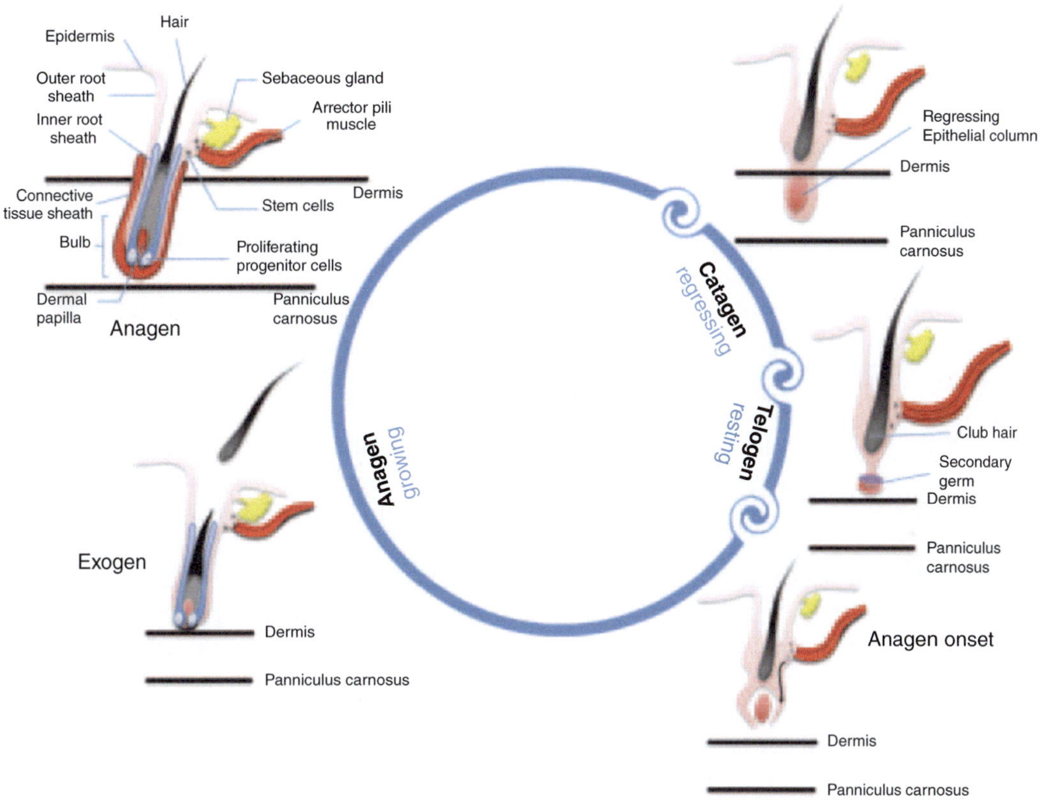

Fig. 4.1 Anatomy of the HF and the hair cycle

Alopecia

There are three main types of alopecia; androgenetic alopecia (AGA), alopecia areata (AA) and chemotherapy-induced alopecia (CIA). All these types of alopecia have different causations and molecular mechanisms of pathogenesis.

Androgenetic Alopecia

AGA affects the majority of males as they age, and the distinctive pattern of hair loss is often called "male pattern baldness" [32]. The most important predisposing factors are genetic and hormonal, and a balance between two androgen steroids, testosterone and 5α-dihydrotestosterone (DHT). This balance depends on the activity of the enzyme, 5α-reductase in the scalp. Differences in expression or polymorphisms in the androgen receptor gene in the HF may also be involved [33]. The precise androgen responsive genes in the HF responsible for AGA have yet to be fully identified. Women can also suffer from AGA which involves similar molecular mechanisms, but the visible pattern of hair loss on the head is different [34].

The only widely-employed approved drug therapies for AGA are topical minoxidil (Rogaine) and oral finasteride (Propecia). In 1988, the FDA approved 2% minoxidil topical solution (Rogaine®) for use in treating AGA in men [35]. A 2% solution for women became available in 1991, and a 5% solution became available over the counter for use in men in 1997. In 1997, finasteride (Propecia) was approved by the FDA for the treatment of male AGA at a dose of 1 mg/day. This medication is a competitive inhibitor of 5α-reductase that inhibits the conversion of testosterone to DHT, which is involved in miniaturizing the HF in AGA [36].

There has been increasing interest in the injection of autologous platelet-rich plasma (PRP) into the scalp as a treatment for AGA [37–39]. The mechanism is proposed to involve the effect of growth factors released from platelets, including vascular endothelial growth factor (VEGF), epidermal growth factor (EGF), insulin like growth factor 1 (IGF-1), fibroblast growth factor (FGF), platelet-derived growth factor (PDGF), and transforming growth factor β1 and β2 (TGF-β) [37]. THE PRP may be activated by calcium chloride before injection to increase the release of growth factors [40]. Injections of a few mL of PRP are usually given at 2 weekly or monthly intervals for 3 months [41].

Alopecia Areata

AA is thought to be an auto-immune disease, in which host T-cells attack the HFs. Autoantibodies that bind to epitopes in anagen HFs have been detected both in human AA patients and experimental mouse models of AA [42]. Biopsies obtained from affected individuals have been shown to display an inflammatory infiltrate around the anagen HFs consisting of activated CD4 and CD8 T lymphocytes [43]. Studies have shown that transplantation of AA tissue into normal mice can induce AA, but if a monoclonal antibody against CD44v10, was injected into the normal mice shortly after transplantation, this was avoided [44]. Similar studies have shown that in vivo depletion of CD4+ cells using a cell-depleting OX-35/OX-38 antibody partially restored hair growth in AA-affected rats [45]. In humans AA is sometimes known as spot-baldness with coin shaped areas of hair loss. AA can progress to alopecia totalis (whole scalp) or alopecia universalis (whole body). Individuals with AA are more likely to have another autoimmune disease, and in about 20% of cases there is a family history of AA [46].

There is currently no universally effective therapy for AA that induces and sustains remission. Ito [47] suggested that since spontaneous remission occurs in 80% of patients within 1 year, and not all patients require intensive therapy, that no therapy at all (watchful observation) could be the best option. Topical corticosteroids remain the cornerstone of initial treatment, as indeed they are for many other inflammatory skin disorders.

Chemotherapy-Induced Alopecia

CIA is one of the best-known side effects of chemotherapy for cancer. Cancer chemotherapy triggers apoptosis in rapidly dividing cancer cells, but also affects rapidly dividing cells in other tissues, such as the hematopoietic system, the gastrointestinal epithelial lining, as well as the HFs. Chemotherapy-induced apoptosis depends on the expression of p53, which accumulates in dividing cells after DNA damage, resulting in growth arrest or induction of programmed cell death [48]. Many p53-responsive genes are up-regulated by chemotherapy, such as Fas, IGF-BP3 and Bax [49]. Chemotherapy affects the rapidly proliferating keratinocytes in the bulb region of the anagen HF that are responsible for producing the hair shaft. The HF then enters a dystrophic catagen stage and the hair falls out.

The most often used intervention for CIA is scalp-cooling [50]. One study reported that use of a scalp-cooling device in women with breast cancer receiving anthracycline and/or taxane based chemotherapy, applied from 30 min before to 90 min after each chemotherapy infusion, preserved hair in 48 out of 95 subjects in the active group and in 0 out of 47 subjects in the sham group [51].

Mechanisms of Action of PBM in Alopecia

Androgenetic Alopecia

The results of PBM for AGA suggest that the proportion of HFs in the anagen phase is increased. This may be due to the ability of PBM to stimulate the mitochondria in the bulge stem cells. Stem cells are quiescent cells that have adapted to survive in their hypoxic niche. One of the most damaging agents to the longevity of cells is oxidative damage to DNA and other biomolecules, caused by the reactive oxygen species (ROS) that are an inevitable by-product of aerobic respiration. Therefore stem cells tend to have an overall anaerobic metabolism characterized by low mitochondrial activity and high expression of glycolytic enzymes [52]. The low metabolic rate of stem cells accounts for their relative quiescence and increased resistance to stress (including oxidative stress). Because stem cells must survive for such a long time, they must minimize the number of cell divisions they undergo because each division carries a small risk of DNA damage.

One hypothesis is that when PBM is delivered to the hypoxic stem cell niche, the rudimentary mitochondria in the stem cells are triggered into action, and then mitochondrial biogenesis can take place producing even more mitochondria [53]. Increased mitochondrial activity is accompanied by an increased demand for oxygen, which is not available in the low-oxygen environment of the stem cell niche. Therefore the stem cells have to leave their niche in pursuit of the oxygen they need to satisfy their new metabolic pathways, involving the upregulation of oxidative phosphorylation (OXPHOS). The burst of intracellular ROS that is observed to follow PBM [54] may also have a role in triggering the differentiation of stem cells [55]. As mentioned above the mobilized stem cells are exposed to naturally occurring cues, when they become progenitor cells, transiently amplifying cells, and finally matrix cells as the HF enters into the anagen phase.

Alopecia Areata

The mechanism of action of PBM in AA has some differences (and some similarities) with that outlined above for AGA. Because AA is an autoimmune disease, the principle molecular signatures are characteristic of a pro-inflammatory environment in the HF [56]. PBM has long been known to have a pronounced anti-inflammatory effect [57], but it is only recently that the possible mechanism for this activity has become apparent. Cells in the macrophage lineage can assume a diversity of phenotypes, and retain the capability to shift their function from one phénotype to another to maintain tissue homeostasis. Macrophages can be activated by LPS (lipopolysaccharide) or IFN-γ (interféron-gamma) to adopt an M1 phenotype, which expresses pro-inflammatory cytokines and is able to kill microbial cells. On the other hand the macrophages can be activated by IL(interleukin)-4/IL-13 to an M2 phenotype, that can carry out the phagocytosis of debris, promote the resolution of inflammation and help tissue repair. Increasing evidence suggests a role for metabolic reprogramming in the regulation of the innate inflammatory response [58]. Studies have demonstrated that the M1 phenotype is often accompanied by a shift from OXPHOS to aerobic glycolysis for energy production in the macrophages [59]. Macrophage activation is involved in the pathogenesis of most autoimmune diseases [60].

Since there is considerable evidence that PBM can alter the mitochondrial metabolism towards OXPHOS, and away from aerobic glycolysis, this is a plausible explanation of why PBM can alter the macrophage phenotype from M1 to M2 [61]. The consequences of this shift would be that the highly pro-inflammatory environment that encourages T-cell attack on the HFs, would switch to a less inflammatory environment that preserves the HFs from attack.

Chemotherapy-Induced Alopecia

The mechanism of PBM in CIA is likely to operate by yet another set of signaling pathways. It has long been known that PBM is able to protect cells at risk of dying. Many in vitro models have been employed to show that PBM can inhibit apoptosis in various cells triggered by a number of different toxic agents. This effect occurs due to the up-regulation of anti-apoptotic proteins, possibly within the mitochondria [62]. The increase in anti-apoptotic proteins in HFs exposed to PBM would be expected to preserve them from the toxic effects of chemotherapy. Another group of chromophores has been identified in the HF, namely opsins [63]. Opsins are blue-light responsive signaling molecules, that were shown to be responsible for reducing apoptosis and prolonging the anagen phase in ex vivo HFs that were treated with 3.2 J/cm^2 of 453 nm LED light.

Photobiomodulation for Alopecia

Devices and Parameters

Most of the marketed devices have been based on low power (5 mW) red laser diodes, while some devices contain LEDs in addition to lasers. The red wavelengths have usually been between 630 and 660 nm. These devices can be divided into four broad types, (a) hand held combs or brushes; (b) head bands; (c) caps or helmets; (d) stationary hoods (see Fig. 4.2 for examples). The total number of laser diodes incorporated into each of the delivery devices determines the total optical power administered to the head, and hence the time required to deliver the desired dose to the affected regions of the scalp. Dosimetry is usually measured as an energy density (J/cm^2) with a value of 4 J/cm^2 frequently quoted as optimum. The time of application is usually between 10 and 20 min, which can be calculated because the desired fluence of 4 J/cm^2 divided by a usual power density of 5 mW/cm^2 equals 800 s. The treatment repetition for a home use device is usually once per day, but once every 2 days is also possible. The advantages of a comb or a band device over a cap or a hood, are that the teeth of the laser comb part the hair allowing the light to penetrate better down to the HFs within the scalp.

All the available evidence suggests that NIR light (800–900 nm) as well as red LEDs as opposed to red lasers would perform as well as the traditionally employed red laser light, but so far these wavelengths have not been much tested, although in one case a combination of 655 and 808 nm was used [64]. A recent study looked at different wavelengths of LED (415, 525, 660, 830 nm) on the stimulation of human dermal papilla cells and the elongation of ex vivo HFs [65]. All four wavelengths showed positive effects, but overall 660 nm was the most efficient. There was significantly increased expression of mRNAs for β-catenin, Axin2, Wnt3a, Wnt5a and Wnt10b. LED irradiation significantly increased the expression of β-catenin and cyclin D, and the phosphorylation of MAPK and extracellular signal-regulated kinase (ERK) as determined by Western blot.

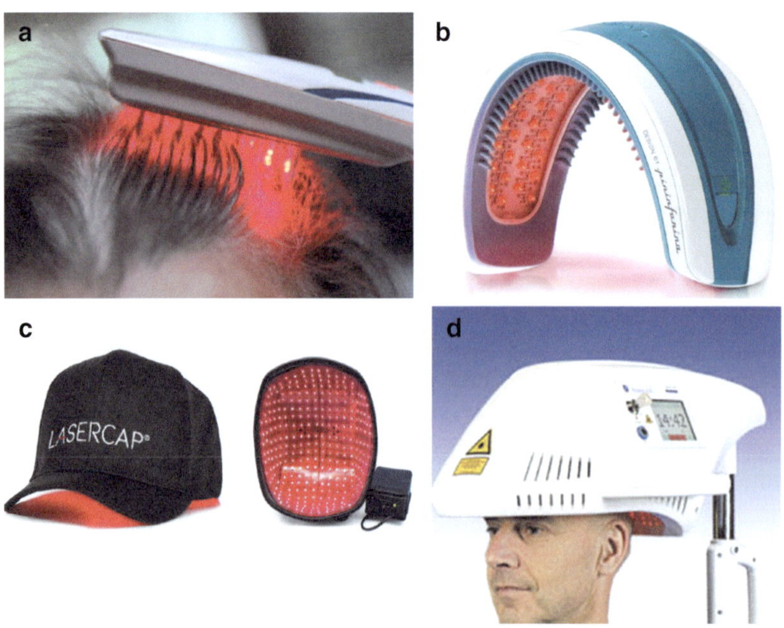

Fig. 4.2 Examples of PBM devices for alopecia. (**a**) HairMax LaserComb (Lexington Int, Boca Raton, FL); (**b**) HairMax LaserBand 82 (Lexington); (**c**) LaserCap HD+ (LaserCap Company, Highland Heights, OH); (**d**) Revage 670 Laser Hood (Apira Science, Boca Raton, FL)

Animal Studies

Mester's original study [5] involved delivering 1 J of pulsed light from a ruby laser at 694-nm (1 ms pulse duration) with a 1 cm^2 spot to the depilated abdominal area of black C57BL/6 and white Balb/c mice every week for up to 11 weeks. Before each successive treatment the skin was again depilated. Increased hair growth in the irradiated spot was observed in all black animals between the fifth and seventh treatment. This reaction continued up to the ninth treatment. In white mice no effect on hair growth was detected up to the eighth irradiation, but thereafter hair growth was stimulated to a lesser extent compared to black mice.

Wikramanayake et al. reported that PBM could have beneficial effects in a mouse model of AA [66]. The model involves topical application of focal heat to the skin of C3H/HeJ mice leading to hair loss accompanied by intra-follicular and peri-follicular mononuclear cell infiltrates in the anagen HF [67]. Affected regions of mouse skin were treated with a 655 nm laser for 20 s daily, three times per week for 6 weeks. Hair regrowth was first observed in the PBM group after 2 weeks of laser treatment and at 6 weeks there was complete hair regrowth in all six mice. In the sham group there was no regrowth of hair at 6 weeks.

The same group (Wikramanayake et al) also reported the use of PBM to treat CIA in a rat model [68]. The chemotherapy agents, cyclophosphamide, etoposide, or a combination of cyclophosphamide and doxorubicin were administered to 2-week old rats to induce whole body alopecia 7–10 days later. The rats received PBM (655 nm laser) for 1 min once daily for 10 days. Rats receiving laser treatment regrew hair 5 days earlier than rats receiving chemotherapy alone or sham laser treatment. The authors checked that the PBM treatment did not protect subcutaneously injected cancer cells from the effects of the chemotherapy.

Clinical Studies

Most clinical trials on PBM for alopecia so far reported have been carried out for AGA in either men or women. One of the first reports used the HairMax Laser Comb (655 nm laser) in a double-blind, sham-controlled, multicenter, 26-week trial with 110 randomized males with Norwood-Hamilton classes IIa-V AGA. Patients were treated for 15 min three times per week for 26 weeks [69]. Subjects receiving active PBM showed a mean increase in hair density (+17.3 ± 11.9 hairs/cm^2) while those receiving sham had a decrease (−8.9 + 11.7), $p < 0.0001$. Kim et al. used a helmet type device containing 630 and 660 nm LEDs and 650 nm laser diodes [70]. They recruited both men (Norwood-Hamilton III-VII) and women (Ludwig I-III) with AGA. Subjects were treated for 15 min once every day for 24 weeks. Subjects receiving active treatment showed a mean increase in hair density of +17.2 + 12.1 while subjects receiving sham showed a decrease of −2.1 + 18.3, $p = 0.003$. There was also a significant increase in hair thickness in active treated subjects. Lanzafame et al. published a pair of papers describing trials of a helmet device consisting of 655 nm LEDs and 655 nm lasers on men [71] and women [72]. Patients were treated for 25 min every 2 days for 16 weeks. The men showed a 62.5% increase in hair counts in the active group versus a 37% increase in sham group (p = 0.003) [71]. The women showed a 48% increase in the active group versus a 11% increase in the sham group ($p < 0.001$) [72].

Other groups have reported significant improvements in hair regrowth in both men and women using a HairMax Laser Comb [73], and in females using a laser cap device [74]. Barikbin et al. compared the effects of a 655 nm laser cap and a laser scanner combining 655 and 808 nm [64]. Both devices significantly improved hair counts, but the 655/808 nm combination was slightly better. In all cases, the incidence of side effects was rare (<10%), tolerable and transient [75]. Dry skin, irritation, pruritis and mild headache were the most often reported.

Scarpim et al. treated 25 male AGA patients with a 660 nm laser twice a week for 10 weeks [76].

The hair density was significantly higher at 5 and 10 weeks.

There have been some recent systematic reviews and meta-analysis studies that have confirmed the effectiveness of PBM for hair regrowth in AGA [77–79].

There have been some studies that have tested various combinations of PBM with other therapeutic approaches. For instance, Esmet et al. compared topical minoxidil 5% with PBM using an iGrow helmet and the combination of both therapies in women with AGA [80]. Topical minoxidil was applied twice daily, and PBM was used for 25 min 3 days a week for 16-week study duration. All groups were effective, but the combination group (PBM + minoxidil) showed a benefit earlier (at 2 months) compared to the monotherapies. On the other hand Ferrera et al. also tested the combination of PBM with topical minoxidil, but did not find that PBM produced any additional hair growth compared to minoxidil alone, which was highly effective [81].

Choi and Park tested a combination of PBM (660 nm 80 mW plus 808 nm 50 mW laser for 15 min) immediately followed by pulsed electromagnetic fields (76.6 and 60 Hz for 10 min) [82]. They conducted a 24-week, randomized, double-blind sham device-controlled trial on 80 subjects with AGA. The subjects were treated every week for 12 weeks, and every other week for the next 8 weeks. At 24 weeks the mean hair density was 139.37 (±31.4)/cm^2 in the treatment group but only 119.78 (±31.92)/cm^2 in the control group ($p < 0.05$).

There were two reports suggesting that PBM could be combined with microneedling for AGA in men or women, but no results confirming the combination was better than either treatment alone have yet been published [83, 84].

There have been only relatively few clinical trials of PBM for alopecia areata. One trial conducted by Yamazaki et used a "SuperLizer" device that emits linear polarized light over a wavelength range of 600–1600 nm [85]. Fifteen patients with patchy hair loss, were treated on some areas for 3 min once every 1 or 2 weeks for up to 5 months, while other areas acted as controls. 46.7% of the treated areas showed hair regrowth, 1.6 months earlier than the non-irradiated areas ($p = 0.003$).

Tawfik et al. conducted a trial on thirty patients, each having three separate patches of AA [86]. Patches were assigned randomly to receive treatment either with injection of PRP or with PBM, while the third patch served as an untreated control. PRP was injected once weekly, whereas PBM was done 3 sessions/week for 6 weeks. The patients were followed up at 1 and 3 months. Both the PRP and PBM treated patches showed improvements in the thickness and density of hair, but the PRP patches (40%) were more likely to improve than PBM patches (32%). The improvements were sustained during the 12 weeks follow up in most of the patients.

Waiz et al. carried out PBM with a pulsed 904 nm laser (weekly for 4 weeks) to treat 16 patients with 34 resistant AA patches [87]. In patients with multiple patches, one patch was left as a control for comparison. Regrowth of hair was observed in 32 PBM treated patches (94%), while no regrowth of hair was observed in the control patches. Palma et al. [88] reported a single case of AA in an adult female that completely resolved after 7 daily treatments with PBM (660 nm laser).

Lodewijckx and colleagues reported a randomized controlled trial of PBM to treat CIA [89]. A total of 32 breast cancer patients receiving an anthracycline and taxane-containing chemotherapy regimen at the Jessa Hospital, Hasselt, Belgium were randomized into a control group or a PBM group (three PBM sessions each week for 12 weeks, starting on the last day of chemotherapy) and then followed up at 1, 2, and 3 months. Significantly higher hair regrowth scores were obtained in the PBM group at 1-month post-chemotherapy compared to baseline, and they scored their global health significantly higher at all time points compared to the control group.

Patient selection should take account of the following points. Both men and women with AGA respond very well to PBM. However because men generally have higher levels of DHT (and testosterone) compared to women, the continuing pressure exerted by hormonal effects is more pronounced in men. Therefore the PBM is constantly fighting against the influence of DHT, and may have to be periodically used throughout the entire lifetime. This consideration may explain why some trials of PBM have shown somewhat better results in women compared to men. Due to the rather gradual benefits of PBM for alopecia, it makes a lot of sense to commence treatment sooner rather than later. Ideally treatment should commence at the earliest stage of self-perceived thinning hair. In shiny bald scalps as are seen in some men, the HF are gone forever, and no amount of PBM will bring them back from the dead. The question is sometimes raised about different pigmentation levels of hair and skin and whether this affects the benefits of PBM. Undoubtedly hair is a barrier to light penetration, and thick dark hair is a considerable barrier. However since the light is most necessary in areas of hair loss, this may not be a big problem in reality. As regards pigment levels in skin, it is believed that dark skin (Fitzpatrick skin types IV-VI) require higher doses of light (longer exposure to a PBM device) compared to light skin (Fitzpatrick skin types I-III), although this hypothesis has not yet been fully tested in a clinical trial. The study showing an increased benefit of combining topical minoxidil with PBM [80] suggests further combination studies should be explored. The use of PBM in combination with hair transplantation surgery has been discussed, but as yet there are no published studies. PBM is proposed to be able to encourage the integration of the transplanted hair grafts and also to hasten the healing of the donor sites. Moreover some investigators are considering the combination of PBM with platelet rich plasma (PRP). PRP is a growing technology for treatment of AGA involving the injection into the scalp of autologous PRP at monthly intervals for 3 months [90]. In some cases the PRP can be activated before injection using calcium chloride [91], and PBM has been proposed as an alternative method to activate PRP.

The use of PBM in cases of AA has not been investigated to anything like the same level as PBM for AGA. This is probably because AA is fairly rare, while AGA affects the majority of the population at some point in their life.

The use of PBM should be tested in patients undergoing chemotherapy for cancer (probably women with breast cancer). It is suggested that consideration should be given to commencing PBM a few days before initiation of chemotherapy as well as during the infusion itself, to give the HF a chance to upregulate the anti-apoptotic proteins.

Conclusion

The use of PBM for hair regrowth still remains contentious both in medical practice and in the general population. This lack of acceptance persists despite an ever-growing number of clinical trials reporting positive results, mainly in AGA. Perhaps one reason for this lack of universal acceptance, is the fact that PBM requires fairly prolonged regular applications over a period of months to achieve the optimal effects. This regimen was probably unrealistic when PBM was often applied in clinics or salons. Some individuals probably gave up when they did not see rapid results, or else expected PBM to work in relatively advanced cases of AGA. Moreover some companies have marketed PBM in an unrealistic fashion, encouraging over-optimistic expectations. Now that home use PBM devices are becoming widely available and affordable, and also the fact that LED devices are becoming more common, perhaps we can expect that the public acceptance will increase. Well-controlled clinical trials of PBM in patients with AA and CIA are urgently required.

References

1. Mester A, Mester A. The history of photobiomodulation: endre mester (1903–1984). Photomed Laser Surg. 2017;35(8):393–4.
2. Mester E, Szende B, Tota JG. Effect of low intensity laser radiation, repeatedly administered over a long period, on the skin and inner organs of mice. Radiobiol Radiother (Berl). 1969;10(3):371–7.
3. Mester E, Jaszsagi-Nagy E. Biological effects of laser radiation. Radiobiol Radiother (Berl). 1971;12(3):377–85.
4. Mester E, Szende B, Spiry T, Scher A. Stimulation of wound healing by laser rays. Acta Chir Acad Sci Hung. 1972;13(3):315–24.
5. Mester E, Szende B, Gartner P. The effect of laser beams on the growth of hair in mice. Radiobiol Radiother (Berl). 1968;9(5):621–6.

6. Anders JJ, Lanzafame RJ, Arany PR. Low-level light/laser therapy versus photobiomodulation therapy. Photomed Laser Surg. 2015;33(4):183–4.
7. Heiskanen V, Hamblin MR. Photobiomodulation: lasers vs. light emitting diodes? Photochem Photobiol Sci. 2018;17(8):1003–17.
8. Lubart R, Wollman Y, Friedmann H, Rochkind S, Laulicht I. Effects of visible and near-infrared lasers on cell cultures. J Photochem Photobiol B. 1992;12(3):305–10.
9. Gupta A, Dai T, Hamblin MR. Effect of red and near-infrared wavelengths on low-level laser (light) therapy-induced healing of partial-thickness dermal abrasion in mice. Lasers Med Sci. 2014;29(1):257–65.
10. Wu Q, Xuan W, Ando T, Xu T, Huang L, Huang YY, et al. Low-level laser therapy for closed-head traumatic brain injury in mice: effect of different wavelengths. Lasers Surg Med. 2012;44:218–26.
11. Wong-Riley MT, Liang HL, Eells JT, Chance B, Henry MM, Buchmann E, et al. Photobiomodulation directly benefits primary neurons functionally inactivated by toxins: role of cytochrome c oxidase. J Biol Chem. 2005;280(6):4761–71.
12. Karu TI. Multiple roles of cytochrome c oxidase in mammalian cells under action of red and IR-A radiation. IUBMB Life. 2010;62(8):607–10.
13. Lane N. Cell biology: power games. Nature. 2006;443:901–3.
14. Chung H, Dai T, Sharma SK, Huang YY, Carroll JD, Hamblin MR. The nuts and bolts of low-level laser (light) therapy. Ann Biomed Eng. 2012;40(2):516–33.
15. Narita K, Asano K, Morimoto Y, Igarashi T, Hamblin MR, Dai T, et al. Disinfection and healing effects of 222-nm UVC light on methicillin-resistant Staphylococcus aureus infection in mouse wounds. J Photochem Photobiol B. 2018;178:10–8.
16. Avci P, Gupta GK, Clark J, Wikonkal N, Hamblin MR. Low-level laser (light) therapy (LLLT) for treatment of hair loss. Lasers Surg Med. 2014;46(2):144–51.
17. Darwin E, Arora H, Hirt PA, Wikramanayake TC, Jimenez JJ. A review of monochromatic light devices for the treatment of alopecia areata. Lasers Med Sci. 2018;33(2):435–44.
18. Darwin E, Heyes A, Hirt PA, Wikramanayake TC, Jimenez JJ. Low-level laser therapy for the treatment of androgenic alopecia: a review. Lasers Med Sci. 2018;33(2):425–34.
19. Delaney SW, Zhang P. Systematic review of low-level laser therapy for adult androgenic alopecia. J Cosmet Laser Ther. 2018;20(4):229–36.
20. Gupta AK, Daigle D. The use of low-level light therapy in the treatment of androgenetic alopecia and female pattern hair loss. J Dermatolog Treat. 2014;25(2):162–3.
21. Gupta AK, Lyons DC, Abramovits W. Low-level laser/light therapy for androgenetic alopecia. Skinmed. 2014;12(3):145–7.
22. Semalty M, Semalty A, Joshi GP, Rawat MS. Hair growth and rejuvenation: an overview. J Dermatolog Treat. 2011;22(3):123–32.
23. Statista. 2017. https://www.statista.com/statistics/489025/value-of-the-global-hair-loss-treatment-market/.
24. Gokalp H. Psychosocial aspects of hair loss. In: Kutlubay Z, Serdaroglu S, editors. Hair and scalp disorders. London: IntechOpen; 2016.
25. Paus R, Muller-Rover S, Van Der Veen C, Maurer M, Eichmuller S, Ling G, et al. A comprehensive guide for the recognition and classification of distinct stages of hair follicle morphogenesis. J Invest Dermatol. 1999;113(4):523–32.
26. Burg D, Yamamoto M, Namekata M, Haklani J, Koike K, Halasz M. Promotion of anagen, increased hair density and reduction of hair fall in a clinical setting following identification of FGF5-inhibiting compounds via a novel 2-stage process. Clin Cosmet Investig Dermatol. 2017;10:71–85.
27. Peus D, Pittelkow MR. Growth factors in hair organ development and the hair growth cycle. Dermatol Clin. 1996;14(4):559–72.
28. Sano S, Kira M, Takagi S, Yoshikawa K, Takeda J, Itami S. Two distinct signaling pathways in hair cycle induction: Stat3-dependent and -independent pathways. Proc Natl Acad Sci U S A. 2000;97(25):13824–9.
29. Rishikaysh P, Dev K, Diaz D, Qureshi WM, Filip S, Mokry J. Signaling involved in hair follicle morphogenesis and development. Int J Mol Sci. 2014;15(1):1647–70.
30. Andl T, Reddy ST, Gaddapara T, Millar SE. WNT signals are required for the initiation of hair follicle development. Dev Cell. 2002;2(5):643–53.
31. Harris PJ, Takebe N, Ivy SP. Molecular conversations and the development of the hair follicle and basal cell carcinoma. Cancer Prev Res (Phila). 2010;3(10):1217–21.
32. Ellis JA, Sinclair R, Harrap SB. Androgenetic alopecia: pathogenesis and potential for therapy. Expert Rev Mol Med. 2002;4(22):1–11.
33. Ellis JA, Stebbing M, Harrap SB. Polymorphism of the androgen receptor gene is associated with male pattern baldness. J Invest Dermatol. 2001;116(3):452–5.
34. Herskovitz I, Tosti A. Female pattern hair loss. Int J Endocrinol Metab. 2013;11(4):e9860.
35. Rossi A, Cantisani C, Melis L, Iorio A, Scali E, Calvieri S. Minoxidil use in dermatology, side effects and recent patents. Recent Patents Inflamm Allergy Drug Discov. 2012;6(2):130–6.
36. Rittmaster RS. Finasteride. N Engl J Med. 1994;330(2):120–5.
37. Abdin R, Zhang Y, Jimenez JJ. Treatment of androgenetic alopecia using PRP to target dysregulated mechanisms and pathways. Front Med. 2022;9:843127.
38. Gupta AK, Cole J, Deutsch DP, Everts PA, Niedbalski RP, Panchaprateep R, et al. Platelet-rich plasma as a treatment for androgenetic alopecia. Dermatol Surg. 2019;45(10):1262–73.

39. Singhal P, Agarwal S, Dhot PS, Sayal SK. Efficacy of platelet-rich plasma in treatment of androgenic alopecia. Asian J Trans Sci. 2015;9(2):159.
40. Gentile P, Garcovich S. Autologous activated platelet-rich plasma (AA-PRP) and non-activated (A-PRP) in hair growth: a retrospective, blinded, randomized evaluation in androgenetic alopecia. Expert Opin Biol Ther. 2020;20(3):327–37.
41. Kramer ME, Keaney TC. Systematic review of platelet-rich plasma (PRP) preparation and composition for the treatment of androgenetic alopecia. J Cosmet Dermatol. 2018;17(5):666–71.
42. Tobin DJ. Characterization of hair follicle antigens targeted by the anti-hair follicle immune response. J Investig Dermatol Symp Proc. 2003;8(2):176–81.
43. Gilhar A, Paus R, Kalish RS. Lymphocytes, neuropeptides, and genes involved in alopecia areata. J Clin Invest. 2007;117(8):2019–27.
44. Guo H, Cheng Y, Shapiro J, McElwee K. The role of lymphocytes in the development and treatment of alopecia areata. Expert Rev Clin Immunol. 2015;11(12):1335–51.
45. McElwee KJ, Spiers EM, Oliver RF. Partial restoration of hair growth in the DEBR model for Alopecia areata after in vivo depletion of CD4+ T cells. Br J Dermatol. 1999;140(3):432–7.
46. Spano F, Donovan JC. Alopecia areata: Part 1: pathogenesis, diagnosis, and prognosis. Can Fam Physician. 2015;61(9):751–5.
47. Ito T. Advances in the management of alopecia areata. J Dermatol. 2012;39(1):11–7.
48. Borges HL, Linden R, Wang JY. DNA damage-induced cell death: lessons from the central nervous system. Cell Res. 2008;18(1):17–26.
49. Botchkarev VA, Komarova EA, Siebenhaar F, Botchkareva NV, Komarov PG, Maurer M, et al. p53 is essential for chemotherapy-induced hair loss. Cancer Res. 2000;60(18):5002–6.
50. Ross M, Fischer-Cartlidge E. Scalp cooling: a literature review of efficacy, safety, and tolerability for chemotherapy-induced alopecia. Clin J Oncol Nurs. 2017;21(2):226–33.
51. Nangia J, Wang T, Osborne C, Niravath P, Otte K, Papish S, et al. Effect of a scalp cooling device on alopecia in women undergoing chemotherapy for breast cancer: the SCALP randomized clinical trial. JAMA. 2017;317(6):596–605.
52. Simsek T, Kocabas F, Zheng J, Deberardinis RJ, Mahmoud AI, Olson EN, et al. The distinct metabolic profile of hematopoietic stem cells reflects their location in a hypoxic niche. Cell Stem Cell. 2010;7(3):380–90.
53. Tatmatsu-Rocha JC, Tim CR, Avo L, Bernardes-Filho R, Brassolatti P, Kido HW, et al. Mitochondrial dynamics (fission and fusion) and collagen production in a rat model of diabetic wound healing treated by photobiomodulation: comparison of 904nm laser and 850nm light-emitting diode (LED). J Photochem Photobiol B. 2018;187:41–7.
54. Chen AC, Arany PR, Huang YY, Tomkinson EM, Sharma SK, Kharkwal GB, et al. Low-level laser therapy activates NF-kB via generation of reactive oxygen species in mouse embryonic fibroblasts. PLoS One. 2011;6(7):e22453.
55. Owusu-Ansah E, Banerjee U. Reactive oxygen species prime Drosophila haematopoietic progenitors for differentiation. Nature. 2009;461(7263):537–41.
56. Jabbari A, Cerise JE, Chen JC, Mackay-Wiggan J, Duvic M, Price V, et al. Molecular signatures define alopecia areata subtypes and transcriptional biomarkers. EBioMedicine. 2016;7:240–7.
57. Hamblin MR. Mechanisms and applications of the anti-inflammatory effects of photobiomodulation. AIMS Biophys. 2017;4(3):337–61.
58. Orihuela R, McPherson CA, Harry GJ. Microglial M1/M2 polarization and metabolic states. Br J Pharmacol. 2016;173(4):649–65.
59. Haschemi A, Kosma P, Gille L, Evans CR, Burant CF, Starkl P, et al. The sedoheptulose kinase CARKL directs macrophage polarization through control of glucose metabolism. Cell Metab. 2012;15(6):813–26.
60. Ushio A, Arakaki R, Yamada A, Saito M, Tsunematsu T, Kudo Y, et al. Crucial roles of macrophages in the pathogenesis of autoimmune disease. World J Immunol. 2017;7(1):1–8.
61. Fernandes KP, Souza NH, Mesquita-Ferrari RA, Silva DF, Rocha LA, Alves AN, et al. Photobiomodulation with 660-nm and 780-nm laser on activated J774 macrophage-like cells: effect on M1 inflammatory markers. J Photochem Photobiol B. 2015;153:344–51.
62. Yin K, Zhu R, Wang S, Zhao RC. Low-level laser effect on proliferation, migration, and antiapoptosis of mesenchymal stem cells. Stem Cells Dev. 2017;26(10):762–75.
63. Buscone S, Mardaryev AN, Raafs B, Bikker JW, Sticht C, Gretz N, et al. A new path in defining light parameters for hair growth: discovery and modulation of photoreceptors in human hair follicle. Lasers Surg Med. 2017;49(7):705–18.
64. Barikbin B, Khodamrdi Z, Kholoosi L, Akhgri MR, Haj Abbasi M, Hajabbasi M, et al. Comparison of the effects of 665 nm low level diode Laser Hat versus and a combination of 665 nm and 808nm low level diode Laser Scanner of hair growth in androgenic alopecia. J Cosmet Laser Ther. 2017; https://doi.org/10.1080/14764172.2017.1326609.
65. Joo HJ, Jeong KH, Kim JE, Kang H. Various wavelengths of light-emitting diode light regulate the proliferation of human dermal papilla cells and hair follicles via WNT/beta-catenin and the extracellular signal-regulated kinase pathways. Ann Dermatol. 2017;29(6):747–54.
66. Wikramanayake TC, Rodriguez R, Choudhary S, Mauro LM, Nouri K, Schachner LA, et al. Effects of the Lexington LaserComb on hair regrowth in the C3H/HeJ mouse model of alopecia areata. Lasers Med Sci. 2012;27(2):431–6.
67. Wikramanayake TC, Alvarez-Connelly E, Simon J, Mauro LM, Guzman J, Elgart G, et al. Heat treatment

increases the incidence of alopecia areata in the C3H/HeJ mouse model. Cell Stress Chaperones. 2010;15(6):985–91.
68. Wikramanayake TC, Villasante AC, Mauro LM, Nouri K, Schachner LA, Perez CI, et al. Low-level laser treatment accelerated hair regrowth in a rat model of chemotherapy-induced alopecia (CIA). Lasers Med Sci. 2013;28(3):701–6.
69. Leavitt M, Charles G, Heyman E, Michaels D. HairMax LaserComb laser phototherapy device in the treatment of male androgenetic alopecia: a randomized, double-blind, sham device-controlled, multicentre trial. Clin Drug Investig. 2009;29(5):283–92.
70. Kim H, Choi JW, Kim JY, Shin JW, Lee SJ, Huh CH. Low-level light therapy for androgenetic alopecia: a 24-week, randomized, double-blind, sham device-controlled multicenter trial. Dermatol Surg. 2013;39(8):1177–83.
71. Lanzafame RJ, Blanche RR, Bodian AB, Chiacchierini RP, Fernandez-Obregon A, Kazmirek ER. The growth of human scalp hair mediated by visible red light laser and LED sources in males. Lasers Surg Med. 2013;45(8):487–95.
72. Lanzafame RJ, Blanche RR, Chiacchierini RP, Kazmirek ER, Sklar JA. The growth of human scalp hair in females using visible red light laser and LED sources. Lasers Surg Med. 2014;46(8):601–7.
73. Jimenez JJ, Wikramanayake TC, Bergfeld W, Hordinsky M, Hickman JG, Hamblin MR, et al. Efficacy and safety of a low-level laser device in the treatment of male and female pattern hair loss: a multicenter, randomized, sham device-controlled, double-blind study. Am J Clin Dermatol. 2014;15(2):115–27.
74. Friedman S, Schnoor P. Novel approach to treating androgenetic alopecia in females with photobiomodulation (low-level laser therapy). Dermatol Surg. 2017;43(6):856–67.
75. Liu KH, Liu D, Chen YT, Chin SY. Comparative effectiveness of low-level laser therapy for adult androgenic alopecia: a system review and meta-analysis of randomized controlled trials. Lasers Med Sci. 2019;34(6):1063–9.
76. Scarpim AC, Baptista A, Magalhães DSF, Nunez SC, Navarro RS, Frade-Barros AF. Photobiomodulation effectiveness in treating androgenetic alopecia. Photobiomodul Photomed Laser Surg. 2022;40(6):387–94.
77. Gupta AK, Bamimore MA. Factors influencing the effect of photobiomodulation in the treatment of androgenetic alopecia: a systematic review and analyses of summary-level data. Dermatol Ther. 2020;33(6):e14191.
78. Zhang Y, Su J, Ma K, Fu X, Zhang C. Photobiomodulation therapy with different wavebands for hair loss: a systematic review and meta-analysis. Dermatol Surg. 2022;48(7):737–40.
79. Meng X, Xie F, Wang W, Wang R, Lin B, Zhao Z, et al. Effects of photobiomodulation therapy for androgenic alopecia: a meta-analysis of randomized controlled trials. J Laser Appl. 2020;32(2):021201.
80. Esmat SM, Hegazy RA, Gawdat HI, Abdel Hay RM, Allam RS, El Naggar R, et al. Low level light-minoxidil 5% combination versus either therapeutic modality alone in management of female patterned hair loss: a randomized controlled study. Lasers Surg Med. 2017;49(9):835–43.
81. Ferrara F, Kakizaki P, de Brito FF, Contin LA, Machado CJ, Donati A. Efficacy of minoxidil combined with photobiomodulation for the treatment of male androgenetic alopecia. A double-blind half-head controlled trial. Lasers Surg Med. 2021;53(9):1201–7.
82. Choi MS, Park BC. The efficacy and safety of the combination of photobiomodulation therapy and pulsed electromagnetic field therapy on androgenetic alopecia. J Cosmet Dermatol. 2023;22(3):831–6.
83. da Silveira SP, Moita SRU, da Silva SV, Rodrigues MFSD, da Silva DFT, Pavani C. The role of photobiomodulation when associated with microneedling in female pattern hair loss: a randomized, double blind, parallel group, three arm, clinical study protocol. Medicine. 2019;98(12):e14938.
84. Gentile P, Garcovich S, Lee S-I, Han S. Regenerative biotechnologies in plastic surgery: a multicentric, retrospective, case-series study on the use of microneedling with low-level light/laser therapy as a hair growth boost in patients affected by androgenetic alopecia. Appl Sci. 2021;12(1):217.
85. Yamazaki M, Miura Y, Tsuboi R, Ogawa H. Linear polarized infrared irradiation using super lizer is an effective treatment for multiple-type alopecia areata. Int J Dermatol. 2003;42(9):738–40.
86. Tawfik AA, Mostafa I, Soliman M, Soliman M, Abdallah N. Low level laser versus platelet-rich plasma in treatment of alopecia areata: a randomized controlled intra-patient comparative study. Open Access Macedonian J Med Sci. 2022;10(B):420–7.
87. Waiz M, Saleh AZ, Hayani R, Jubory SO. Use of the pulsed infrared diode laser (904 nm) in the treatment of alopecia areata. J Cosmet Laser Ther. 2006;8(1):27–30.
88. Palma LF, Campos L, Álvares CMA, Serrano RV, de Moraes LOC. Photobiomodulation with a continuous wave red laser (660 nm) as monotherapy for adult alopecia areata: a case presentation. J Lasers Med Sci. 2023;14:e21.
89. Lodewijckx J, Robijns J, Claes M, Pierson M, Lenaerts M, Mebis J. The use of photobiomodulation therapy for the management of chemotherapy-induced alopecia: a randomized, controlled trial (HAIRLASER trial). Support Care Cancer. 2023;31(5):1–11.
90. Ferneini EM, Beauvais D, Castiglione C, Ferneini MV. Platelet-rich plasma in androgenic alopecia: indications, technique, and potential benefits. J Oral Maxillofac Surg. 2017;75(4):788–95.
91. Ince B, Yildirim MEC, Dadaci M, Avunduk MC, Savaci N. Comparison of the efficacy of homologous and autologous platelet-rich plasma (PRP) for treating androgenic alopecia. Aesthet Plast Surg. 2018;42(1):297–303.

5 The Evolution of Photobiomodulation for the Treatment of Hair Loss

Robert Haber

Hair loss has been a persistent concern for humanity throughout history. From ancient remedies to modern medical innovations, various approaches have been explored to address this cosmetic issue. One such innovative approach is light-based therapy, which involves the use of specific wavelengths of light to stimulate hair follicles and promote hair growth. Over the years, light-based therapy for hair loss has undergone significant evolution, merging ancient wisdom with cutting-edge technology. This chapter will explore the development of light-based therapy for hair loss, from its early roots to its contemporary applications.

The use of light as a therapeutic agent traces back to ancient civilizations. Historical records indicate that ancient Egyptians and Greeks recognized the potential of sunlight in promoting general health and treating various ailments, including hair loss. The concept of heliotherapy, or sun therapy, prevailed as a practice to enhance well-being. Although these early civilizations didn't have a precise understanding of the underlying mechanisms, their observations laid the groundwork for future developments.

In ancient India, Ayurvedic medicine emphasized the holistic approach to health and healing. Ayurvedic texts mentioned techniques involving massage, herbal remedies, and sun exposure to address hair loss. The holistic philosophy of Ayurveda recognized the interconnectedness of the body, mind, and spirit, which contributed to the integration of light-based therapies in the treatment of hair-related issues.

The scientific understanding of light and its effects on biological systems progressed significantly in the nineteenth and twentieth centuries. Pioneers like Niels Finsen, a Danish physician, won the Nobel Prize in Physiology or Medicine in 1903 for his work on light therapy for diseases like lupus vulgaris, a skin tuberculosis. Finsen's research laid the foundation for comprehending the therapeutic potential of light in medical applications.

In the mid-twentieth century, the concept of low-level laser therapy (LLLT) began to emerge. The Hungarian researcher Endre Mester conducted experiments on mice, demonstrating that low-level laser irradiation could stimulate hair growth and wound healing [1]. Mester's findings sparked interest in exploring the potential of lasers for hair loss treatment.

The late twentieth century witnessed significant advancements in laser technology, enabling the development of devices specifically designed for hair loss treatment. Laser hair combs and helmets became commercially available, offering individuals a non-invasive approach to address hair thinning and balding. These devices utilized low-level lasers or light-emitting diodes (LEDs) to deliver controlled light energy to the scalp.

R. Haber (✉)
Clinical Professor of Dermatology, Case Western Reserve University School of Medicine, Cleveland, OH, USA

P. J. Panagotacos, H. Maibach (eds.), *Hair Loss*, Updates in Clinical Dermatology,
https://doi.org/10.1007/978-3-031-74314-6_5

Eventually, clinical studies sought to establish the efficacy of light-based therapy for hair loss. Rigorous research methodologies were employed to evaluate the benefits of these treatments. Several studies demonstrated positive outcomes, showing increased hair density and improved hair growth in participants who underwent light-based therapy.

The accumulating clinical evidence led to regulatory approvals from organizations such as the U.S. Food and Drug Administration (FDA). Laser devices for hair loss treatment gained recognition as safe and effective options for individuals seeking non-pharmacological interventions. These approvals provided a significant boost to the credibility and acceptance of light-based therapy within the medical community.

During the formative years of this field of study, non-specific and inaccurate terminology was introduced and entered mainstream use, including low level laser therapy and low level light therapy, among many others. A more scientifically accurate terminology was needed, and as early as 2003 Juanita Anders, PhD along with her scientific team coined the more accurate term photobiomodulation. Unfortunately, it was not until 2016 that photobiomodulation therapy was added to the National Library of Medicine's MeSH database as a search term, following an article published by Dr. Anders et al. the prior year [2].

Photobiomodulation (PBM) is the mechanism by which non-ionizing optical radiation in the visible and near-infrared spectral range is absorbed by endogenous chromophores to elicit photo-physical and photo-chemical events at various biological scales.

Photobiomodulation therapy (PBMT) is a photon therapy based on the principles of PBM. It involves the use of non-ionizing forms of light sources including lasers, LED's, and broadband light, in the visible and infrared spectrum to cause physiological changes and therapeutic benefits. The putative target for PBM is the mitochondria, the cellular engine critical for cell health and survival. Any cell with mitochondrial downregulation will not function properly, and PBM, by targeting mitochondrial chromophores, upregulates this structure resulting in improved cellular function. Hair follicle cells, due to their proximity to the skin surface, can be reached by externally applied light sources, thus the role of PBM in the treatment of hair loss.

While there is a wide assortment of therapeutic devices available for consumer use, there remains a paucity of scientific data regarding the ideal treatment wavelength, power output and duration of therapy. As clinicians, we are asked by our patients if PBM actually works, and if it does, which devices and protocols are best. The field of hair loss treatment has also long been tarnished by unethical practitioners hawking ineffective remedies, so it is incumbent upon ethical practitioners to be aware of the development of treatment devices and justifications for treatment recommendations.

The goal of a clinician reading a chapter about PBM is to glean information that can be applied in the office setting. Clinicians are bombarded with claims of superiority when it comes to light based devices, whether it be wavelength, power, comfort, efficacy or some combination, and our patients expect us to distill these claims into a specific recommendation.

Ideally, data would exist to scientifically specify the ideal wavelength, power and treatment time. Unfortunately, such data does not in fact exist, in spite of the high level research that has been performed by experts such as Mike Hamblin and Juanita Anders among others, and it's possible that some questions will never be answered. Therefore, to utilize PBM we must instead rely on partial data and personal experience.

All clinicians experienced with photobiomodulation have responders and non-responders, and the proportion of each will color our enthusiasm for this treatment modality. As with many treatments, patient selection is important, but just as the ideal treatment parameters are unknown, so are ideal patient characteristics unknown.

Hair loss specialists have a limited selection of treatments to choose from, and thus PBM, even with all of its unknowns, will be used since it is well documented to provide benefits to the correct patient population. It's also cost effective, as it's the only treatment that gets cheaper the longer one uses it as there are no consumables associated with its use. PBM also has good peer reviewed support in the literature. In fact, there is more peer reviewed support for photobiomodulation than for platelet rich plasma (PRP) treatments, another popular hair loss treatment [3–16].

Photobiomodulation first became commercially available to clinicians in the 1990's in the form of large office-based devices from companies such as Sunetics (Sunetics International Marketing Group LLC, Dallas, Texas) (Fig. 5.1). Patients were required to visit an office several times each week to undergo treatments (Fig. 5.2). This was inconvenient, but at the time there was no alternative.

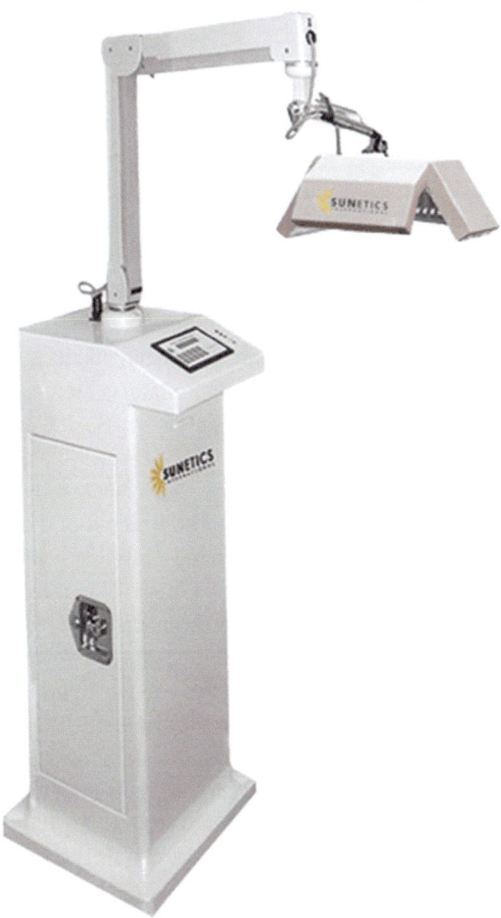

Fig. 5.1 Example of large, office based Sunetics PBM device

In 2003, the first helmet-based device appeared on the market (iRestore Laser, Irvine, CA) (Fig. 5.3), but this was cumbersome and not discrete, and had limited consumer acceptance. The Lasercomb was introduced in 2004 containing a small linear array of laser diodes, and instructions directed the user to move the device on the scalp every 4 s for a 15 min period (Fig. 5.4). This translates to 225 movements per treatment session, and while effective if performed properly, long term compliance was very difficult to achieve outside of a research environment. In 2008 the Theradome was introduced (Theradome, Inc. Pleasanton, California) which functionally and visually added little to the available devices and was certainly not something a patient would wear in public (Fig. 5.5).

While all of these devices were functional, each had features that negatively impacted compliance and patient acceptance. The field needed

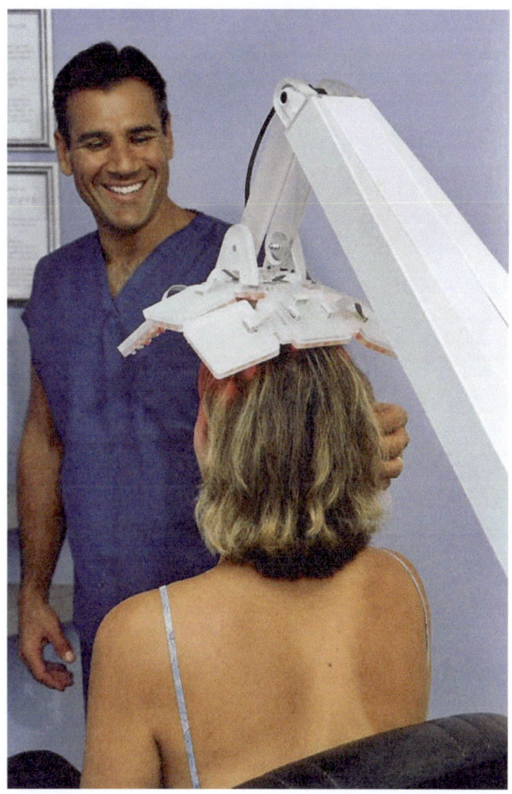

Fig. 5.2 Office based devices require patients to visit the office several times each week for treatments. Image courtesy of Dr. Robert Leonard

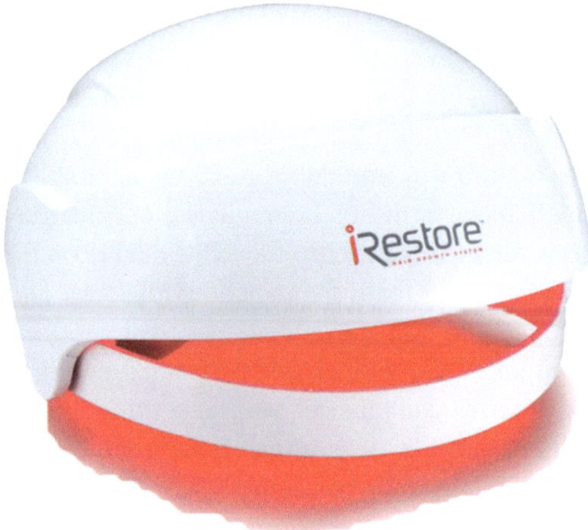

Fig. 5.3 The iRestore device has a hard shell resembling a bicycle helmet

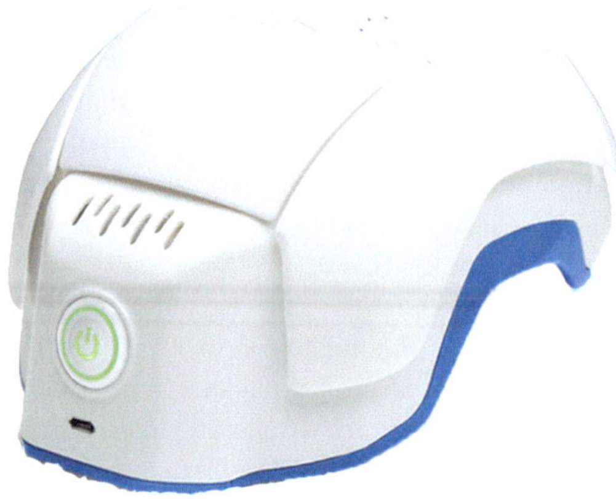

Fig. 5.5 The Theradome is another hard shelled device resembling a bicycle helmet

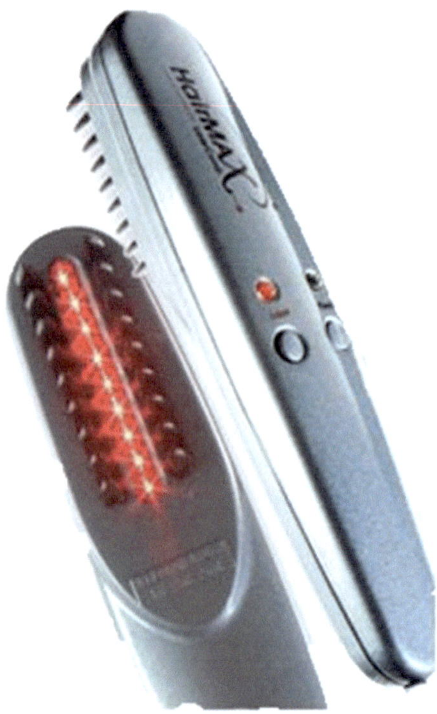

Fig. 5.4 The HairMax Lasercomb requires frequent hand movements during each treatment session

something disruptive, and two important advancements happened in 2009. First, Leavitt, et al. published the first peer reviewed report presenting a PBM device granted 510(k) clearance by the FDA [3]. This groundbreaking study of the Lasercomb (Lexington Intl., LLC, Boca Raton, Fl) set the stage for all subsequent treatment devices. Second was the introduction of the LaserCap (Transdermal Cap, Inc., Highland Heights, Ohio) which was the first discrete, powerful wearable device to deliver photobiomodulation therapy (Fig. 5.6). The device could fit inside any ballcap or other hat, was powered by a belt mounted battery, and thus could deliver high energy while the wearer was performing other routine activities. The LaserCap changed the entire industry, and its success spawned a series of imitators including Capillus in 2013, followed by Kiierr, Bosley and others over the next decade.

As mentioned previously, there is no proven ideal treatment wavelength, power output or duration of therapy. However, sound scientific principles can be used to make treatment recommendations. Importantly, the depth of penetration into the skin is determined purely by wavelength and is not affected by power or treatment duration. And as the hair follicles are fairly superficial, deeply penetrating wavelengths do not offer therapeutic advantages. Red light lasers and diodes emitting in the 650 nm wavelength range are readily available and penetrate to the hair follicle depth, and thus are the most commonly used in consumer devices. Devices offering additional wavelengths do so for marketing benefit and generally without data to support those wavelengths.

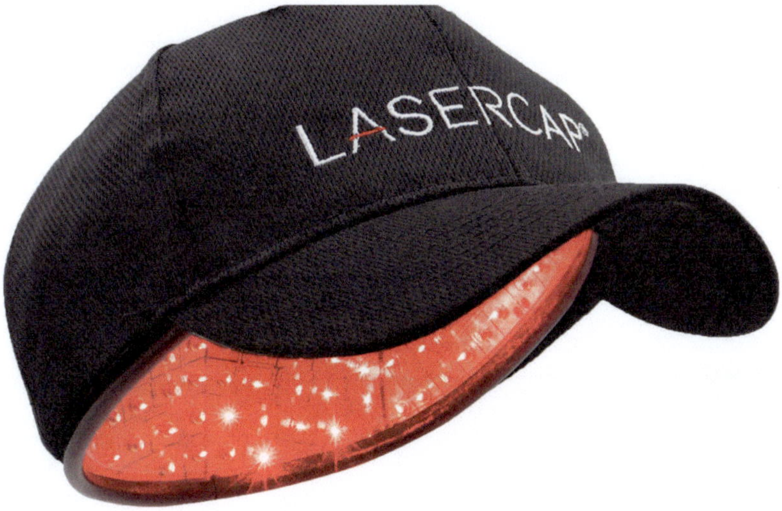

Fig. 5.6 The LaserCap administers higher laser power than other devices, and is discrete when worn

Power and duration are important, as the mitochondria need to receive sufficient energy to undergo upregulation, even if the exact amount of energy is not known. Most experts recommend treatments of 30 min duration every other day. It is possible to expose the mitochondria to too much energy and this will result in an inhibitory effect. Therefore, patients should be discouraged from utilizing these devices on a daily basis, or for many hours at a time. Devices that recommend treatment durations of less than 10 min are most likely underdosing and often these devices also provide lower power output.

As with all hair loss therapies, most patients will benefit from reduced shedding and subsequent stabilization of hair loss. A small percentage will enjoy increased visible density. Subtle results are all we can sometimes expect with photobiomodulation, generally seen as a reduction in part width, a common clinical assessment of treatment efficacy (Fig. 5.7a–c). Patients will often also report subjective improvements in hair texture and shine, and this along with the increased density generally results in high patient satisfaction.

Research in this field continues to expand, investigating optimal wavelengths, energy doses, and treatment protocols. In addition, further understanding of the mechanism of action of PBM may reveal effects on blood circulation and nutrient delivery to the scalp, as well as promoting cell proliferation and reducing inflammation. Photobiomodulation may also play a role in reducing inflammation and accelerating hair growth after hair restoration surgery.

The landscape of light-based therapy for hair loss continues to evolve with advancements in technology and scientific understanding. Today, a wide array of devices, ranging from wearable helmets to handheld combs, is available for consumers. These devices often combine different wavelengths of light and innovative features to enhance treatment outcomes.

Moreover, researchers are exploring the synergistic effects of light-based therapy with other treatments, such as topical medications and regenerative therapies. The combination of multiple modalities aims to maximize hair growth potential and provide comprehensive solutions for individuals experiencing hair loss.

The journey of light-based therapy for hair loss encompasses a rich historical tapestry, from ancient civilizations recognizing the healing power of sunlight to modern-day clinical applications backed by scientific evidence. This innovative approach bridges tradition and technology, offering individuals an alternative avenue for managing hair loss. As technology continues to advance and research deepens our understanding, the future holds promise for further refinement and customization of light-based therapy, providing hope for those seeking effective solutions to hair loss.

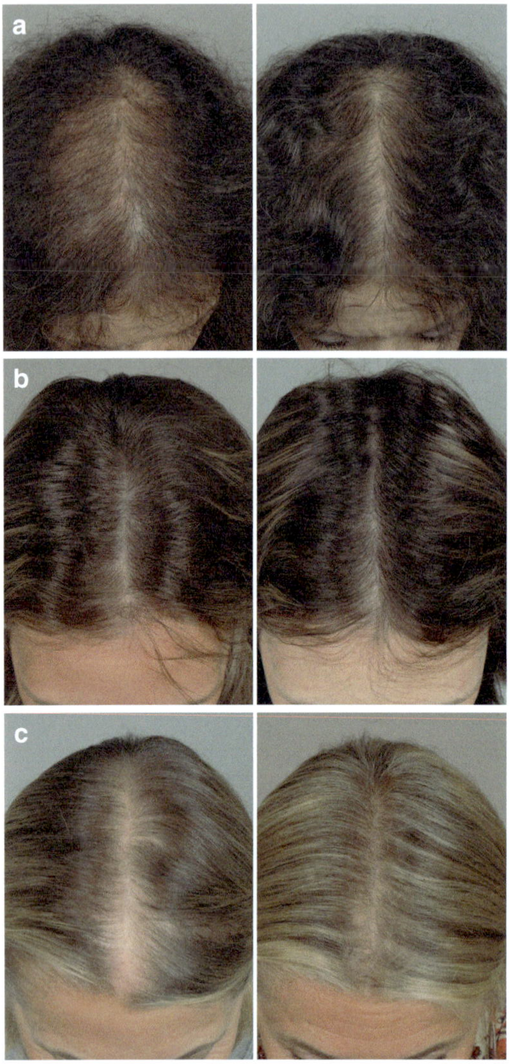

Fig. 5.7 (**a–c**) In each of the examples, a significant reduction in part width can be seen after therapy with the LaserCap

References

1. Mester E, Szende B, Tota JG. Effect of laser on hair growth of mice. Kiserl Orvostud. 1967;19:628–31.
2. Anders JJ, Lanzafame RJ, Arany PR. Low-level light/laser therapy versus photobiomodulation. Ther Photomed Laser Surg. 2015;33(4):183–4.
3. Leavitt M, Charles G, Heyman E, Michaels D. HairMax LaserComb laser phototherapy device in the treatment of male androgenetic alopecia: a randomized, double-blind, sham device-controlled, multicentre trial. Clin Drug Investig. 2009;29(5):283–92.
4. Afifi L, Maranda EL, Zarei M, Delcanto GM, et al. Low-level laser therapy as a treatment for androgenetic alopecia. Lasers Surg Med. 2016;49:27–39.
5. Mignon C, Botchkareva NV, Uzunbajakava NE, Tobin DJ. Photobiomodulation devices for hair regrowth and wound healing: a therapy full of promise but a literature full of confusion. Exp Dermatol. 2016;25(10):745–9.
6. Jimenez JJ, Wikramanayake TC, Bergfeld W, Hordinsky M, Hickman JG, Hamblin MR, Schachner LA. Efficacy and safety of a low-level laser device in the treatment of male and female pattern hair loss: a multicenter, randomized, sham device-controlled, double-blind study. Am J Clin Dermatol. 2014;15(2):115–27.
7. Avci P, Gupta GK, Clark J, Wikonkal N, Hamblin MR. Low-level laser (light) therapy (LLLT) for treatment of hair loss. Lasers Surg Med. 2014;46(2):144–51.
8. Gupta AK, Daigle D. The use of low-level light therapy in the treatment of androgenetic alopecia and female pattern hair loss. J Dermatolog Treat. 2014;25:162–3.
9. Lanzafame RJ, Blanche RR, Bodian AB, Chiacchierini RP, Fernandez-Obregon A, Kazmirek ER. The growth of human scalp hair mediated by visible red light laser and LED sources in males. Lasers Surg Med. 2013;45(8):487–95.
10. Kim H, Choi JW, Kim JY, Shin JW, Lee SJ, Huh CH. Low-level light therapy for androgenetic alopecia: a 24-week, randomized, double-blind, sham device-controlled multicenter trial. Dermatol Surg. 2013;39(8):1177–83.
11. Wikramanayake TC, Villasante AC, Mauro LM, Nouri K, Schachner LA, Perez CI, Jimenez JJ. Low-level laser treatment accelerated hair regrowth in a rat model of chemotherapy-induced alopecia (CIA). Lasers Med Sci. 2013;28(3):701–6.
12. Kalia S, Lui H. Utilizing electromagnetic radiation for hair growth: a critical review of phototrichogenesis. Dermatol Clin. 2013;31:193–200.
13. Wikramanayake TC, Rodriguez R, Choudhary S, Mauro LM, Nouri K, Schachner LA, Jimenez JJ. Effects of the Lexington LaserComb on hair regrowth in the C3H/HeJ mouse model of alopecia areata. Lasers Med Sci. 2012;27(2):431–6.
14. Shukla S, Sahu K, Verma Y, Rao KD, Dube A, Gupta PK. Effect of helium-neon laser irradiation on hair follicle growth cycle of Swiss albino mice. Skin Pharmacol Physiol. 2010;23(2):79–85.
15. Chung PS, Kim YC, Chung MS, Jung SO, Ree CK. The effect of low-power laser on the murine hair growth. J Korean Soc Plastic Reconstruct Surg. 2005;32(2):149–54.
16. Satino JL, Markou M. Hair regrowth and increased hair tensile strength using the HairMax LaserComb for low-level laser therapy. Int J Cosmetic Surg Aesth Dermatol. 2003;5:113–7.

6 Alopecia Areata: JAK Inhibitors—PRP and Exosomes

Doris Day

Description

Alopecia Areata typically manifests as one or several round or oval non-scarring patches of hair loss. The skin appears normal, without signs of inflammation or scarring [1]. A tell-tale sign of alopecia areata are "exclamation point hairs, which are short, broken hairs that are narrower near the scalp and wider at the broken or tapered end, resembling an exclamation point" [2]. They are often seen at the edges of the bald patches in individuals with alopecia areata.

Exclamation point hairs are considered a clinical sign of active hair loss and are indicative of the disease's autoimmune nature. They result from inflammation and damage to the hair follicles in alopecia areata, causing the hair to become weak and break off at the scalp [2].

Over time, multiple patches can occur, coalesce, or expand, leading to more widespread hair loss. Alopecia Totalis (AT). This form is characterized by the complete loss of all hair on the scalp. It can emerge as a progression from the patchy form, or it can present as the initial manifestation. Alopecia Universalis (AU) the most severe form, involves hair loss across the entire body, including eyebrows, eyelashes, and even nasal and ear hair [3]. This condition often signifies a broader and more aggressive autoimmune response.

D. Day (✉)
NYU Langone Health, New York, NY, USA
e-mail: drday@dorisdaymd.com

Diagnosis

The diagnosis for AA, AT, and AU primarily remains clinical, but more extensive presentations might require more intensive investigations to rule out associated autoimmune disorders or underlying triggers and to ascertain if there are concomitant autoimmune conditions.

Clinical Examination

Pull Test: Gentle traction is applied to affected areas. Positive results indicate active disease.

Dermoscopy: This can reveal yellow dots (dilated follicular orifices filled with keratin), black dots (broken hairs), and short vellus hairs [2, 4].

Biopsy and Histology

When clinical features are ambiguous, a 4-mm punch biopsy is performed where the hair is sparsest within the alopecic patch [5]. In AA, early lesions show peribulbar lymphocytic inflammation ("swarm of bees") around anagen-phase hair follicles. Advanced lesions may exhibit fibrosis [6].

P. J. Panagotacos, H. Maibach (eds.), *Hair Loss*, Updates in Clinical Dermatology,
https://doi.org/10.1007/978-3-031-74314-6_6

Pathophysiology

The onset and progression from AA to AT or AU depend on a complex interplay of genetic factors, immune dysregulation, and potentially environmental triggers. The hair follicles in the anagen phase become the target of immune cells, with the exact trigger remaining elusive.

Molecular Mechanisms

At the molecular level, AA is characterized by the presence of autoreactive T cells which target the hair follicles, primarily in their active growth (anagen) phase. This immune-mediated attack leads to the disruption of the hair growth cycle.

Immune Cell Infiltration

Histological analysis of AA lesions commonly reveals a peri-follicular lymphocytic infiltrate. CD8+ NKG2D+ effector T cells target the hair follicle, releasing pro-inflammatory cytokines such as IFN-γ and TNF-α, culminating in hair loss.

Cytokine Disruption

There's an upregulation of the Th1 cytokines (like IFN-γ) in the affected scalp areas. This cytokine milieu pushes hair follicles from the anagen (growth) phase to the telogen (rest) phase, inhibiting hair growth.

Genetic Predisposition

Genetic factors undeniably play a role. Genome-wide association studies have identified several potential genes located on various chromosomes that may heighten susceptibility to hair loss [7].

Treatment Paradigms

Modern treatments encompass traditional methods and cutting-edge technologies and techniques.

The treatment goal for all forms of AA, including AT and AU, is to suppress the immune response against the hair follicles and promote hair regrowth [8]. The treatment goal for all forms of AA, including AT and AU, is to suppress the immune response against the hair follicles and promote hair regrowth [9].

Topical Treatments

Topical corticosteroids: Corticosteroids: Act by suppressing the local immune response.

Topical Steroids: Patient Selection: Ideal for those with <25% scalp involvement.

Application: Potent corticosteroid cream/ointment is applied to bald patches once or twice daily.

Duration: Continued for a few weeks then intermittently as needed, with regular follow up to ensure no atrophy noted.

Localized treatments

Intralesional Corticosteroids: Patient Selection: Those with limited patchy AA or patients in which topical treatments are ineffective.

Drug Selection: Triamcinolone acetonide 0.1% (2–5 mg/ml).

Administration: Injected into the mid-to-upper dermal layer. Repeat treatments at 4–6-week intervals as needed.

Systemic treatments

Oral Corticosteroids and Immunosuppressants: These suppress the overarching immune response, sometimes offering relief in more extensive cases.

Broad-spectrum immunosuppressants: Methotrexate, cyclosporine, or azathioprine can be useful, especially in treatment-resistant cases.

Cutting-Edge Therapeutic Interventions

JAK Inhibitors: These represent the newest class of FDA-approved drugs that interrupt the Janus kinase-signal transducer and activator of transcription (JAK-STAT) signaling pathway. The JAK-STAT pathway is a critical intracellular signaling pathway involved in various cellular processes, including immune responses and inflammation [10]. Cytokines, such as interleukins and interferons, bind to their respective receptors on cell surfaces, initiating the JAK-STAT pathway. JAK enzymes (JAK1, JAK2, JAK3, and TYK2) are activated upon cytokine binding and phosphorylate STAT (Signal Transducer and Activator of Transcription) proteins. Phosphorylated STAT proteins form dimers and translocate to the nucleus, where they regulate gene expression [11]. This pathway plays a crucial role in immune cell activation, cytokine production, and inflammatory responses. There are now class 1, 2 and 3 JAK inhibitors available: Tofacitinib, Ruxolitinib, Baricitinib:

Ruxolitinib primarily inhibits JAK1 and JAK2. It is more selective for these two JAK enzymes.

JAK1 and JAK2 are involved in several cytokine signaling pathways, including those associated with interleukins (IL-2, IL-6, IL-12, IL-23) and interferons (IFN-γ) [10]. These pathways are implicated in inflammatory and autoimmune conditions:

Baricitinib primarily inhibits JAK1 and JAK2, but it has a greater affinity for JAK1.

JAK1 is associated with multiple cytokine receptor pathways, including those of IL-6, IL-12, IL-23, and granulocyte-macrophage colony-stimulating factor (GM-CSF) (Fig. 6.1). These pathways play critical roles in immune responses and inflammatory processes [12].

Both ruxolitinib and baricitinib work by suppressing these JAK pathways, leading to the downregulation of pro-inflammatory signaling and immune responses. These medications are used to treat autoimmune and inflammatory conditions such as rheumatoid arthritis and alopecia areata, where excessive immune activation is a contributing factor. The selective inhibition of JAK enzymes helps to modulate the immune system and reduce inflammation.

Tofacitinib is a Janus kinase (JAK) inhibitor that primarily inhibits multiple JAK enzymes,

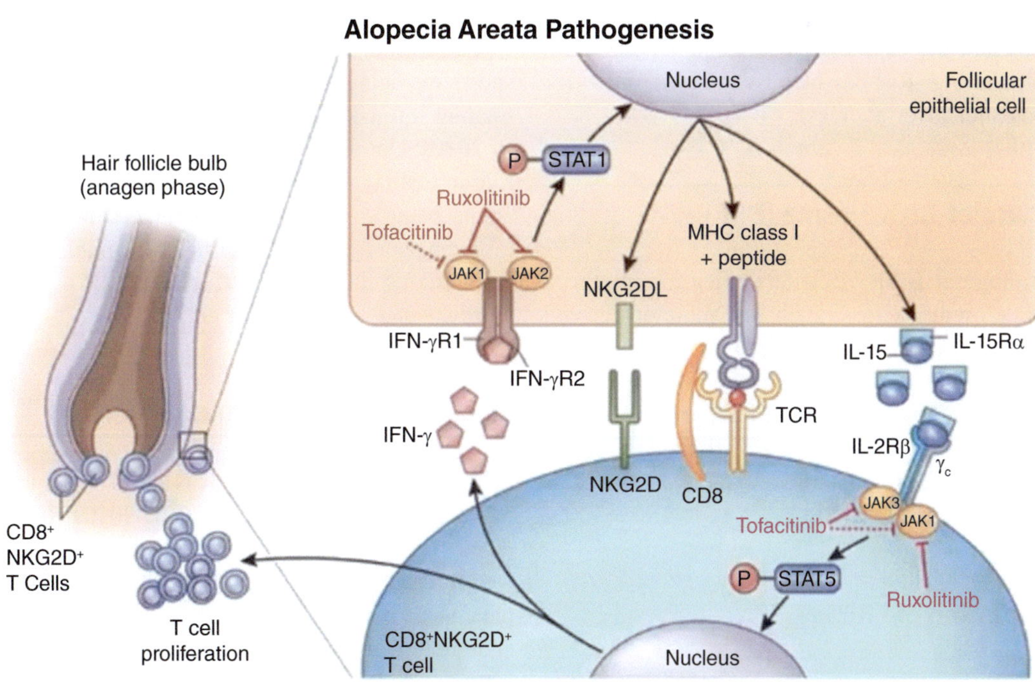

Fig. 6.1 Alopecia. *IFN* interferon, *MSH* melanocyte-stimulating hormone, *TGF-β1* human transforming growth factor beta 1, *IGF-1* insulin-like growth factor 1, *HLA-DR* HLA-D-related, *Treg* T regulatory (cells), *MHC* major histocompatibility complex, *CD* cluster of differentiation, *Th1* T helper type 1 (cells), *ICAM-1* intercellular adhesion molecule-1 (Source: Divito SJ, et al. *Nat Med.* 2014;20(9):989–90; Xing L, et al. *Nat Med.* 2014;20(9):1043–49)

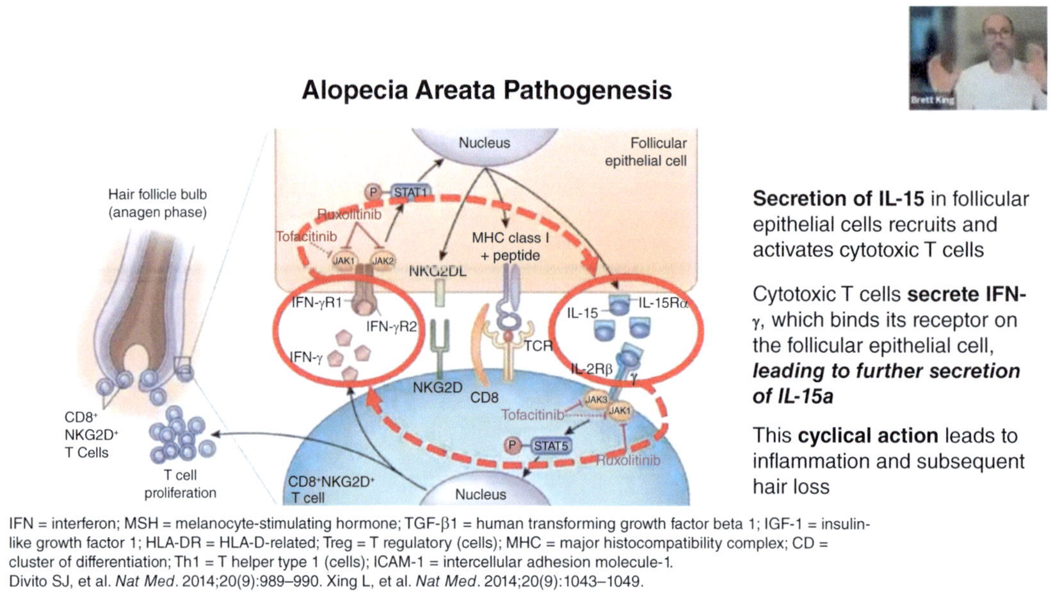

Fig. 6.2 Secretion of IL-15 in follicular epithelial cells recruits and activates cytotoxic T cells. Cytotoxic T cells secrete IFN-y, which binds its receptor on the follicular epithelial cell, leading to further secretion of IL-15. This cyclical action leads to inflammation and subsequent hair loss

including JAK1 and JAK3 (Fig. 6.2). This interferes with cytokine signaling and downstream immune responses, leading to immunomodulation and the suppression of inflammation [12]. Monitoring: Regular blood tests to monitor for potential adverse effects.

Platelet-Rich Plasma (PRP)

Biological Basis: Platelets release a plethora of growth factors such as platelet-derived growth factor (PDGF), transforming growth factor (TGF), vascular endothelial growth factor (VEGF), and epidermal growth factor (EGF). These molecules are believed to stimulate hair follicle stem cells, enhancing hair regrowth [13].

Evolution of PRP

1980s: The therapeutic potential of PRP was first recognized in hematology. Its role in promoting wound healing after surgical procedures, especially in maxillofacial surgeries, became evident.

1990s: Orthopedic surgeons started using PRP for bone grafting procedures, noting its potential in improving bone healing.

Early 2000s: Its application expanded to sports medicine and orthopedics, especially for treating soft tissue injuries.

2010s: Dermatologists began exploring PRP's role in treating various conditions, with alopecia areata being one of the prime targets. Multiple research papers and clinical trials were published, emphasizing the positive effects of PRP in hair regrowth and increased hair density.

Mechanism of Action Rediscovery

While the init'ial use of PRP was based on empirical evidence, further studies in the 2010s elucidated the mechanism behind its efficacy. PRP was found to be rich in growth factors, such as platelet-derived growth factor (PDGF), vascular endothelial growth factor (VEGF), and transforming growth factor-beta (TGF-β). These growth factors, when introduced to the scalp, enhanced blood flow stimulated hair follicle stem cells, promoting hair regrowth.

Procedure

Blood Collection: Around 20 ml of patient's blood is drawn.

Centrifugation: Double-spin method to extract PRP.

Activation: With calcium chloride or autologous thrombin.

Administration: Injected into areas of alopecia at 1 cm intervals.

Frequency: Monthly sessions for 3 months, followed by maintenance sessions.

Exosomes

Initial Discovery

- 1980s: Exosomes were initially considered cellular waste, tiny vesicles released by cells without any perceived significant function.
- 1990s: Their role in intercellular communication began to be understood, with exosomes being recognized as carriers of proteins, lipids, and RNA.
- 2000s: It was identified that exosomes play a critical role in various biological processes, including immune response modulation, pathogenesis of diseases, and even tumor progression.
- Emergence in Dermatology
- 2010s: The therapeutic potential of exosomes started being explored in regenerative medicine and dermatology. Exosomes derived from mesenchymal stem cells (MSCs) were found to carry growth factors, cytokines, and genetic material that could modulate hair growth and potentially reverse the autoimmune responses seen in alopecia areata.
- Late 2010s & 2020s: Clinical trials commenced, investigating the safety and efficacy of exosome therapy in alopecia areata. These trials found that MSC-derived exosomes, when introduced into the scalp, can enhance hair regrowth, strengthen existing hair follicles, and even modulate local immune responses, reducing the autoimmune attack on hair follicles.

Mechanism: Exosomes are nano-sized extracellular vesicles that contain proteins, lipids, and nucleic acids. When derived from mesenchymal stem cells (MSCs) and introduced into AA sites, they might promote hair regrowth by modulating the immune response or stimulating hair follicle activity [14]. This could be due to the immunomodulatory proteins, mRNAs, and microRNAs they carry. They might also directly stimulate hair follicles, promoting growth.

Efficacy: Preliminary studies on exosomes in hair regrowth are promising, though more extensive clinical trials are needed to establish their efficacy.

Supportive and Cosmetic Therapies

With AT and AU, complete regrowth is challenging, and can have a significant psychological impact. From wigs and hairpieces to topical camouflage solutions, the emphasis is on improving aesthetic appearances and boosting patient morale. These can be custom designed to match the patient's original hair [15]. Cosmetic solutions for eyebrows and eyelashes include cosmetic tattoos or specific makeup techniques to help restore the appearance of hair.

Psychosocial Implications and Support

Psychological therapy is equally paramount, addressing the mental and emotional strain of AA, as the transition from AA to AT or AU can be emotionally traumatizing. Patients often grapple with issues of identity, self-esteem, and societal acceptance [16]. Tailored psychological support, counseling, and patient support groups become paramount. Addressing these concerns holistically can greatly improve the overall quality of life [16]. Support structures, both formal (therapists, counselors) and informal (support groups), can make this journey more manageable.

Conclusion

Alopecia Areata and its extensive forms, Totalis and Universalis, symbolize the complexities of autoimmune disorders. With evolving treatments, from traditional methods to groundbreaking techniques like JAK inhibitors, PRP and exosomes, there is renewed hope for patients.

While therapeutic advancements offer hope for hair regrowth, the emotional and psychological well-being of patients remains equally crucial. A multi-dimensional approach, combining medical interventions with emotional support, ensures the best outcomes for those navigating the challenges of alopecia in its various forms.

References

1. Gilhar A, Etzioni A, Paus R. Alopecia areata. N Engl J Med. 2012;366(16):1515–25. https://doi.org/10.1056/NEJMra1103442.
2. Olsen EA, Roberts J, Sperling L, Tosti A, Shapiro J, McMichael A, Bergfeld W, Callender V, Mirmirani P, Washenik K, Whiting D, Cotsarelis G, Hordinsky M. Objective outcome measures: collecting meaningful data on alopecia areata. J Am Acad Dermatol. 2018;79(3):470–478.e3. https://doi.org/10.1016/j.jaad.2017.10.048.
3. Ludwig E. Classification of the types of androgenetic alopecia (common baldness) occurring in the female sex. Br J Dermatol. 1977;97(3):247–54. https://doi.org/10.1111/j.1365-2133.1977.tb15179.x.
4. Tosti A, Whiting D, Iorizzo M, Pazzaglia M, Misciali C, Vincenzi C, Micali G. The role of scalp dermoscopy in the diagnosis of alopecia areata incognita. J Am Acad Dermatol. 2008;59(1):64–7. https://doi.org/10.1016/j.jaad.2008.03.031.
5. JAAD. 2023;89(2):Supplement S16-S19.
6. Marwah M, Nadkarni N, Patil S. 'Ho-ver'ing over alopecia areata: histopathological study of 50 cases. Int J Trichology. 2014;6(1):13–8. https://doi.org/10.4103/0974-7753.136749.
7. McDonagh AJ, Tazi-Ahnini R. Epidemiology and genetics of alopecia areata. Clin Exp Dermatol. 2002;27(5):405–9. https://doi.org/10.1046/j.1365-2230.2002.01077.x.
8. Jabbari A, Nguyen N, Cerise JE, Ulerio G, de Jong A, Clynes R, Christiano AM, Mackay-Wiggan J. Treatment of an alopecia areata patient with tofacitinib results in regrowth of hair and changes in serum and skin biomarkers. Exp Dermatol. 2016;25(8):642–3. https://doi.org/10.1111/exd.13060.
9. Strand V, Ahadieh S, French J, Geier J, Krishnaswami S, Menon S, Checchio T, Tensfeldt TG, Hoffman E, Riese R, Boy M, Gómez-Reino JJ. Systematic review and meta-analysis of serious infections with tofacitinib and biologic disease-modifying antirheumatic drug treatment in rheumatoid arthritis clinical trials. Arthritis Res Ther. 2015;17:362. https://doi.org/10.1186/s13075-015-0880-2.
10. Curtis JR, Lee EB, Kaplan IV, Kwok K, Geier J, Benda B, Soma K, Wang L, Riese R. Tofacitinib, an oral Janus kinase inhibitor: analysis of malignancies across the rheumatoid arthritis clinical development programme. Ann Rheum Dis. 2016;75(5):831–41. https://doi.org/10.1136/annrheumdis-2014-205847.
11. Craiglow BG, Liu LY, King BA. Tofacitinib for the treatment of alopecia areata and variants in adolescents. J Am Acad Dermatol. 2017;76(1):29–32. https://doi.org/10.1016/j.jaad.2016.09.006.
12. Kennedy Crispin M, Ko JM, Craiglow BG, Li S, Shankar G, Urban JR, Chen JC, Cerise JE, Jabbari A, Winge MC, Marinkovich MP, Christiano AM, Oro AE, King BA. Safety and efficacy of the JAK inhibitor tofacitinib citrate in patients with alopecia areata. JCI Insight. 2016;1(15):e89776. https://doi.org/10.1172/jci.insight.89776.
13. Stevens J, Khetarpal S. Platelet-rich plasma for androgenetic alopecia: a review of the literature and proposed treatment protocol. Int J Womens Dermatol. 2018;5(1):46–51. https://doi.org/10.1016/j.ijwd.2018.08.004.
14. Hu S, Zhang J, Ji Q, Xie S, Jiang J, Ni H, He X, Yang Y, Wu M. Exosomes derived from uMSCs promote hair regrowth in alopecia areata through accelerating human hair follicular keratinocyte proliferation and migration. Cell Biol Int. 2024;48(2):154–61. https://doi.org/10.1002/cbin.12099.
15. Messenger AG, Sinclair R. Follicular miniaturization in female pattern hair loss: clinicopathological correlations. Br J Dermatol. 2006;155(5):926–30. https://doi.org/10.1111/j.1365-2133.2006.07409.x.
16. Whiting DA. Chronic telogen effluvium: increased scalp hair shedding in middle-aged women. J Am Acad Dermatol. 1996;35(6):899–906.

Nutraceuticals in the Treatment of Hair Loss

7

Nicole Rogers

Introduction

Most would agree that the ideal of beauty and health includes a head of thick, healthy, lustrous hair. And yet, numerous forces work against us as we age, including factors that affect the quality of our hair. Although hair is a constantly regenerating organ, it is still subject to weathering from the environment in the form of ultraviolet light, pollution, wind, and humidity. Individual grooming habits can also take a toll on the health and quality of the hair shaft. Such habits include chemical relaxing or straightening, as well as high-temperature devices such as flat irons and blow dryers. Repetitive use of these chemicals and heating elements together can result in trichorhexxis nodosa (breakage) or bubble hair (formation of air bubbles when wet hair is flat ironed) (Fig. 7.1) [1].

Persons with a family history of hair loss may also notice a gradual hair thinning or loss, typical for male and female pattern hair loss (androgenetic alopecia, or AGA). Although we have a number of pharmaceutical options for hair regrowth including minoxidil, finasteride, dutasteride, and spironolactone (women only), many patients do not want to take drugs and prefer a more natural option. Even patients who undergo hair surgery may ask about more natural products that can enhance the appearance of their new hair. The use of nutraceuticals, or foods containing medicinal benefits, can be applied toward the treatment of hair loss with surprising patient adherence.

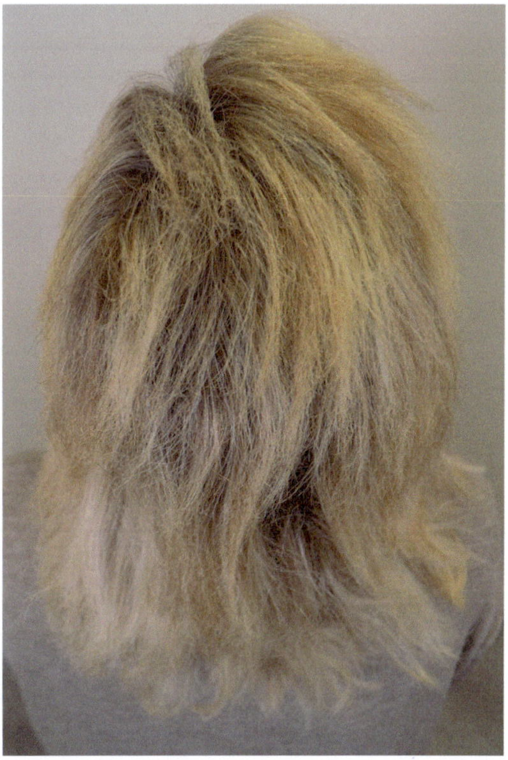

Fig. 7.1 Severe trichorrhexis nodosa from combined hair bleaching and flat iron use

N. Rogers (✉)
Metairie, LA, USA

Tulane Department of Dermatology, New Orleans, LA, USA

P. J. Panagotacos, H. Maibach (eds.), *Hair Loss*, Updates in Clinical Dermatology,
https://doi.org/10.1007/978-3-031-74314-6_7

As physicians we must understand as much as we can about the basic science of these ingredients and help guide patients toward products that may help them. Although most such ingredients are lacking multi-center, placebo-controlled clinical hair growth trials, we can learn their mechanisms of action from the medical literature. In this chapter we will cover the steps patients can take to prevent hair aging and cover some key nutraceuticals that may help retain the health and vitality of their hair.

How Can We Prevent Hair Aging?

Perhaps the most obvious steps one can take are to avoid those environmental factors that can be damaging to the hair shaft. Avoid excessive UV exposure by wearing a hat at all times. A number of protective hair sprays and conditioners now include SPF ingredients. By limiting use of chemicals to straighten or highlight the hair, its structure and integrity will remain intact. By washing hair less often, there may be less damage to the hair cuticle. And by avoiding excessive use of hot styling tools there will be less breakage overall.

There is some evidence that a diet rich in antioxidants may help improve hair quality. In one hospital-based case control study in Italy, 104 males with AGA were compared with 108 controls not affected by AGA. After controlling for age, education, body mass index, family history of AGA, the researchers found there were protective effects for AGA with high consumption (>3× weekly) of raw vegetables and fresh herbs (>3× weekly) [2].

Supplements represent an easier way for patients who do not want to make major lifestyle changes. A number of supplements covered here are touted for their anti-oxidant effects, which can translate to a positive effect on the hair follicles. Likewise, some are known for their anti-apoptotic effects, because they can slow the senescence or aging of the hair follicle. Table 7.1 provides a listing of the important mechanisms affecting hair growth are described. In addition, many hair growth supplements specifically touted to improve androgenetic alopecia, can block 5α-reductase, the enzyme responsible for converting testosterone to di-hydro testosterone (DHT). By lowering DHT levels some of these supplements can represent plant-based alternatives to finasteride or dutasteride. Table 7.2 provides a listing of plant ingredients with known 5α-reductase inhibiting properties. Most of the nutraceutical ingredients we discuss appear to have multiple mechanisms by which they exert their effect on hair follicles.

Table 7.1 Known mechanisms affecting hair growth

Positive regulators	Negative regulators
Epidermal growth factor (EGF)	Bone morphogenetic proteins (BMPs)
Hepatocyte growth factor (HGF)	MicroRNA (miR)
Insulin-like growth factor-1 (IGF-1)	Fibroblast growth factor (FGF)
Vascular endothelial growth factor (VEGF)	
Wnt/β-catenin	Transforming growth factor-β, TGF-β1, TGF-β2, TGF-β3
Epithelial sonic hedgehog (SHH)-promotes Noggin	TNF-α
Noggin (inhibits BMP2/BMP4)	IL-1α, IL-1β
Erk and Akt activation	
Bcl-2 expression (anti-apoptotic)	Bax expression (pro-apoptotic)
Protein kinase C	

Table 7.2 Summary of plant-derived 5α-reductase inhibitors

Plant	Latin name	Bioactive components
Pumpkin seed oil	*Cucubita pepo*	Oleic and linoleic acids
Saw palmetto	*Serenoa repens*	Lauric and myristic acids
Red ginseng	*Panax ginseng*	Triterpine saponins
Rosemary oil	*Rosmarinus officialis*	12-methoxycarnosic acid
Green tea	*Camellia sinensis*	Epigallocatechin-4-gallate (EGCG)
Dried root of plant	*Sophora flavescens*	Unknown
Black pepper	*Piper nigrum leaf*	Active lignin 1&2
		Piperine (high in linoleic, oleic, and palmitic acids)
Japanese false nettle	*Boehmeria nipononivea*	α-linoleic acid, elaidic and stearic acids
Safflower	*Carthamus tinctorius L.*	Carthamin, Carthamidin, Isocarthamidin
Red babyberry	*Murica rubra*	Myricanol, myricanone
Lingzhi mushroom	*Ganoderma lucidum*	Triterpenoids
Japanese climbing fern	*Lygodii Spora*	Oleic, linoleic, palmitic acids
White cedar seed	*Thujae occidentalis*	Unknown
Amarvela (Parasitic herb)	*Cuscuta reflexa Roxb*	Unknown

Polyphenols: Proanthocyanidins

Proanthocyanidins are considered a species of polyphenol compounds, that exist as polymers or oligomers, built of flavan-3-ol units. These species are known for anti-microbial, anti-oxidant, anti-fungal, anti-viral, and anti-tumor promoting effects, to name a few. These molecules were first identified and proposed for the treatment of hair loss in 1998 by a group of Japanese researchers. They were identified among 1000 different types of plant extracts and found to be present in dry grape seeds (Chardonnay variety), apple juice (procyanidin B-2), and barley husk (procyanidin B-3), with the ability to convert telogen hairs to anagen hairs in C_3H mice [3] (Fig. 7.2). Specifically, they found that procyanidin dimer and trimer exhibited greater hair growth-promoting activity than monomer, with procyanidin B-2 about 300% relative to controls (=100%), and procyanidin C-1 about 220% relative to controls [4]. Procyanidin B-2 was shown to be safe and with no symptoms of mutagenicity or topical irritation in rabbits or guinea pigs [5].

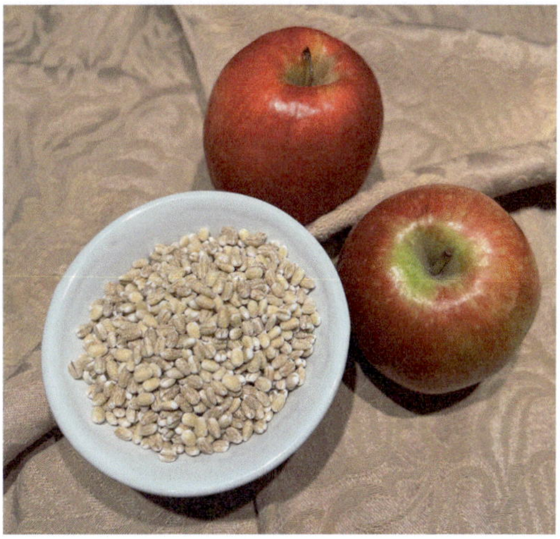

Fig. 7.2 Apples and barley contain procyanidins

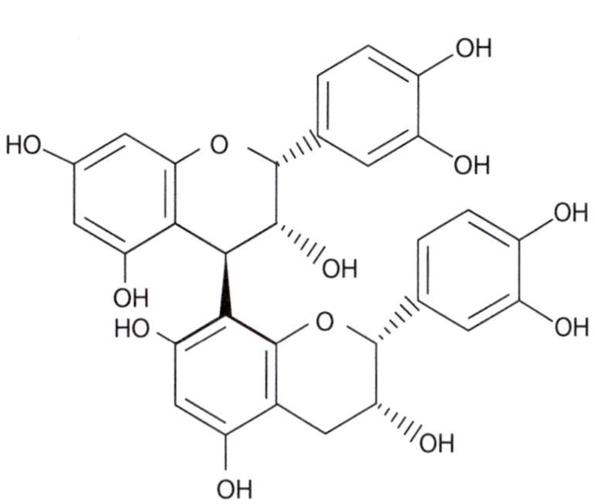

Fig. 7.3 Chemical structure of Procyanidin B-2

After the initial in vitro and in vivo success of procyanidin B-2 was demonstrated, a 1% tonic was developed for use in humans (Fig. 7.3). It showed promise in a double-blind, placebo-controlled study where 19 men with AGA who applied the topical treatment had significantly greater hair counts after 6 months than the ten men who served as controls [6, 7]. Subsequently a larger double-blind study tested the application of a 0.7% apple procyanidin oligomers (2 ml, twice daily) in 21 men with AGA vs. 22 controls. They found statistically greater hair counts in the treatment group after 6 months, with continued improvement seen at the 12-month extension [8].

The polyphenolic content of different apple varieties was found to be highest in the fruits of *Malus pumila Miller cv. Annurca* (AFA), native to southern Italy. The same research group developed the first gastro-protected oral formulation of procyanidin-B2 combined with selenium, zinc, and biotin called AppleMets (Oscar Green, Naples Italy), and demonstrated that it could improve hair growth in as little as 8 weeks treatment in healthy volunteers with AGA [9]. In Korea, this same *Annurca* apple extract was given orally to 6-week old C57BL/6 mice with the observation of improved hair length, thickness, weight, and density [10].

At first, it was proposed that procyanidins may work by inhibiting protein kinase C, which plays a role in cell regulation, differentiation, and proliferation [11, 12]. However, procyanidins (B-3) have also been shown in cell culture to counteract the growth-inhibiting effects of TFG-β1 and TGF-β2, as well as to possibly upregulate expression of MAPK/ERK kinase [13, 14]. There is some evidence that procyanidins may inhibit several NADPH dependent reactions but stimulate mitochondrial respiration, β-oxidation, and subsequent keratin production in hair follicles [15]. When it was given orally in mice, there was upregulated gene expression of VEGF-A and FGF-7, as well as suppression of type 1 5α-reductase [10].

Polyphenols (Botanical 5-Alpha Reductase Inhibitors): Saw Palmetto, Pumpkin Seed Oil Etc.

Just as finasteride was first developed for prostate enlargement but serendipitously shown to cause hair growth, saw palmetto and pumpkin seed oil are two plant-based ingredients that have shown some efficacy in treating both benign prostatic hypertrophy (BPH) and hair loss. In fact, a number of such supplements are already marketed over the counter either alone or in combination for the treatment of both conditions. The mechanism by which these ingredients work is to block 5α-reductase, the enzyme that converts testosterone to dihydrotestosterone (DHT). Pattern hair loss develops in patients with increased sensitivity to DHT, and the therapeutic lowering of DHT levels can help reverse this hair miniaturization process.

A number of reports have demonstrated the efficacy of saw palmetto (*Serenoa repens*) in treating BPH with the advantage of no known sexual side effects [16–18]. Based on the success of its active ingredient beta-sitosterol in treating BPH [19], saw palmetto was first investigated for the treatment of androgenetic alopecia in a randomized, double-blind, placebo-controlled trial in 19 males between the ages of 23 and 64 with androgenetic alopecia [20]. The treatment arm was given 50 mg of β-sitosterol with 200 mg saw palmetto extract, and after 21 weeks 60% of patients had an 'improved outcome' versus just 11% of patients in the control group. Although blinded investigators were asked to rate the hair from −3 to +3, no standardized hair counts or hair weights were conducted.

Subsequently, an open label study of 100 men with AGA compared one group receiving *Serenoa repens* 320 mg daily with a second group receiving finasteride 1 mg daily for 2 years [21]. Using standardized global photos, it was found that only 38% of the saw palmetto group had an increase in hair growth, compared with 68% of the men treated with finasteride. The researchers also found that the growth was more pronounced in both the frontal scalp and vertex with finasteride, but only the vertex with saw palmetto.

A topical regimen of *Serenoa repens* demonstrated improved hair counts in 50 male patients after 12 and 24 weeks but the results leveled off presumably due to the cessation of the more concentrated serum after the first 4 weeks [22]. There is evidence that nanoliposomes loaded with carbon dioxide may enhance the topical delivery of saw palmetto for hair growth [23]. There is also evidence that liquid saw palmetto supplements contain significantly higher concentrations of total fatty acids and phytosterols than powders or tinctures [24].

Pumpkin seed oil, extracted from the seeds of *Cucubita pepo,* is touted for its anti-inflammatory, antimicrobial, anti-tumor, anti-parasitic, antiviral, and analgesic health benefits [25]. It contains more unsaturated than saturated fatty acids, with oleic acid and linoleic acid in greatest quantities. However, it also contains polyphenols and phytosterols, which impart its anti-oxidant properties. In particular, β-sitosterol is the most prevalent sterol [26], but the content can be influenced by processing methods such as roasting or by storage conditions [27].

Like saw palmetto, pumpkin seed oil has been proven beneficial in the treatment of BPH without any evident side effects [28]. So far, we have only had a single study investigating its treatment of male pattern hair loss. This randomized, double-blind, placebo-controlled trial enrolled 76 men who were given either 400 mg pumpkin seed oil or placebo daily for 24 weeks. The treatment group showed a 40% increase in hair counts at 24 weeks versus just a 10% increase in the placebo group ($p < 0.001$). Also, patients had higher rates of self-reported improvement in the treatment group [29]. It is widely available over the counter in gel capsules of dosages up to 1000 mg. Topical delivery of pumpkin seed oil is being investigated with the use of niosomes [30].

Green tea was observed to inhibit 5α-reductase when the gallate ester in epigallocatechin-3-gallate (EGCG) was replaced with a long-chain fatty acid, such as lauric (10 carbon chain), myristic (12 chain carbon), or stearic acid (16-carbon chain), and the most potent inhibitor of 5α-reductase was formed with the addition of palmitic acid (14-carbon chain) [31]. When EGCG was studied on dermal papilla cells in vitro and in vivo, it was found to upregulate the phosphorylation of Erk and Akt, and to increase the ratio of Bcl-2/Bax [32]. This research suggests that EGCG has both proliferative and anti-apoptotic effects.

Other lesser-known plant ingredients can also help block 5α-reductase. *Sophora flavescens* is a plant used in Chinese medicine that can promote conversion of telogen to anagen when applied to the backs of C57BL/6 mice. RT-PCR analysis showed that it could induce mRNA levels of growth factors such as IGF-1 and KGF in dermal papilla cells, and that the extract could inhibit type II 5α-reductase [33]. The extract of black pepper (*Piper nigrum*) has demonstrated anti-androgenic activity *in vivo*. Piperine is a major alkaloid amide found in the *P. nigrum* fruit and this can inhibit 5α-reductase [34].

In a study investigating various Thai plants, safflower (*Carthamus tinctorius L.*) was found to have the greatest ability to block 5α-reductase and to promote hair growth in C57BL/C mice [35]. Other plants that can inhibit 5α-reductase include Japanese false nettle [36], white cedar seed [37], Japanese climbing fern [38], red bayberry bark [39], lingzhi mushroom [40], and a parasitic herb called *Cuscuta reflexa* [41]. The list of plants in Table 7.2 is not meant to be exhaustive, as new 5α-reductase inhibitors are certainly being identified every day.

Collagen and Peptides

There is great interest in the consumption of collagen for its presumed benefits to skin and hair. Non-medical bloggers on Youtube and Instagram are touting its benefits, but with little scientific data to support their claims [42]. At the present time, there are no clinical studies in humans demonstrating improved hair growth with collagen ingestion. However, there is some basic science data supporting the use of collagen peptides (smaller, hydrolyzed collagen molecules) as signaling molecules to help promote hair growth. Collagen peptides are made of up individual amino acids and can selectively interact with cell receptors.

Marine-sourced collagen has emerged as an alternative to bovine or porcine collagen, appearing in many commercially available hair supplements. One study using collagen peptides extracted from the scales of Mozambique tilapia examined the in vitro effects on human dermal papilla cells and the in vivo effects after oral administration to C57BL/6 mice [43]. The collagen peptides enhanced hair regrowth in the human dermal papilla cells and increased expression of hair growth factors IGF-1, VEGF, and Ki67 among others. They decreased the growth of inhibitory factor TGF-β1. The collagen peptides were also shown to upregulate the Wnt/β--catenin pathways and downregulate the BMP pathways. The authors concluded that these collagen peptides could be used as food supplements and nutraceuticals for hair loss prevention and hair regrowth.

Biomimetic peptides are synthetic versions of collagen peptides that have been created to interact with growth factors and provide anti-aging effects. They have been widely used in the beauty industry and can regulate synthesis of proteins in Ki-67 in cell cultures of human fibroblasts [44]. In one study looking at 30 women with telogen effluvium, a treatment group applied a lotion containing biomimetic peptides (decapeptide-18, oligopeptide-54, decapeptide-10, octapeptide-2, decapeptide-19, oligopeptide-71, decapeptide-28) followed by microneedling, and a control group applied normal saline followed by microneedling. Punch biopsies taken before and after the intervention demonstrated increased expression of growth promoters VEGF, EGF, and decreased expression of the growth inhibitor TGF-β1 [45]. This improved regrowth was also seen on trichoscopy and phototrichography.

Researchers in Seoul found that the adiponectin protein (APN) promotes hair growth and can induce mRNA expression of the growth factors IGF-1, VEGF, and HGF [46]. This same group went on to develop a small transdermally deliverable pentapeptide from the original sequence of endogenenous APN called (GLYFF;P5) that can bind to adiponectin receptor 1 (AdipoR1) to promote hair growth and suppress hair loss symptoms [47]. Their studies confirmed that P5 molecule induced anagen hair cycle in vivo mouse models, suggesting promise for use in human studies.

A number of topical peptides have been developed for their anti-aging effects in dermatology. These can be divided into signaling peptides, neurotransmitter-affecting peptides, and carrier peptides. The most commonly encountered carrier peptide is used to stabilize and deliver copper into cells [48]. As cosmeceuticals, copper peptides are thought to improve skin firmness and texture, fine lines, and hyperpigmentation. They also have some data supporting their use for the treatment of hair loss [49, 50]. Copper and other biomimetic peptides have been incorporated into a number of commercially available shampoos, conditioners, and post-hair-transplant care kits.

Red Ginseng

Ginseng has been used for thousands of years in Asian medicine for its proclaimed antioxidant, antitumor, hepatoprotective, and anti-inflammatory properties. It is grown and sold as supplements and candies all over South Korea, China, and Japan (Fig. 7.4). Ginseng has bioactive compounds collectively called saponins, which are made up of 40 different ginsenosides, including Rb1, Rb2, Rc, Rd., Re, Rf, Rg1, Rg2, Rg3, Rh1 and -Ro. Depending on the number of hydroxyl groups available for glycosylation, they are classified as protopanaxadiol (PPD) or protopanaxatriol (PPT) [51]. It appears that we are just now learning the benefits it may have related to hair growth and its numerous mechanisms of action.

Interest in its possible role in hair growth came about after one study demonstrated a protective effect of *Panax ginseng* against ionizing radiation in the hair follicles of mice. Mice that

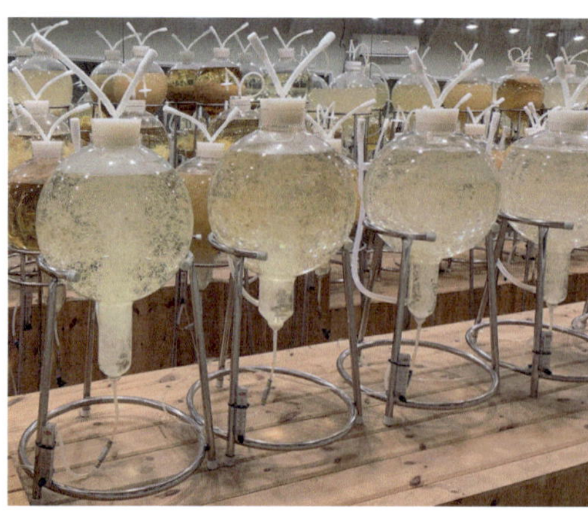

Fig. 7.4 Ginseng in a fermentation lab in South Korea

were pre-treated with the ingestion of a water fraction of ginseng had fewer apoptotic hair medullary cells after radiation than the control group [52]. Based on previous reports that red ginseng had more bioactive components than white ginseng, it was proven that red also had superior activity over white ginseng in promoting the growth of cultured mouse vibrissal hair follicles [53]. Further work investigating the effects of Korean red ginseng demonstrating that it could help prevent cisplatin-induced ototoxicity [54] and gentamicin-induced hearing loss in rats [55].

So far, we have only two studies demonstrating an *in vivo* benefit of red ginseng for androgenetic alopecia in humans. Forty patients with androgenetic alopecia were randomly assigned to either take 3000 mg/day Korean red ginseng for 24 weeks, or placebo. Changes in hair counts, thickness, and density were evaluated with a Folliscope®, and the results found that the treatment group had effectively increased hair density and thickness. Patients in the treatment group were satisfied and photographs evaluated by dermatologists also confirmed its effectiveness [56]. However, it was a small study and it is not clear whether the patients and/or researchers were blinded.

The second study compared 41 patients with female pattern hair loss, half of whom were treated with topical 3% minoxidil and half of whom were treated with topical 3% minoxidil plus an oral Korean red ginseng capsule containing Rb1, Rb2, Rc, Rd., Re, Rf, Rg1, Rg2, Rg3 and other minor ginsenosides [57]. Both groups showed a significant improvement in hair thickness from baseline, but only the combination treatment group showed a significant increase in hair density over baseline ($p < 0.05$). The combination group did have improved hair density and thickness over the minoxidil-only group, but the results were not statistically significant.

Ginseng appears to have a variety of effects on hair follicles. Its promotional mechanisms appear to be through the induction of p63 in follicular keratinocytes [58], upregulation of vascular endothelial growth factor (VEGF) [59], activation of ERK and AKT signaling pathways [60], and upregulation of β-catenin/WNT signaling [61, 62]. It also has anti-apoptotic effects, in that it was found to enhance Bcl-2 expression and decrease Bax expression in cultured human dermal papilla cells [63], as well as to inhibit transforming growth factor β signaling cascades [64]. It can also antagonize the effects of WNT-inhibitor DKK-1 [65].

Interestingly, red ginseng may also inhibit 5α-reductase activity. Ginsenoside-Rg3 was found to inhibit the transcriptional activities of androgen receptors and downregulate androgen receptors in a prostate cancer cell line [66]. Based on the finding that it contained largely linoleic acid and β-sitosterol (plant-based 5α-reductase inhibitors), one group demonstrated the ability of red ginseng oil to restore hair regenerative capacity in mice treated with testosterone [67].

Melatonin

Melatonin (N-acetyl-5-methoxy-tryptamine) is an indole hormone produced naturally by the pineal gland in humans and most other mammal species. Recent research has demonstrated that it can also be produced in a number of extra-pineal sites including the skin, bile, bone marrow, cerebrospinal fluid, and gastric mucosa. Its lipophilic nature allows it to easily penetrate cell membranes and organelles where it can protect against oxidative damage. It has specifically been shown to provide better protection against ultraviolet-induced skin erythema when applied as a 0.5% lotion prior to skin irradiation, compared with melatonin 0.05% or just vehicle [68].

Much of what we know about the influence of melatonin on hair follicles is garnered from animal research. Cashmere goats from New Zealand, in particular, showed more rapid hair cycle induction under the influence of melatonin [69, 70]. A number of other animals have been studied for the effects of melatonin including other goat species, ferrets, merino sheep, mink, dogs, red deer, and most recently rabbits [71, 72]. Many species have an overcoat and undercoat that are populated by primary and secondary follicles, and their relative densities seem to be modulated by changes in the seasons as well as changes in melatonin production or exposure.

How does melatonin exert this growth-promoting effect on hair follicles? One study demonstrated that melatonin could prevent nicotine-induced oxidative stress, apoptosis, and inflammation affecting cochlear hair cells in vitro. It specifically decreased inflammatory cytokines TNF-α, ILK-6 and IL-1β [73]. In one study of cashmere goats, the group treated with melatonin implantation demonstrated significantly increased expression of Wnt10b and β-catenin at various stages in the hair growth cycle versus controls [74]. Melatonin also seems to stimulate Noggin, which inhibits the negative regulators bone morphogenetic proteins (BMPs) [75].

There is evidence that melatonin can promote human hair growth as well. The first *in vivo* research was a double-blind randomized, placebo-controlled study conducted in 40 women with either female pattern hair loss or diffuse alopecia. Patients who applied a 0.1% melatonin tonic had significantly increased anagen hair rates in the occipital scalp compared with placebo, suggesting a need for further research [76]. Since then a total of 11 human studies have been identified in the medical literature investigating the use of melatonin for hair regrowth. Most of these involve topical use and showed favorable results at doses of 0.0033% to 0.1% melatonin solution, over 90–180 days, in the form of improved scalp hair growth (n = 8), density (n = 4), and hair shaft thickness (n = 2) compared with controls [77, 78].

There may be a role for nanostructured lipid carriers to improve topical delivery of melatonin over a traditional solution [79]. The co-delivery of melatonin with other anti-oxidant ingredients such as vitamin C has also been investigated for treatment of androgenetic alopecia [80].

So far, only one open-label, proof-of-concept study has investigated the use of oral melatonin taken 1.5 mg twice daily for hair growth. Although the results showed improved hair growth as well as a significant increase in terminal hair counts and hair mass index, the product also included several other ingredients (cholecalciferol, omega 3 and 6 fatty acids, antioxidants, and botanical 5α-reductase inhibitors) which may confound the results [81].

Rosemary Oil

A number of over-the-counter remedies containing rosemary oil (*Rosmarinus officinalis L.*) proclaim its ability to enhance hair growth. It is derived from the Latin word *ros* (dew) and *marinus* (sea) to mean 'dew of the sea' [82]. Besides flavoring food, rosemary has long been touted for its health benefits (Fig. 7.5) [83]. It contains a number of phenolic acids and flavonoids which confer antioxidant and anti-inflammatory properties [84, 85]. The primary bioactive ingredients are caffeic acid and rosmarinic acid, but other compounds include camphor and 12-methoxycarnosic acid.

It has been shown to be neuroprotective with the ability to downregulate oxidative stress. In one rat model investigating neuropathic pain, it has been shown to suppress apoptotic factors Bax, caspase 3, and caspase 9 [86]. In another, it was shown to suppress inflammatory markers COX-2, prostaglandin E2 (PGE-2), matrix metallopeptidase 2 (MMP2), and nitric oxide [87]. While one might think a mechanism for hair growth could include increased nitric oxide production (to promote vasodilation), this does not appear to be likely. In fact, one study showed specifically that carnosol in rosemary could suppress nitric oxide production by down-regulating NF-kappa B activation in mouse macrophages [88].

More recent research seems to suggest that rosemary may have properties allowing it to inhibit 5α-reductase. In one study, the topical

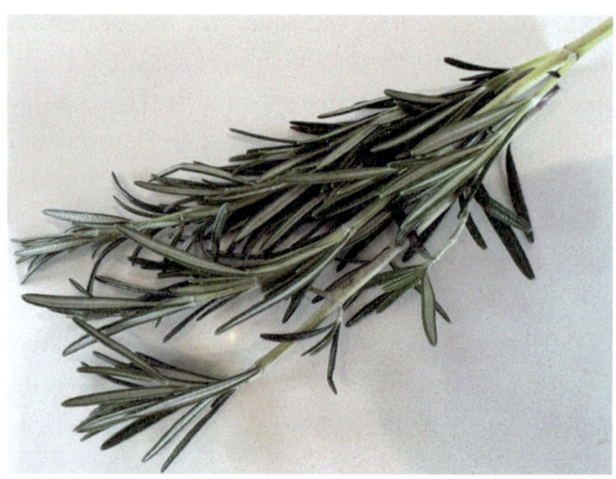

Fig. 7.5 Rosemary grows readily in gardens and can be found in most grocery stores

application of rosemary leaf extract in mice (2 mg/day/mouse) was able to help reverse hair loss induced by testosterone treatment. The authors specifically identified 12-methoxycarnosic acid as the most likely active constituent binding to androgen receptors [89]. So far there has been only one study investigating rosemary oil for hair growth in humans. It was a randomized single-blind comparative trial enrolling 100 patients, half of whom were randomly assigned to apply rosemary oil and half were assigned to apply 2% minoxidil for a period of 6 months [90]. Standardized microphotographic counts were performed at baseline, 3 months, and 6 months. There were no significant differences in counts between the two groups at either 3 months or 6 months, however both groups had significantly greater hair counts at 6 months compared with baseline. These results suggest that topical rosemary oil may be at least as effective as 2% minoxidil.

Caffeine

In addition to its psychostimulant properties, caffeine appears to also have some ability to stimulate hair follicles. This may be counterintuitive, given the fact that it is known for its vasoconstrictive properties. Caffeine is a purine alkaloid that works by blocking the binding of adenosine to the adenosine A receptor, which enhances the release of the neurotransmitter acetylcholine. Caffeine also increases cyclic AMP levels via nonselective inhibition of phosphodiesterase, providing higher energy levels to promote increased metabolic activity and cell proliferation [91]. While there is no recommended daily dose, it is generally recognized as safe by the US FDA, with toxic doses being over 10 grams per day for an adult. Given the average cup of coffee contains 80–175 mg of caffeine, it would take 50–100 cups of coffee to achieve this upper limit.

How does this translate to hair? It was found to have a protective effect against the inhibitory effect of testosterone on hair follicles in vitro. Caffeine enhanced hair shaft elongation, prolonged anagen duration, and stimulated hair matrix keratinocyte proliferation. Specifically, it was found to upregulate IFG-1 gene expression, while TGF-β2 secretion was down-regulated [92]. Further antioxidant properties were demonstrated as caffeine was shown to protect against damaging effects of ultraviolet radiation on the human hair follicle. Whereas UVA + UVB doses induced oxidative damage and cytotoxicity in hair follicles, promoting catagen development and promoting apoptosis of the hair follicle outer root sheath, the topical application of 0.1% caffeine stimulated the expression of IGF-1 in the proximal hair follicle outer root sheath [93].

As a hydrophilic molecule, caffeine has been shown to penetrate more quickly (resulting in higher serum concentrations) through the hair follicles versus when the follicle orifices are blocked [94, 95]. One single-center, double-blind trial in which female patients with androgenetic alopecia were asked to wash with a phyto-caffeine-containing shampoo or a control shampoo found that the treatment group had an improved hair pull test at 6 months, compared with control subjects [96]. Another similar study investigating a caffeine-based shampoo in male androgenetic alopecia, showed reduced hair pull counts at 6 months but there was no control group [97]. Perhaps the most relevant study demonstrated non-inferiority of a 0.2% caffeine solution when compared with topical minoxidil 5% solution studied in 210 males over a 6 month time period [98].

Cannabidiol Oil

Cannabis has been around for centuries, and cannabidiol (CBD) oil has gained widespread interest for medicinal use as a less psychoactive version. Cannabinoids are classified into three groups: endocannabinoids (naturally produced in animal or human bodies), phytocannabinoids (sourced from plants, i.e., *Cannabis sativa/indica*), and synthetic cannabinoids (produced in a lab) [99]. So far, only one human clinical trial has investigated the use of CBD for hair regrowth. In this study, 35 patients with androgenetic alopecia (28 males, 7 females), demonstrated a 93.5% increase in non-vellus hair counts after applying 3–4 g/day of CBD-rich hemp oil over a 6-month period [100]. This topical formation was prepared from ultra-pulverizing *Cannabis sativa* (hemp) flower into a green chalk-like powder (10.78% CBD and 0.21% tetrahydrocannabinol) and then infusing the powder into a lanolin paste and Emu oil carrier [101].

Several theories exist for how CBD may impact the hair follicle. One is that it may help maintain the anagen phase by differentiating dermal progenitor cells into new hair follicles through the Wnt/β-catenin pathway [102]. CBD is a TRPV1 (Vanilloid receptor-1) and TRPV4 (Vanilloid receptor-4) agonist. There is evidence that at high concentrations (10 μM), CBD may reduce hair shaft development and induce apoptosis, but at low concentrations (0.1 μM), it may increase hair shaft elongation via the adenosine receptor [103]. As we have seen with other supplements, there is likely to be a happy medium because excessive use of CBD may in fact impair hair growth [104].

Conclusion

Although the ingredients discussed here have some data to support their use, many questions remain. We clearly need more research on optimal dosing and delivery recommendations.

- How can we achieve optimal absorption when nutraceutical ingredients are taken by mouth?
- How can we achieve optimal penetration, when nutraceutical ingredients are delivered topically?
- Can evidence for hair growth using topical bioactive ingredients translate to success taking them by mouth, and vice-versa?
- Will some people respond better or less well to certain ingredients?
- Is it safe to assume that all ingredients are safe? Specifically, can we give plant-based 5α-reductase inhibitors to women of child-bearing potential without worries of teratogenicity?
- Is there added benefit to combining some ingredients with others? This may be true for ingredients with varying mechanisms of action, but less so for supplements with similar mechanisms. For instance, one study investigating the combined use of saw palmetto with pumpkin seed oil for BPH showed there was no added benefit over using the ingredients by themselves [105].
- And perhaps most importantly of all, how can we make sure the marketing is not ahead of the science?

As clinicians, we must be sensitive to the wishes of our patients and should look for opportunities to combine medical, surgical, and evidence-based nutraceutical therapies for best outcomes.

References

1. Savitha A, Sacchidanand S, Revathy T. Bubble hair and other aquired hair shaft anomalies due to hot ironing on wet hair. Int J Trichology. 2011;3:118–20.
2. Fortes C, Mastroeni S, Mannooranparampil T, Abeni D, Panebianco A. Mediterranean diet: fresh herbs and vegetables decrease the risk of androgenetic alopecia in males. Arch Dermatol Res. 2018;310:71–6.
3. Takahashi T, Kamiya T, Yokoo Y. Proanthocyanidins from grape seeds promote proliferation of mouse hair follicles cells *in vitro* and convert hair cycle *in vivo*. Acta Derm Venereol. 1998;78:428–32.
4. Takahashi T, Kamiya T, Hasegawa A, Yokoo Y. Procyanidin oligomers selectively and intensively promote proliferation of mouse hair epithelial cells in vitro and activate hair follicle growth in vivo. J Invest Dermatol. 1999;112:310–6.
5. Takahashi T, Yokoo Y, Inoue T, Ishii A. Toxicological studies on procyanidin B-2 for external application as a hair growing agent. Food Chem Toxicol. 1999;37:545–52.
6. Kamimura A, Takahashi T, Watanabe Y. Investigation of topical application of procyanidin B-2 from apple to identify its potential use as a hair growing agent. Phytomedicine. 2000;7:529–36.
7. Takahashi T, Kamimura A, Yokoo Y, Honda S, Watanabe Y. The first clinical trial of topical application of procyanidin B-2 to investigate its potential as a hair growing agent. Phytother Res. 2001;15:331–6.
8. Takahashi T, Kamimura A, Kagoura M, Toyoda M, Morohashi M. Investigation of the topical application of procyanidin oligomers from applies to identify their potential use as a hair-growing agent. J Cosmet Dermatol. 2005;4:245–9.
9. Tenore GC, Caruso D, Buonomo G, D'Avino M, Santamaria R, Irace C, Piccolo M, Maisto M, Novellino E. Annurca apple nutraceutical formula-

tion enhances keratin expression in a human model of skin and promotes hair growth and tropism in a randomized clinical trial. J Medicinal Food. 2018;21:90–103.
10. Lee YI, Ham S, Lee SG, Jung I, Suk J, Yoo J, Choi S-Y, Lee JH. An exploratory in vivo study on the effect of Annurca apple extract on hair growth in mice. Curr Issues Mol Biol. 2022;44:6280–9.
11. Takahashi T, Kamimura A, Shirai A, Yokoo Y. Several selective protein kinase C inhibitors including procyanidins promote hair growth. Skin Pharmacol Appl Skin Physiol. 2000;13:133–42.
12. Kamimura A, Takahashi T. Procyanidin B-2, extracted from apples, promotes hair growth: a laboratory study. Br J Dermatol. 2002;146:41–51.
13. Kamimura A, Takahashi T. Procyanidin B-3, isolated from barley and identified as a hair-growth stimulant, has the potential to counteract inhibitory regulation by TGF-β1. Exp Dermatol. 2002;11:532–41.
14. Kamimura A, Takahashi T, Morohashi M, Takano Y. Procyanidin oligomers counteract TGF-β1 and TGF-β2-induced apoptosis in hair epithelial cells: an insight into their mechanisms. Skin Pharmacol Physiol. 2006;19:259–65.
15. Badolati N, Sommella E, Riccio G, Salviati E, Heintz D, Bottone S, Di Cicco E, Dentice M, Tenore G, Campiglia P, Stornaiuolo M, Novellino E. Annurca apply polyphenols ignite keratin production in hair follicles by inhibiting the pentose phosphate pathway and amino acid oxidation. Nutrients. 2018;10:1406.
16. Wilt TJ, MacDonald R, Ishani A. Beta-sitosterol for the treatment of benign prostatic hyperplasia. BJU Int. 1999;83:876–83.
17. Wilt TJ, Ishani A, Stark G, MacDonald R, Lau J, Mulrow C. Saw palmetto extracts for treatment of benign prostatic hyperplasia: a systematic review. JAMA. 1998;280:1604–9.
18. Sudeep HV, Thomas JV, Shyamprasad K. A double blind, placebo-controlled randomized comparative study on the efficacy of phytosterol-enriched and conventional saw palmetto oil in mitigating benign prostate hyperplasia and androgen deficiency. BMC Urol. 2020;20:86.
19. Bracher F. Phytotherapy of benign prostatic hyperplasia. Urologe A. 1997;36:10–7.
20. Prager N, Bickett K, French N, Marcovici G. A randomized, double-blind, placebo-controlled trial to determine the effectiveness of botanically derived inhibitors of 5-α-reductase in the treatment of androgenetic alopecia. J Altern Complem Med. 2002;8:143–52.
21. Rossi A, Mari E, Scarno M, et al. Comparative effectiveness and finasteride vs. serenoa repens in male androgenetic alopecia: a two-year study. Int J Immunopathol Pharmacol. 2012;25:1167–73.
22. Wessagowit V, Tangjaturonrusamee C, Kootiratrakarn T, et al. Treatment of male androgenetic alopecia with topical products containing Serenoa repens extract. Australas J Dermatol. 2016;57:e76–82.
23. Vanti G, Bergonzi MC, Bilia AR. Development of nanoliposomes loaded with carbon dioxide Serenoa repens (Saw palmetto) extract. J Nanosci Nanotechnol. 2021;21:2943–5.
24. Penugonda K, Lindshield BL. Fatty acid and phytosterol content of commercial saw palmetto supplements. Nutrients. 2013;5:3617–33.
25. Samec D, Loizzo MR, Gortzi O, Cankaya IT, Tundis R, Suntar I, Shirooie S, Zengin G, Devkota HP, Reboredo-Rodriguez P, Hassan STS, Manayi A, Kashani HRK, Nabavi SM. The potential of pumpkin seed oil as a functional food-A comprehensive review of chemical composition, health benefits, and safety. Compr Rev Food Sci Food Saf. 2022;21:4422–46.
26. Ryan E, Galvin K, O'Connor TP, Maguire AR, O'Brien NM. Phytosterol, squalene, tocopherol content and fatty acid profile of selected seeds, grains, and legumes. Plant Foods Human Nutr. 2007;62:85–91.
27. Raczyk M, Siger A, Radziejewska-Kubzdela E, Ratusz K, Rudzinska M. Roasting pumpkin seeds and changes in the composition and oxidative stability of cold-pressed oils. Acta Scientiarum Polonorum Technologia Alimentaria. 2017;16:293–301.
28. Zerafatjou N, Amirzargar M, Biglarkhani M, Shobeirian F, Zoghi G. Pumpkin seed oil (Curcubita pepo) versus tamulosin for benign prostatic hyperplasia symptom relief: a single-blind randomized clinical trial. BMC Urol. 2021;21:147.
29. Cho YH, Lee SY, Jeong DW, et al. Effect of pumpkin seed oil on hair growth in men with androgenetic alopecia: a randomized, double-blind, placebo-controlled trial. Evid Based Complement Alternat Med. 2014;2014:1–7.
30. Morakul B, Teeranachaideekul V, Junyaprasert VB. Niosomal delivery of pumpkin seed oil: development, characterization, and physical stability. J Microencapsulation. 2019;36:120–9.
31. Lin SF, Lin Y-H, Lin M, Kao Y-F, Wang R-W, Teng L-W, Chuang S-H, Chang J-M, et al. Synthesis and structure-activity relationship of 3-O-acylated(−) epigallocatechins as 5α-reductase inhibitors. Eur J Med Chem. 2010;45:6068–76.
32. Kwon OS, Han JH, Yoo HG, Chung JH, Cho KH, Eun HC, Kim KH. Human hair growth enhancement in vitro by green tea epigallocatechin-3-gallate (EGCG). Phytomedicine. 2007;14:551–5.
33. Roh SS, Kim CD, Lee M-H, Hwang S-L, Rang M-J, Yoon Y-K. The hair growth promoting effect of *Sophora flavescens* extract and its molecular regulation. J Dermatol Sci. 2002;30:43–9.
34. Hirata N, Tokunaga M, Naruto S, Iinuma M, Matsuda H. Testosterone 5α-reductase inhibitory active constituents of *Piper nigrum* leaf. Biol Pharm Bull. 2007;12:2402.
35. Kumar N, Rungseevijitprapa W, Narkkhong N-A, Suttajit M, Chaiyasut C. 5α-reductase inhibition and

hair growth promotion of some Thai plants traditionally used for hair treatment. J Ethnopharmacol. 2012;139:765–71.
36. Shimizu K, Kondo R, Sakai K, Shoyama Y, Sato H, Ueno T. Steroid 5α-reductase inhibitory activity and hair regrowth effects of an estract from Boehmeria nipononivea. Biosci Biotechnol Biochem. 2000;64:875–7.
37. Park W-S, Lee C-H, Lee B-G, Chang I-S. The extract of *Thujae occidentalis* semen inhibited 5α-reductase and androchronogenetic alopecia of B6CBAF1/J hybrid mouse. J Dermatol Sci. 2003;31:91–8.
38. Matsuda H, Yamazaki M, Naruto S, Asanuma Y, Kubo M. Anti-androgenic and hair growth promoting activities of Lygodii Spora (Spore of *Lygodium japonicum*) I. Active constituents inhibiting testosterone 5α-reductase. Biol Pharm Bull. 2002;25:622–6.
39. Matsuda H, Yamazaki M, Matsuo K, Asanuma Y, Kubo M. Anti-androgenic activity of myricae cortex-Isolation of active constituents from bark of *Myrica rubra*. Biol Pharm Bull. 2001;24:259–63.
40. Liu J, Kurashiki K, Shimizu K, Kondo R. Structure-activity relationship for inhibition of 5α-reductase by triterpenoids isolated from *Ganoderma lucidum*. Bioorgan Medicinal Chem. 2006;14:8654–60.
41. Pandit S, Chauhan NGG, Dixit VK. Effect of *Cuscuta reflexa* Roxb on androgen-induced alopecia. J Cosm Dermatol. 2008;7:199–204.
42. Rustad AM, Nickles MA, McKenney JE, Bilimoria SN, Lio PA. Myths and media in oral collagen supplementation for the skin, nails, and hair: a review. J Cosm Dermatol. 2022;21:438–43.
43. Hwang SB, Park HJ, Lee B-H. Hair-growth-promoting effects of the fish collagen peptide in human dermal papilla cells and C57BL/6 mice modulating Wnt/B-catenin and BMP signaling pathways. Int J Molec Sci. 2022;23:11904.
44. Gazitaeva Z, Drobintseva AO, Chung Y, Polyakova VO, Kvetnoy IM. Cosmeceutical product consisting of biomimetic peptides: antiaging effects in vivo and in vitro. Clin Cosm Inv Dermatol. 2017;10:11–6.
45. Kubano AA, Gallyamova YA, Korableva OA. A randomized study of biomimetic peptides efficacy and impact on the growth factors expression in the hair follicles of patients with telogen effluvium. J Appl Pharm Sci. 2018;8:15–22.
46. Won CH, Yoo HG, Park KY, Shin SH, Park WSS, Park PJ, Chung JH, Kwon OS, Kim KH. Hair growth-promoting effects of adiponectin in vitro. J Invest Dermatol. 2012;132:2849–51.
47. Ohn J, Been KW, Kim JY, Kim EJ, Park T, Yoon H-J, Ji JS, Okada-Iwabu M, Iwabu M, Yamauchi T, Kim YK, Seok C, Kwon O, Kim KH, Lee HH, Chung JH. Discovery of a transdermally deliverable pentapeptide for activating AdipoR1 to promote hair growth. EMBO Molec Med. 2021;13:e13790.
48. Lupo MP, Cole AL. Cosmeceutical peptides. Dermatol Ther. 2007;20:343–9.
49. Pyo HK, Yoo HG, Won CH, et al. The effect of tripeptide-copper complex on human hair growth in vitro. Arch Pharm Res. 2007;30:834–9.
50. Trachy RE, Fors TD, Pickart I, Uno H. The hair follicle-stimulating properties of peptide copper complexes. Results in C3H mice. Ann N Y Acad Sci. 1991;642:468–9.
51. Choi BY. Hair-growth potential of ginseng and its major metabolites: a review on its molecular mechanisms. Int J Mol Sci. 2018;19:2703.
52. Kim SH, Jeong KS, Ryu SY, Kim TH. Panax ginseng prevents apoptosis in hair follicles and accelerates recovery of hair medullary cells in irradiated mice. In Vivo. 1998;12:219–22.
53. Matsuda H, Yamazaki M, Asanuma Y, Kubo M. Promotion of hair growth by ginseng radix on cultured mouse vibrissal hair follicles. Phytother Res. 2003;17:797–800.
54. Im GJ, Chang JW, Choi J, Chae SW, Ko EJ, Jung HH. Protective effect of Korean red ginseng extract on cisplatin ototoxicity in HEI-OCI auditory cells. Phytother Res. 2010;24:614–21.
55. Choung Y-H, Kim SW, Tian C, Min JY, Lee HK, Park S-N, Lee JB, Park K. Korean red ginseng prevents gentamycin-induced hearing loss in rats. Laryngoscope. 2011;121:1294–302.
56. Kim JH, Yi SM, Choi JE, Son SW. Study of the efficacy of Korean red ginseng in the treatment of androgenetic alopecia. J Ginseng Res. 2009;33:223–8.
57. Ryu HJ, Yoo MG, Son SW. The efficacy of 3% minoxidil vs. combined 3% minoxidil and Korean red ginseng in treating female pattern alopecia. Int J Dermatol. 2014;53:e340–2.
58. Li Z, Li J-J L, Zhang D-L, Wang Y-B, Sung C-K. Ginsenosides Rb1 and Rd regulate proliferation of mature keratinocytes through induction of p63 expression in hair follicles. Phytother Res. 2013;27:1095–101.
59. Shin DH, Cha YJ, Yang KE, Jang I-S, Son C-G, Kim BH, Kim JM. Ginsenoside Rg3 up-regulates the expression of vascular endothelial growth factor in human dermal papilla cells and mouse hair follicles. Phytother Res. 2014;28:1088–95.
60. Park G-H, Park K-Y, Cho H, Lee S-M, Han JS, Won CH, Chang SE, Lee MW, Choi JH, Moon KC, Shin H, Kang YJ, Lee DH. Red ginseng extract promotes the hair growth in cultured human hair follicles. J Medicinal Food. 2015;18:354–62.
61. Shin H-S, Park S-Y, Hwang E-S, Lee D-G, Song H-G, Mavlonov GT, Yi T-H. The inductive effect of ginsenoside F2 on hair growth by altering the WNT signal pathway in telogen mouse skin. Eur J Pharmacol. 2014;730:82–9.
62. Truong V-L, Jeong W-S. Hair growth-promoting mechanisms of red ginseng extract through stimulating dermal papilla cell proliferation and enhancing skin health. Prev Nutr Food Sci. 2021;26:275–84.
63. Park S, Shin W-S, Ho J. Fructus panax ginseng extract promotes hair regeneration in C57BL/6 mice. J Ethnopharmacol. 2011;138:340–4.

64. Li Z, Ryu S-W, Lee J, Choi K, Kim S, Choi C. Protopanaxatirol type ginsenoside Re promotes cyclic growth of hair follicles via inhibiting transforming growth factor β signaling cascades. Biochem Biophys Res Comm. 2016;470:924–9.
65. Lee Y, Kim SN, Hong YD, Park BC, Na Y. Panax ginseng extract antagonizes the effect of DKK1-induced catagen-like changes of hair follicles. Int J Mol Med. 2017;40:1194–200.
66. Bae JS, Park HS, Park JW, Li SH, Chun YS. Red ginseng and 20(S)-Rg3 control testosterone-induced prostate hyperplasia by deregulating androgen receptor signaling. J Nat Med. 2012;66:476–85.
67. Truong V-L, Bak MJ, Lee C, Jun M, Jeong W-S. Hair regenerative mechanisms of red ginseng oil and its major components in the testosterone-induced delay of anagen entry in C57BL/6 mice. Molecules. 2017;22:1505.
68. Bangha E, Elsner P, Kistleret GS, et al. Suppression of UV-induced erythema by topical treatment with melatonin (N-acetyl-5-methoxytryptamine). A dose response study. Arch Dermatol Res. 1996;288:522–9.
69. Welch RAS, Gurnsey MP, Betteridge K, Mitchell RJ. Goat fibre response to melatonin given in spring in two consecutive years. Proc NZ Soc Anim Prod. 1990;50:335–8.
70. Nixon AJ, Choy VJ, Parry AL, Pearson AJ. Fiber growth initiation in hair follicles of goats treated with melatonin. J Exp Zool. 1993;267:47–56.
71. Fischer TW, Slominski A, Tobin DJ, Paus R. Mini review: melatonin and the hair follicle. J Pineal Res. 2008;44:1–15.
72. Feng Y, Gun S. Melatonin supplement induced the hair follicle development in offspring rex rabbits. J Anim Physiol Anim Nutr. 2021;105:167–74.
73. Zhou X, Gao Y, Hu Y, Ma X. Melatonin protects cochlear hair cells from nicotine-induced injury through inhibiting apoptosis, inflammation, oxidative stress and endoplasmic reticulum stress. Basic Clin Pharmacol Toxicol. 2021;129:308–18.
74. Liu J, Mu Q, Liu Z, Wang Y, Liu J, Wu Z, Gong W, Lu Z, Zhao F, Zhang Y, Wang R, Su R, Li J, Ziao H, Zhao Y. Melatonin regulates the periodic growth of cashmere by upregulating the expression of Wnt10b and β-catenin in inner Mongolia cashmere goats. Front Genet. 2021;12:1–13.
75. Zhang W, Wang N, Zhang T, Wang M, Ge W, Wang X. Roles of melatonin in goat hair follicle stem cell proliferation and pluripotency through regulating the Wnt signaling pathway. Front Cell Dev Biol. 2021;9:1–13.
76. Fischer TW, Burmeister G, Schmidt HW, Elsner P. Melatonin increases anagen hair rate in women with androgenetic alopecia or diffuse alopecia: results of a pilot randomized controlled trial. Br J Dermatol. 2004;150:341–5.
77. Fischer TW, et al. Topical melatonin for treatment of androgenetic alopecia. Int J Trichology. 2012;4:236–45.
78. Babadjouni A, Reddy M, Zhang R, Raffi J, Phong C, Mesinkovska N. Melatonin and the human hair follicle. J Drugs Dermatol. 2023;22:260–4.
79. Hatem S, Nasr M, Moftah NH, Ragai MH, Geneidi AS, Elkheshen SA. Clinical cosmeceutical repurposing of melatonin in androgenetic alopecia using nanostructured lipid carriers prepared with antioxidant oils. Exp Opin Drug Deliv. 2018;15:927–35.
80. Hatem S, Nasr M, Moftah NH, Ragai MH, Geneidi AS, Elkheshen SA. Melatonin vitamin C-based nanovesicles for treatment of androgenetic alopecia: design, characterization and clinical appraisal. Eur J Pharm Sci. 2018;122:246–53.
81. Nichols AJ, Hughes OB, Canazza A, Zaiac MN. An open-label evaluator blinded study of the efficacy and safety of a new nutritional supplement in androgenetic alopecia: a pilot study. J Clin Aesth Dermatol. 2017;10:52–6.
82. Begum A, Sandhya S, Ali SS, Vinod KR, Reddy S, Banji D. Na in-depth review on the medicinal flora Rosmarinus officinalis (Lamiaceae). Acta Sci Pol Technol Aliment. 2013;12:61–73.
83. Al-Sereiti MR, Abu-Amer KM, Sen P. Pharmacology of rosemary (Rosmarinus officinalis Linn.) and its therapeutic potentials. Indian J Exp Biol. 1999;37:124–30.
84. Raskovic A, Milanovic I, Pavlovic N, Cebovic T, Vukmirovic S, Mikov M. Antioxidant activity of rosemary (Rosmarinus officinalis L.) essential oil and its hepatoprotective potential. Complement Alt Med. 2014;14:225.
85. Nabavi SF, Tenore GC, Daglia M, Tundis R, Loizzo MR, Nabavi SM. The cellular protective effects of rosmarinic acid: from bench to bedside. Curr Neurovasc Res. 2015;12:98–105.
86. Rahbardar MG, Amin B, Mehri S, Mirnajafi-Zadeh SJ, Hosseinzadeh H. Rosmarinic acid attenuates development and existing pain in a rat model of neuropathic pain: an evidence of anti-oxidative and anti-inflammatory effects. Phytomedicine. 2018;40:59–67.
87. Rahbardar MG, Amin B, Mehri S, Mirnajafi-Zadeh SJ, Hosseinzadeh H. Biomed Pharmadother. 2017;86:441–9.
88. Lo A-H, Liang Y-C, Lin-Shiau S-Y, Ho C-T, Lin J-K. Carnosol, an antioxidant in Rosemary, suppresses inducible nitric oxide synthase through down-regulating nuclear factor-kappaB in mouse macrophages. Carcinogenesis. 2002;23:983–91.
89. Murata K, Noguchi K, Kondo M, Onishi M, Watanabe N, Okamura K, Matsuda H. Promotion of hair growth by Rosmarinus officinalis leaf extract. Phytother Res. 2013;27:212–7.
90. Panahi Y, Taghizadeh M, Marzony ET, Sahebkar A. Rosemary oil vs minoxidil 2% for the treatment of androgenetic alopecia: a randomized comparative trial. Skinmed. 2015;13:15–21.
91. Herman A, Herman AP. Caffeine's mechanisms of action and its cosmetic use. Skin Pharmacol Physiol. 2013;26:8–14.

92. Fischer TW, Herczeg-Lisztes E, Fung W, Zillikens D, Biro T, Paus R. Differential effects of caffeine on hair shaft elongation, matrix and outer root sheath keratinocyte proliferation, and transforming growth factor-β2/insulin-like growth factor-1 mediated regulation of the hair cycle in male and female human hair follicles in vitro. Br J Dermatol. 2014;171:1031–43.
93. Gerardini J, Wegner J, Cheret J, Ghatak S, Lehmann J, Alam M, Jimenez F, Fung W, Bohm M, Botchkareva NV, Ward C, Paus R, Bertolini M. Transepidermal UV radiation of scalp skin ex vivo induces hair follicle damage that is alleviated by the topical treatment with caffeine. Int J Cosm Sci. 2019;41:164–82.
94. Otberg N, Patzelt A, Rasulev U, Hagemeister T, Linscheid M, Sinkgraven R, Sterry W, Lademann J. The role of hair follicles in the percutaneous absorption of caffeine. Br J Clin Pharmacol. 2007;65:488–92.
95. Otberg N, Teichmann A, Rasuljev U, Sinkgraven R, Sterry W, Lademann J. Follicular penetration of topically applied caffeine via a shampoo formulation. Skin Pharmacol Physiol. 2007;20:195–8.
96. Bussoletti C, Tolaini MV, Celleno L. Efficacy of a cosmetic phyto-caffeine shampoo in female androgenetic alopecia. G Ital Dermatol Venereol. 2020;155:492–9.
97. Bussoletti C, Mastropietro F, Tolaini MV, Celleno L. Use of a caffein shampoo for the treatment of male androgenetic alopecia. J Appl Cosmetol. 2011;29:167–80.
98. Dhurat R, Chitallia J, May TM, Jayaraaman AM, Madhukara J, Anandan S, Vaidya P, Klenk A. An open-label randomized multicenter study assessing the noninferiority of a caffeine-based topical liquid 0.2% versus minoxidil 5% solution in male androgenetic alopecia. Skin Pharmacol Physiol. 2017;30:298–305.
99. Gupta AK, Talkukder M. Cannabinoids for skin diseases and hair regrowth. J Cosmet Dermatol. 2021;20:2703–11.
100. Smith G, Satino J. Hair regrowth with cannabidiol (CBD)-rich hemp extract. Cannabis. 2021;4:53–9.
101. Gupta AK, Talukder M. A cannabinoid hairy-tale: hair loss or hair gain? J Cosmet Dermatol. 2022;21:6653–60.
102. Vallee A, Lecarpentier Y, Guillevin R, Valle J-N. Effects of cannabidiol interactions with Wnt/β--catenin pathway and PPAR-γ on oxidative stress and neuroinflammation in Alzheimer's disease. Acta Biochem Biophys Sin. 2017;49:853–66.
103. Szabo IL, Lisztes E, Beke G, et al. The phytocannabinoid (CBD) operates as a complex, differential modulator of human hair growth: anti-inflammatory submicromolar versus hair growth inhibitory micromolar effects. J Invest Dermatol. 2020;140:484–8.
104. Telek A, Biro T, Bodo E, et al. Inhibition of human hair follicle growth by endo- and exocannabinoids. FASEB J. 2007;21:3534–41.
105. Hong H, Kim C-S, Maeng S. Effects of pumpkin seed oil and saw palmetto in Korean men with symptomatic benign prostatic hyperplasia. Nutr Res Pract. 2009;3:323–7.

Frontal Fibrosing Alopecia

8

Aaron Chen and Peter J. Panagotacos

Introduction

The signs of FFA may first clinically show up as a band of incomplete hair loss that starts at the anterior hairline and progresses back posteriorly. In some cases, there may also be temporal and occipital involvement. Men may have facial hair that is affected and/or the sideburns. Men and women of all ethnicities can be affected by FFA. Patients that have FFA may have contact allergy to fragrances, regular sunscreen use, hypothyroidism, and autoimmune diseases such as rheumatoid arthritis, vitiligo, or lupus erythematosus. There are different causes that have been suggested in the pathogenesis of FFA which include genetic, autoimmune, hormonal, and environmental. There has also been a study that suggested a link between sunscreen/moisturizer use with development of FFA. There also may be a connection between contact allergy to cosmetics, sunscreen, moisturizers, hair dye that have been suggestive as causes to the development of FFA. Most recently, there was connection between the light stabilizer, ethylhexyl salicylate, found in sunscreens with FFA [1].

A. Chen (✉)
California Skin Institute, San Francisco, CA, USA

P. J. Panagotacos
University of California San Francisco,
San Francisco, CA, USA

Clinical signs to look for in suspected FFA patients that may clue the dermatologist into the diagnosis of FFA is perifollicular erythema and fine scale. FFA in its pattern distribution was described by Zinkernagel and Trüeb as a type of alopecia that shares parallel characteristics with lichen planopilaris and androgenic alopecia. The disease is clinically characterized by progressive miniaturization of the hairs of the central scalp. Important features to note are perifollicular erythema, and follicular hyperkeratosis leading to complete loss of follicular ostia and scarring [2]. During the active stage of disease, patients will sometimes report pruritus and trichodynia. A common area that is affected are the eyebrows (Fig. 8.1a, b) which may be often thinned or absent as seen in this patient that also has non-inflammatory facial papules characteristic of FFA. In the photos of a 57-year-old patient (Fig. 8.2), one can also appreciate the perifollicular erythema and diffuse erythema that this patient has. There is also progressive hair loss along the anterior hairline and the eyebrows. Clinical signs include a linear band of hair loss that is seen across the front and sides of the hair margin. This results in a receding anterior hair line. There are also atypical patterns of FFA which may be involvement of both the front and back hairlines and diffuse patterned hair loss. The skin affected by FFA is seen in areas that lack actinic damage on the forehead. The appearance is a shiny, scarred appearance, without vis-

P. J. Panagotacos, H. Maibach (eds.), *Hair Loss*, Updates in Clinical Dermatology,
https://doi.org/10.1007/978-3-031-74314-6_8

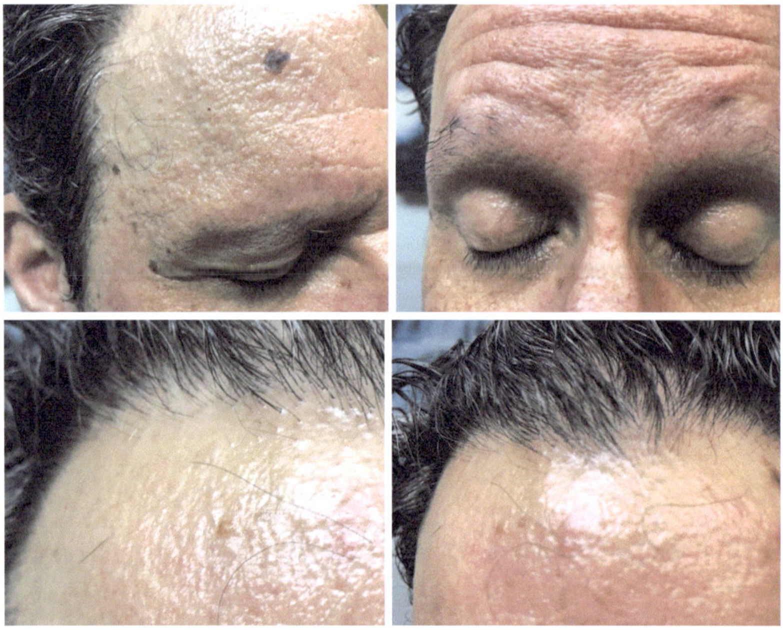

Fig. 8.1 (**a, b**) Courtesy of Peter J. Panagotacos, MD

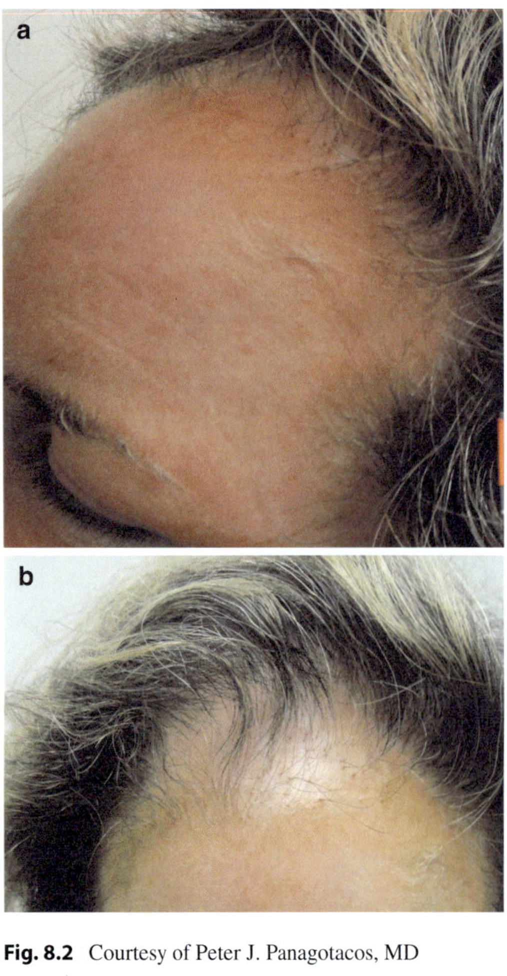

Fig. 8.2 Courtesy of Peter J. Panagotacos, MD

ible hair follicle openings which one can appreciate with dermoscopy. Classic findings are eyebrow thinning or madarosis which may precede the hair loss seen on the scalp. Hair loss can also involve other parts of the body, beard, and/or sideburns. Loss of hair can be confined to one site which is atypical. Commonly, frontal fibrosing alopecia is misdiagnosed as androgenetic alopecia.

On histology, the features that will typically be seen on biopsy specimens are hair follicle miniaturization with a lymphocytic inflammatory cell infiltrate in the region of the isthmus and the infundibulum (Fig. 8.3a, b). The lesions that have progressed are characterized by perifollicular lamellar fibrosis and fibrous follicular tracts. Typically, the best biopsies to diagnose FFA are those that have been guided by dermoscopy. Of note, these histologic changes are not confined to the scalp but can be seen on the eyebrows, face, and upper limbs in asymptomatic patients that have FFA [3, 4].

Patients that are of African descent or darker skin colors present differently than lighter skin-colored patients. The redness and scale are less obvious and present differently. Redness may present as a violaceous hue or hyperpigmented. These types of patients may present earlier and have speckled pigmentation of hair follicles along the margins of the hair with use of dermoscopy. Therefore, a careful history and physical examination is essential to correct diagnosis of this unfortunate condition. To make the diagnosis, there have been diagnostic criteria that has been set forth. Part of the major criteria in diagnosing FFA are scarring hair loss of eyebrows, scarring hair loss of the frontal scalp, and/or frontotemporal/temporal scalp involvement. While minor criteria are; classic histology on biopsy, noninflammatory facial papules, itch/pain preceding or concurrently at sites of involvement, redness and scale around hair follicles/"lonely" hair seen on dermoscopy. Diagnosis using the proposed criteria requires 2 major criteria or one major and two minor criteria (Table 8.1) [4].

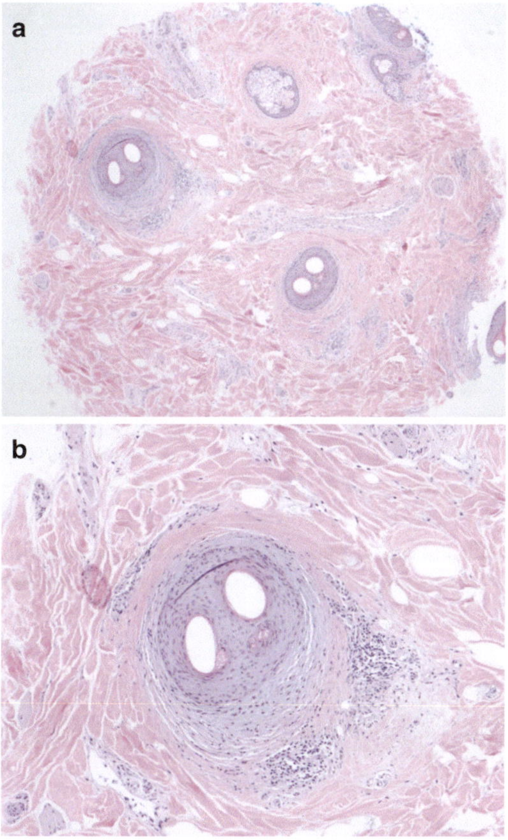

Fig. 8.3 (**a**, **b**) Courtesy of UCSF Dermatopathology Department

Facial involvement in some cases may precede alopecia which may be often easier to visualize on dermoscopy. Common findings on trichoscopy include yellow dots, vellus hairs, tapering and/or dystrophic hairs. In skin of color patients, some findings are subtler such as erythema that presents as violaceous, pink, or brown and in contrast to lighter skin color which may appear pink or red [5, 6].

Diagnosis of early frontal fibrosing alopecia can be differentiated from female pattern hair loss with pruritus as a common symptom. Perifollicular erythema and scale also are clues that can help with diagnosis. Skin biopsy is sometimes performed to exclude other forms of cicatricial alopecia and will demonstrate perifollicular fibrosis and lymphocytic infiltrate that is similar to lichen planopilaris. Along with punch biopsy one can consider ordering thyroid studies to rule out hypothyroidism. Often other hair con-

Table 8.1 FFA diagnostic criteria: requires 2 major criteria or 1 major and 2 minor criteria

Major criteria
1. Cicatricial alopecia of the frontal, temporal, or frontotemporal scalp on examination, in absence of follicular keratotic papules on the body
2. Diffuse bilateral eyebrow cicatricial alopecia
Minor criteria:
1. Perifollicular erythema, perifollicular hyperkeratosis, or solitary hairs on physical or trichoscopic examination in a field of frontal/frontotemporal cicatricial alopecia
2. Histopathologic features of cicatricial alopecia in the pattern of FFA or LPP on biopsy; Peri-infundibular and peri-isthmal lymphocytic inflammation, interface changes at the infundibular-isthmal epithelium, peri-infundibular and peri-isthmal fibrosis, increased hair in the catagen and telogen phases, and polytrichia
3. Involvement (hair loss, perifollicular erythema, or perifollicular hyperkeratosis) of additional FFA sites: occipital area, facial hair, sideburns, or body hair
4. Noninflammatory facial papules
5. Preceding or concurrent symptoms, such as pruritus or pain, at areas of involvement

Source: Tolkachjov SN, Chaudhry HM, Imhof RL, Camilleri MJ, Morgerson RR. Reply to: "Updated diagnostic criteria for frontal fibrosing alopecia". *J Am Acad Dermatol*. 2018;78(1):e23–e24

ditions such as androgenetic alopecia and traction alopecia can co-exist. Other types of cicatricial alopecia need to be considered, however they tend to not share the same band-like pattern seen in frontal fibrosing alopecia [7–10].

Treatment of frontal fibrosing alopecia is difficult as there is no therapy that has been established as a gold standard treatment. Therapies that help may stop or slow progression of the hair loss but typically do not lead to new hair regrowth. Treatment typically involves multiple modalities such as topical, intralesional, and systemic. Topical corticosteroids have been used but have not been shown to be completely effective in stopping hair loss. Topical calcineurin inhibitors and intralesional steroids may help produce eyebrow regrowth. Intralesional steroids are also administered into active areas on the scalp which will diminish inflammation and is an important adjunctive therapy. The patient should be counseled on risk of hypopigmentation and atrophy which is diminished when the appropriate concentration of intralesional steroid is injected. The 5-α-reductase-inhibitors such as oral dutasteride or finasteride that is often used in treatment of androgenetic alopecia has also been shown to be efficacious in treatment of FFA according to some systematic reviews. Some believe the main problem resides in the sebaceous gland and that Dutasteride is the drug that works best to calm this condition. It is an indolent condition, and it is difficult to determine when it has burned itself out. Hair transplantation as a treatment has led to dismal failure in several reported cases [11]. Females of childbearing potential should be counseled on mandatory contraception due to effects of dutasteride/finasteride. Hydroxychloroquine may be also an effective treatment. Some oral tetracycline antibiotics such as doxycycline/minocycline may be helpful in reducing inflammation. Oral prednisone may help halt the rapid progression of some cases of FFA. Methotrexate, mycophenolate mofetil have shown mixed results in the treatment of FFA. The use of intramuscular steroids may be of some benefit but also have mixed results. The off-label treatment of FFA with use of diabetic drug pioglitazone (PPAR-γ agonist) has been reported to reduce progression and inflammation but more studies are needed to support the use of this [7, 8].

Another treatment that has been promoted recently is low-dose oral minoxidil. However, patients should be carefully counseled on the risks and side effects such as cardiovascular effects (hypotension, pericarditis, pericardial effusion). Recently, low-dose oral minoxidil has recently been widely promoted as a treatment for non-scarring alopecia and scarring alopecia. However, there are studies showing topical minoxidil is as effective as the low-dose oral minoxidil [12]. Therefore, "Is it worth the risk especially when used in scarring alopecia when the scarred hair follicle is already dead? Oral minoxidil may not be as safe as everyone says it is" As said by Dr. Panagotacos who has lectured nationally and internationally at ISHRS conferences most recently in 2022. Other reported novel treatments include rituximab and adalimumab. There have been some case studies with improvement of refractory FFA with treatment using topical/oral JAK inhibitor that may reduce perifollicular erythema, scale, and hair loss. Aside from hair loss, patients concerned about the cosmetic appearance of the coinciding facial papules can be treated with oral isotretinoin or energy devices such as laser resurfacing. Once hair disease has stabilized and burned out, hair transplant may be considered but the patient should be counseled that there is a risk of decreased hair graft survival due to unpredictable flares of FFA. Photography of affected areas is important to track disease progress and control of FFA as with any other alopecia. To conclude, the clinician needs to be careful with diagnosis of androgenetic alopecia/traction alopecia as there may be signs of FFA which would change the course of management of the patient [7, 8, 13].

References

1. Pastor-Nieto MA, et al. Sensitization to ethylhexyl salicylate: another piece of the frontal fibrosing alopecia puzzle. Contact Dermatitis. 2023;90(4):402–10. https://doi.org/10.1111/cod.14463.
2. Kossard S, Lee MS, Wilkinson B. Postmenopausal frontal fibrosing alopecia: a frontal variant of lichen planopilaris. J Am Acad Dermatol. 1997;36:59–66.
3. Chew AL, Bashir SJ, Wain EM, et al. Expanding the spectrum of frontal fibrosing alopecia: a unifying concept. J Am Acad Dermatol. 2010;63(4):653–60.

4. Tolkachjov SN, Chaudhry HM, Imhof RL, Camilleri MJ, Morgerson RR. Reply to: "Updated diagnostic criteria for frontal fibrosing alopecia". J Am Acad Dermatol. 2018;78(1):e23–4.
5. Miteva M, Whiting D, Harries M, et al. Frontal fibrosing alopecia in black patients. Br J Dermatol. 2012;167:208–10.
6. Poblet E, Jiménez F, Pascual A, Piqué E. Frontal fibrosing alopecia versus lichen planopilaris: a clinicopathological study. Int J Dermatol. 2006;45:375–80.
7. Banka N, Mubki T, Bunagan MJ, et al. Frontal fibrosing alopecia: a retrospective clinical review of 62 patients with treatment outcome and long-term follow-up. Int J Dermatol. 2014;53:1324–30.
8. Rácz E, Gho C, Moorman PW, et al. Treatment of frontal fibrosing alopecia and lichen planopilaris: a systematic review. J Eur Acad Dermatol Venereol. 2013;27:1461–70.
9. Donati A, Molina L, Doche I, et al. Facial papules in frontal fibrosing alopecia: evidence of vellus follicle involvement. Arch Dermatol. 2011;147:1424–7.
10. Fernandez-Flores A, Manjón JA. Histopathology of keratotic papules of the limbs in frontal fibrosing alopecia. J Cutan Pathol. 2016;43:468–71.
11. Porriño-Bustamante ML, et al. Frontal fibrosing alopecia: a review. J Clin Med. 2021;10(9):1805. https://doi.org/10.3390/jcm10091805.
12. Randolph M, Tosti A. Oral Minoxidil treatment for hair loss: a review of efficacy and safety. J Am Acad Dermatol. 2021;84(3):737–46. https://doi.org/10.1016/j.jaad.2020.06.1009.
13. Vañó-Galván S, Molina-Ruiz AM, Serrano-Falcón C, et al. Frontal fibrosing alopecia: a multicenter review of 355 patients. J Am Acad Dermatol. 2014;70:670–8.

9 Trichoscopy

Lily Park, Aaron Chen, and Martin Zaiac

Introduction

Trichoscopy allows for a thorough examination of peri and interfollicular patterns and hair shaft thickness and shapes to aid us with recognition of a hair condition or pattern on the scalp, eyebrows, and other hairy areas [1]. It also allows for visualization of vessels (better with non-contact polarized dermoscopy at higher magnification) and follicular patterns and helps us determine an optimal biopsy site. While a hand-held dermotoscope provides a magnification of 10×, a videodermatoscope (Fig. 9.1) can provide a magnification of 10× to 1000× on a high-resolution monitor screen and allow storage of the images for comparison at follow-ups for serial assessment of the progression of diseases or treatments [2].

L. Park (✉)
College of Osteopathic Medicine, Touro University California, Vallejo, CA, USA

Berman Skin Institute, Roseville, CA, USA

A. Chen
College of Osteopathic Medicine, Touro University California, Vallejo, CA, USA

California Skin Institute, San Francisco, CA, USA

M. Zaiac
Department of Dermatology, Herbert Wertheim College of Medicine, Florida International University, Miami, FL, USA

Greater Miami Skin and Laser Center, Mount Sinai Medical Center, Miami Beach, FL, USA

The concept of trichoscopy as a tool for examining hair and scalp disorders is a relatively recent advancement in dermatology. Ross and his associates were the first to introduce the term 'trichoscopy' in their article in 2006, defining it as the use of videodermoscopy to analyze hair and scalp for diagnosing hair loss [3]. Before that, Lacarrubba and colleagues published the first clinical study that described the videodermoscopic features of alopecia areata in 2004 [4].

A trichoscopy exam usually starts with dry trichoscopy performed without immersion fluid, to examine scales (for scarring alopecia, psoriasis, and seborrheic dermatitis) or foreign materials on the scalp. However, the standard trichoscopy technique involves non-polarized contact trichoscopy using immersion fluid. Application of immersion fluid such as 70% isopropyl alcohol displaces air, reducing light penetration into the skin, and minimizing glare from the stratum corneum. Polarized light neutralizes the reflection from the stratum corneum, allowing most of the light to reflect off the deeper skin layers, especially from the blood vessels and collagen [2].

P. J. Panagotacos, H. Maibach (eds.), *Hair Loss*, Updates in Clinical Dermatology,
https://doi.org/10.1007/978-3-031-74314-6_9

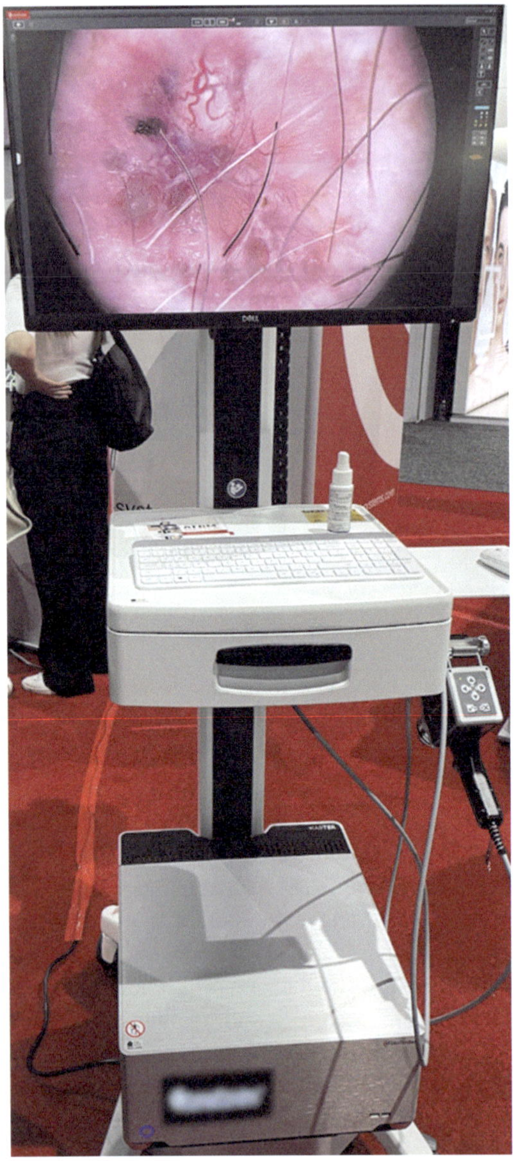

Fig. 9.1 Videodermoscopy machine by FotoFinder Systems GmbH, Bad Birnbach, Germany

Trichoscopy of Noncicatricial Alopecia

Pinpoint white dots (Fig. 9.2) are openings of sweat glands and follicles and are present in the normal scalp but can be seen in all alopecias [5].

Exclamation mark hairs (Fig. 9.3) are characterized by a narrower proximal end and a wider distal end and are pathognomonic in alopecia areata [6].

Yellow dots (Fig. 9.3) are round to polycyclic yellow dots with or without broken hair shafts or vellus hairs, representing dilated follicular infundibula with sebum and keratin, that are visible in most skin types I-III but not in darker skin types. Yellow dots are seen in alopecia areata, androgenetic alopecia, discoid lupus erythematosus, and dissecting cellulitis [7].

Black dots (Figs. 9.3 and 9.5), refer to follicular openings filled with the remnants of dark pigmented hairs that have broken off at the level of the scalp. Black dots can be present in a variety of scalp pathologies including alopecia areata, trichotillomania, tinea capitis, central centrifugal cicatricial alopecia, syphilitic alopecia, and pressure-induced alopecia.

Circle hairs (Fig. 9.4), also known as pigtail hairs, are thin, coiled hairs that can be seen in alopecia areata and androgenetic alopecia. A high count of coiled hairs strongly indicates the presence of alopecia areata [8].

V-signs and tulip hairs (Fig. 9.5) can also be seen in trichotillomania. V-signs are characterized by multiple hairs of equal length exiting from a single follicular opening, resulting from their concurrent breakage upon being pulled. On the other hand, tulip hairs, distinguishable by their short length and darker, tulip-shaped ends, form as a result of the hair shaft breaking at an angle [7].

Trichoscopy of androgenetic alopecia shows a variation in hair shaft thickness, known as anisotrichosis, with a variation of more than 20% for males and over 10% for females, attributed to hair follicle miniaturization. There is a higher count of individual hairs emerging from each follicular unit (Fig. 9.6). Yellow dots (Fig. 9.7) are also a characteristic finding in androgenetic alopecia (Fig. 9.8) although they can be found in other conditions [9].

Trichoscopy findings of telogen effluvium include short regrowing hairs with thinner ends and thicker bases. Other non-specific findings such as vertical hair regrowth and yellow dots are common (Fig. 9.9).

In traction alopecia (Fig. 9.10), decreased hair density, reduced variety in hair diameter, and empty follicles are often observed [10].

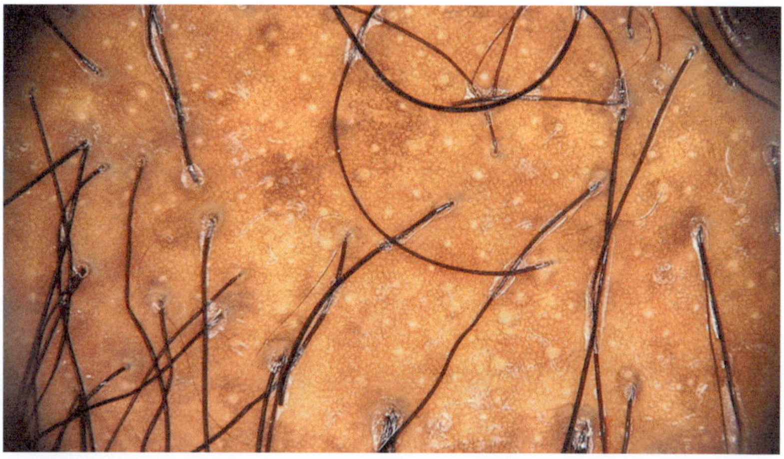

Fig. 9.2 White dots (20×)

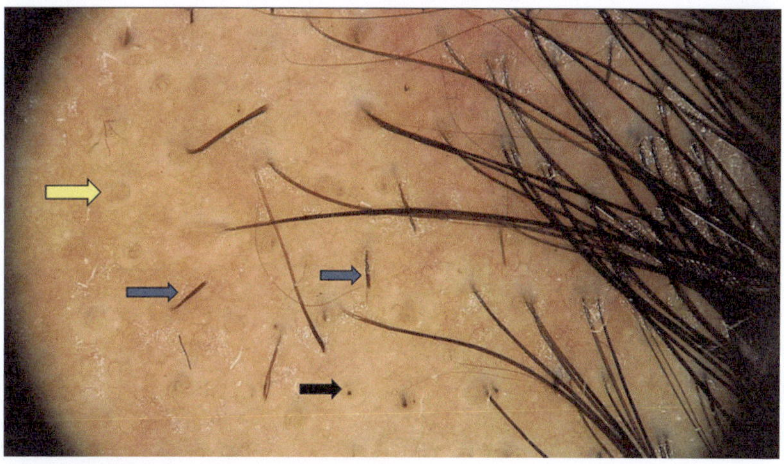

Fig. 9.3 Alopecia areata. exclamation mark hair shafts (see blue arrows), yellow dots (yellow arrow), and black dots (black arrow) (20×)

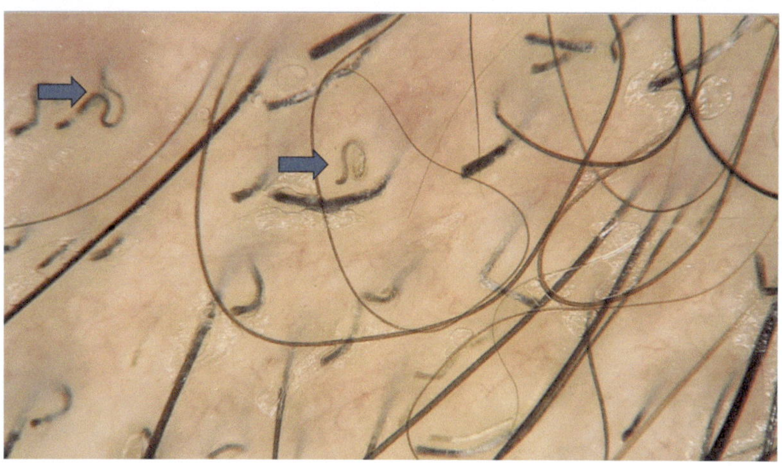

Fig. 9.4 Alopecia areata. Circle hairs (blue arrows) (50×)

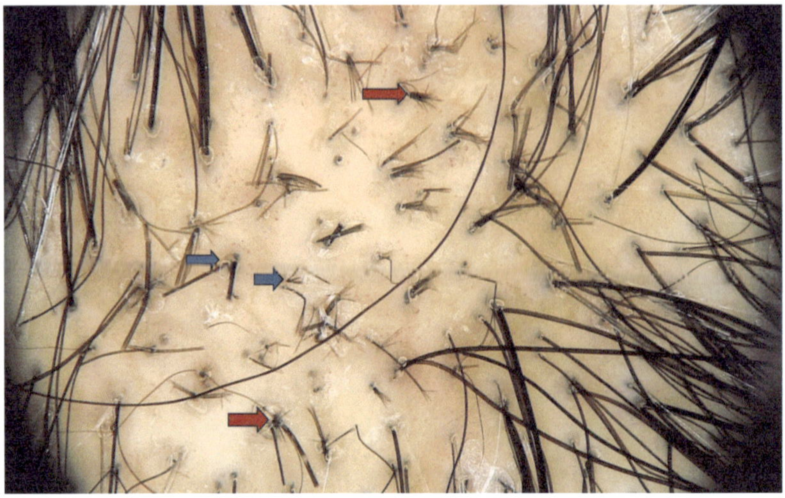

Fig. 9.5 Trichotillomania. black dots, V-signs (blue arrows), tulip signs (red arrows), and hairs broken at varying lengths (20×)

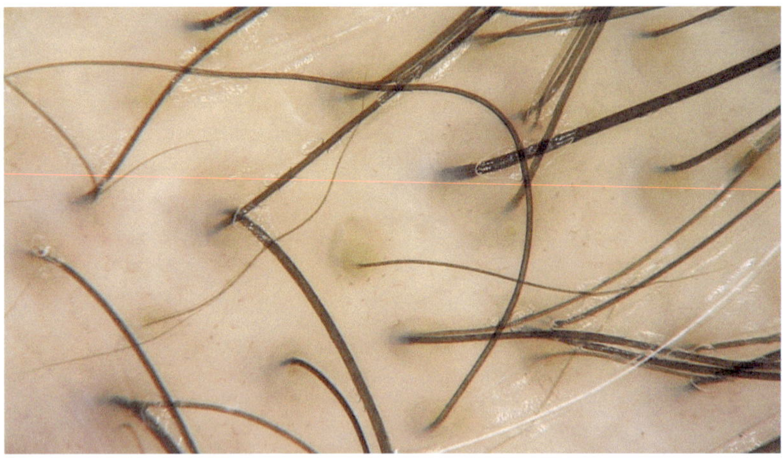

Fig. 9.6 Androgenetic alopecia. anisotrichosis and increased number of single hairs per follicular unit (50×)

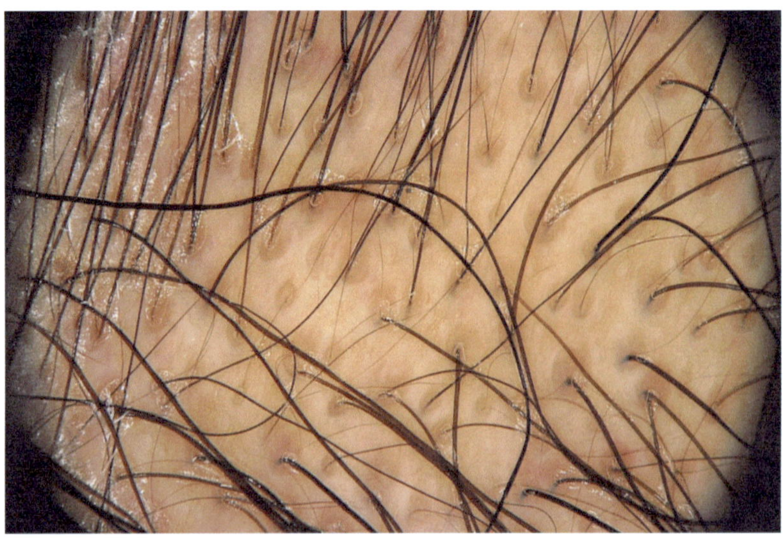

Fig. 9.7 Androgenetic Areata. Yellow dots

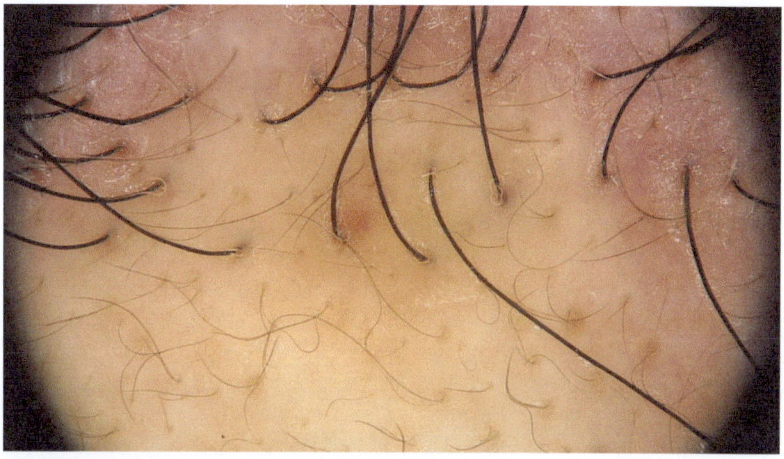

Fig. 9.8 Androgenetic Alopecia. Thicker transplanted hairs amongst vellus hairs

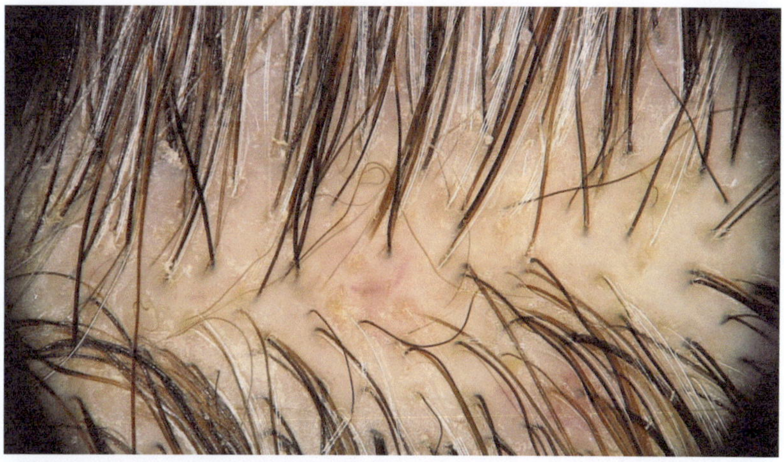

Fig. 9.9 Telogen effluvium. Note short regrowing hairs

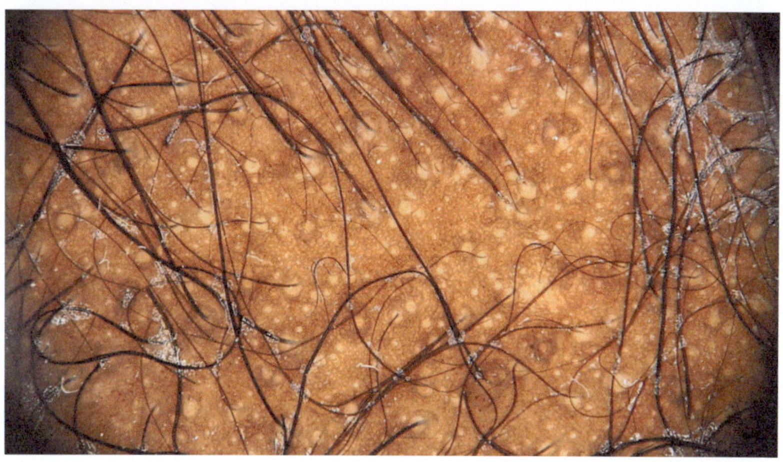

Fig. 9.10 Traction alopecia. Diminished hair density and abundance of empty follicles

Trichoscopy of Cicatricial Alopecia

White patches are frequently seen in cicatricial alopecia (Fig. 9.11), including frontal fibrosing alopecia (Fig. 9.12) and lichen planopilaris (Fig. 9.13) in skin of color. White patches are characterized by a lack of hairs and follicular ostia and represent dermal fibrosis. Irregular distribution of follicular ostia are also seen in cicatricial alopecia. Perifollicular erythema may be a sign of an active disease. Hair tufts with fewer than four hair shafts per follicular ostium may be present [6].

Gray-white peripilar halos, indicative of lamellar perifollicular fibrosis, mark the outer root sheaths of affected follicles. These halos can encircle a single hair or a cluster of two to three hairs emerging from an ostium, a characteristic feature of central centrifugal cicatricial alopecia (Figs. 9.14 and 9.15).

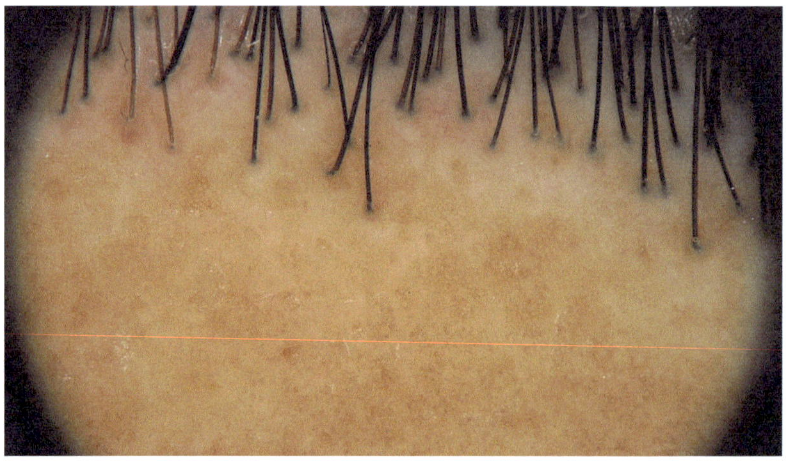

Fig. 9.11 Cicatricial alopecia. White patches in frontal fibrosing alopecia

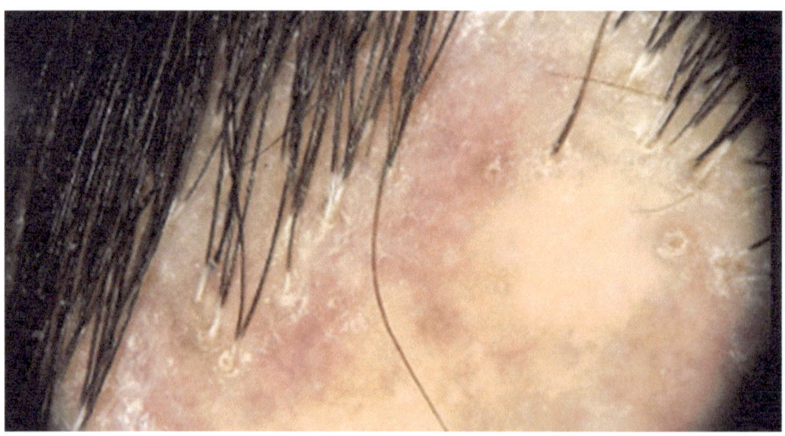

Fig. 9.12 Frontal fibrosing alopecia. Milky white patches

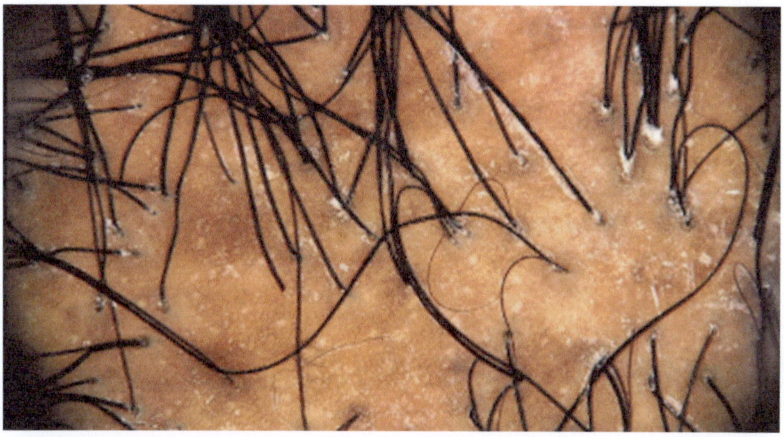

Fig. 9.13 Lichen planopilaris. White patches, irregular distribution of follicular ostia, and perifollicular scales

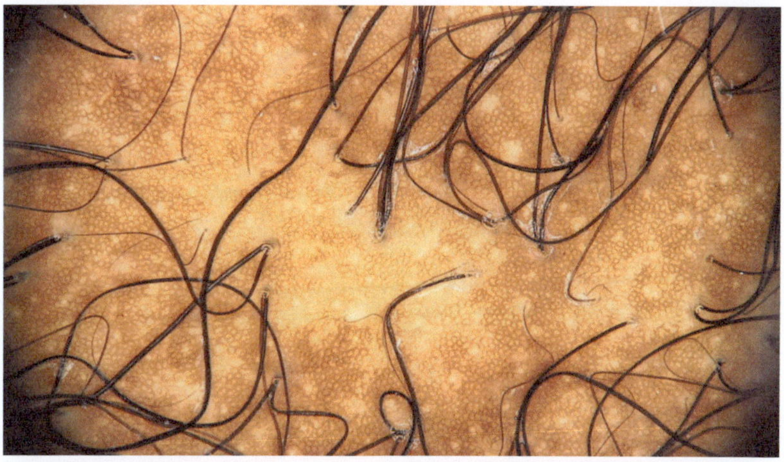

Fig. 9.14 Central centrifugal cicatricial alopecia (20×)

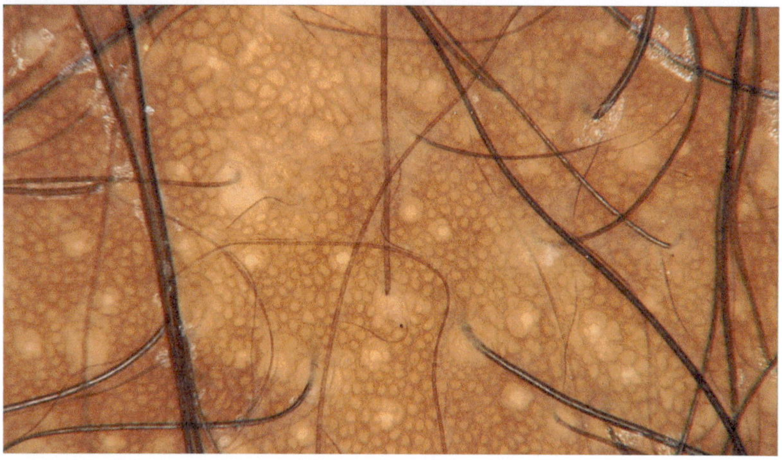

Fig. 9.15 Central centrifugal cicatricial alopecia (50×)

Trichoscopy of Localized Cicatricial Alopecia

Hair tufting, indicative of cicatricial alopecia, is defined by the emergence of multiple hairs from a single follicular ostium. The presence of more than six hair shafts in one follicle is a hallmark of folliculitis decalvans (Fig. 9.16) [6].

White scales on the scalp can be best appreciated with dry trichoscopy. Perifollicular and peripilar scales occur in conditions such as folliculitis decalvans (Fig. 9.17), discoid lupus, lichen planopilaris, frontal fibrosing alopecia [7].

Initial stages of dissecting cellulitis (Fig. 9.18) features noncicatricial alopecia similar to alopecia areata, including empty follicles, short hairs that are regrowing or broken, and yellow and black dots. As the condition advances, erythema, follicular pustules, and keratotic plugs become more noticeable. In its late stages, dissecting cellulitis is characterized by white patches devoid of hair follicles and skin fissures through which hairs emerge.

In cases of discoid lupus erythematosus (Fig. 9.19), keratotic plugs, erythema, and scales are present. Red dots representing inflammatory infiltration around hair follicles with extravasation of red blood cells are often seen in early acute discoid lupus erythematosus. Thick arborizing vessels may be seen as well. Hair tufts featuring less than four hair shafts per follicular opening may be found. Milky-red patches and the disappearance of follicular openings are seen in the late stages. In darker skin color, pigment loss from the inflammation disrupting the pigment network may lead to speckled patterns of blue-gray dots.

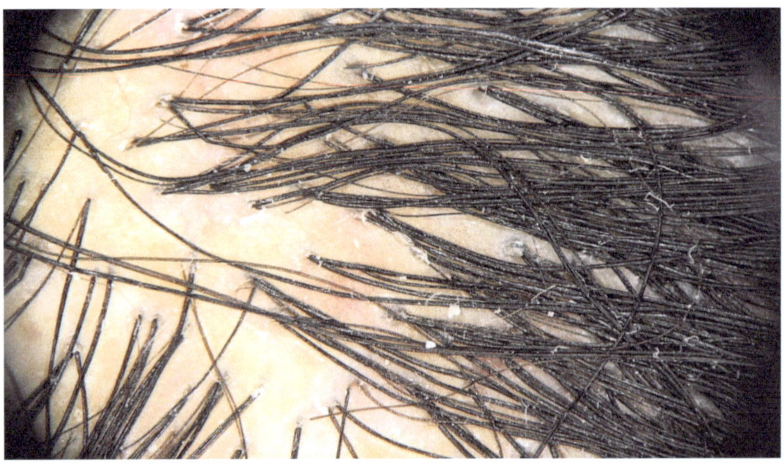

Fig. 9.16 Folliculitis decalvans. Hair tufts and white scales

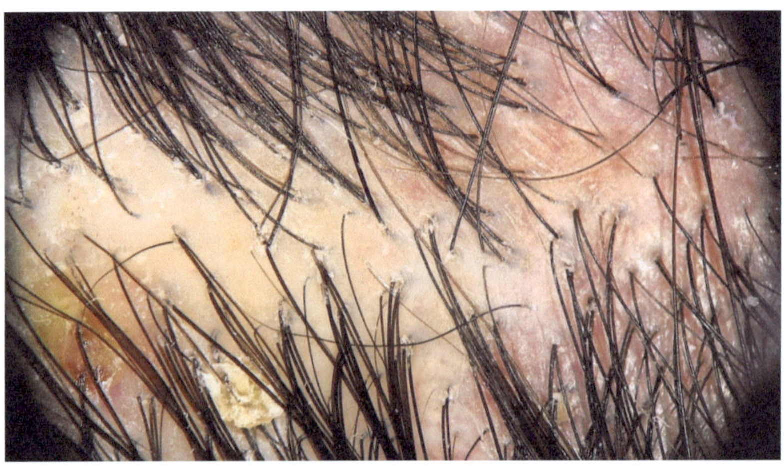

Fig. 9.17 Folliculitis decalvans. Perifollicular and peripillar scales

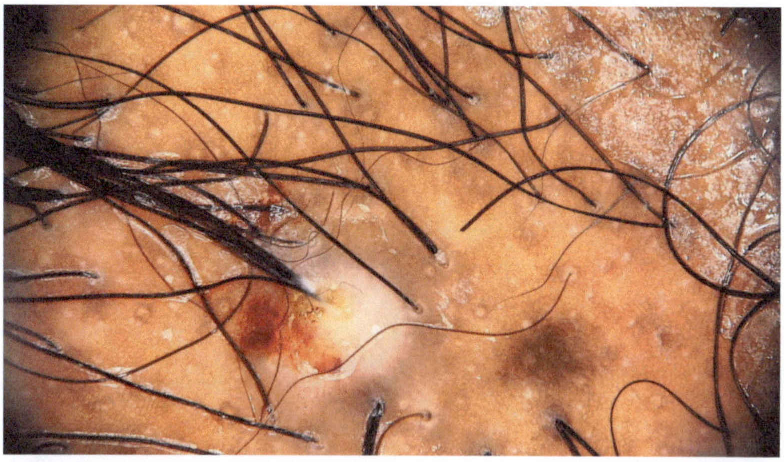

Fig. 9.18 Dissecting cellulitis. Empty follicles, short hairs, and white patches

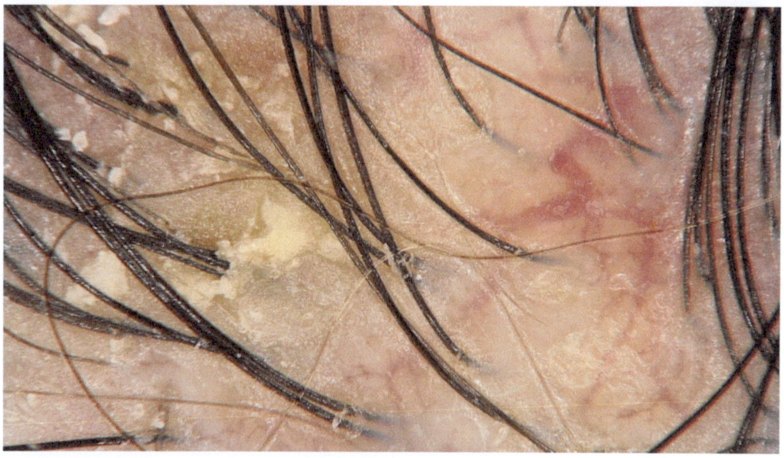

Fig. 9.19 Discoid lupus erythematous. Interfollicular, peripilar, and perifollicular scales, hair tufts, and dilated thick arborizing vessels

Trichoscopy of Inflammatory Conditions

White scales and twisted or glomerular-like vessels arranged into rings are characteristic features seen in psoriasis (Figs. 9.20 and 9.21). Hair casts, defined as scales surrounding a hair shaft, are also frequently observed in psoriasis, although also seen in various other conditions including lichen planopilaris, discoid lupus, frontal fibrosing alopecia, traction alopecia, tinea capitis, and folliculitis decalvans.

Trichoscopy of seborrheic dermatitis (Fig. 9.22) will frequently demonstrate arborizing vessels, adherent yellow scales and interfollicular white scales, oily material, and yellow dots.

In cases of keratosis pilaris (Fig. 9.23), varying degrees of perifollicular erythema accompanied by keratotic plugs are observed.

The main trichoscopic characteristics of scalp dermatomyositis (Fig. 9.24) include the presence of arborizing vessels, giant vessels or dilated tortuous vessels, diffuse and perifollicular scales, and interfollicular or perifollicular pigmentation [11].

Follicular mucinosis, also known as alopecia mucinosa, is accompanied by perifollicular whitish rims, indicative of mucin accumulation, alongside interfollicular brownish-yellow dots (Fig. 9.25). Mucin casts (Fig. 9.26) encircling the hair shafts are also a notable feature. Furthermore, the presence of red dots and dilated capillary vessels can be observed [12].

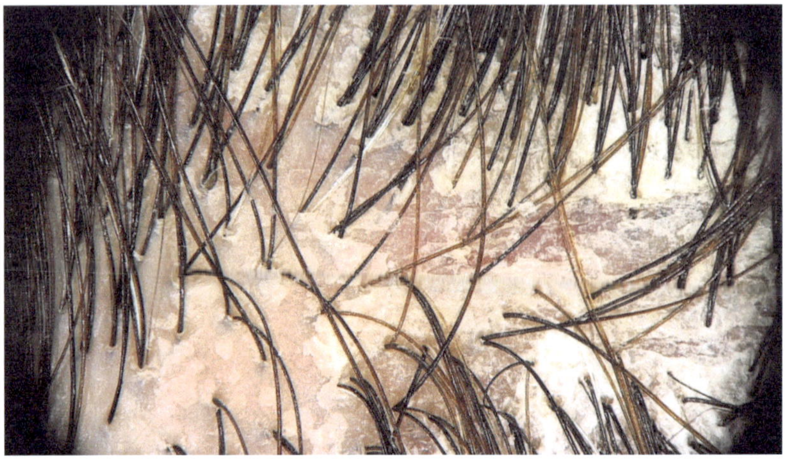

Fig. 9.20 Psoriasis. Thick white scales

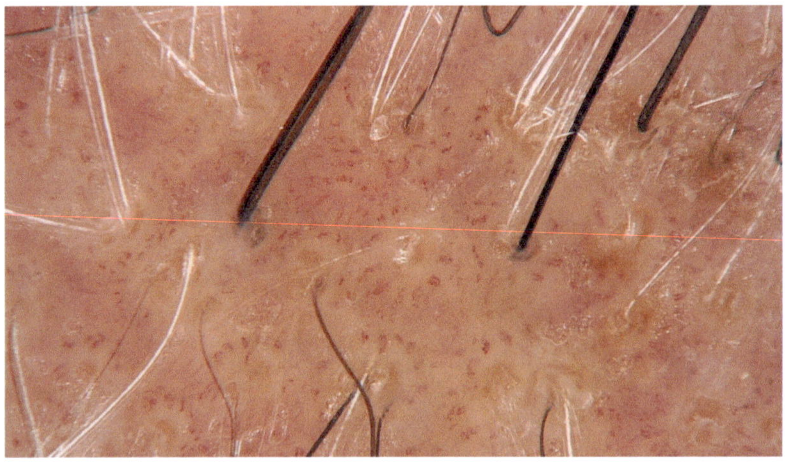

Fig. 9.21 Psoriasis. twisted red loops and dotted (glomerular) vessels

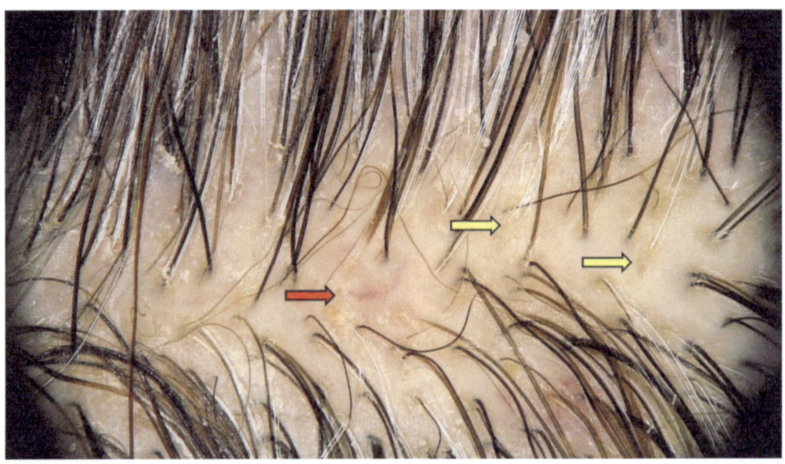

Fig. 9.22 Seborrheic dermatitis. A serpentine vessel (red arrow) and perifollicular oily yellow dots (yellow arrows)

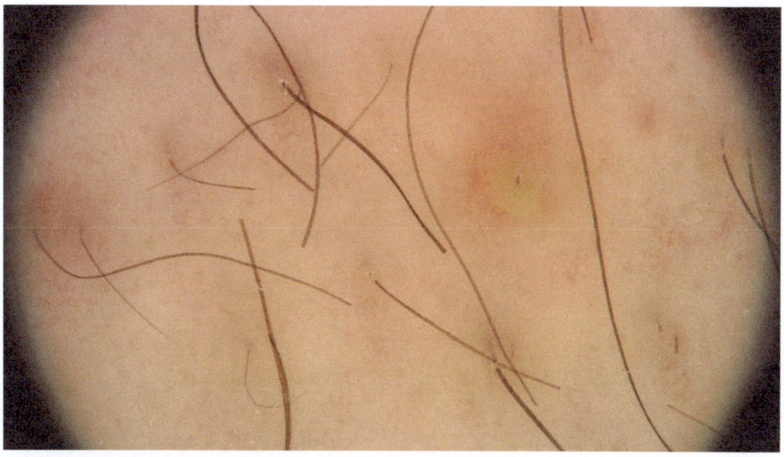

Fig. 9.23 Keratosis pilaris. Follicular erythema

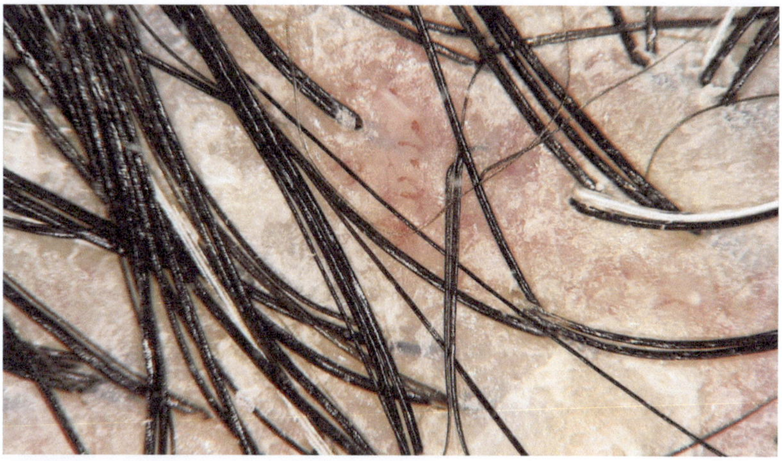

Fig. 9.24 Dermatomyositis. perifollicular and peripillar scales with tortuous vessels, 50×

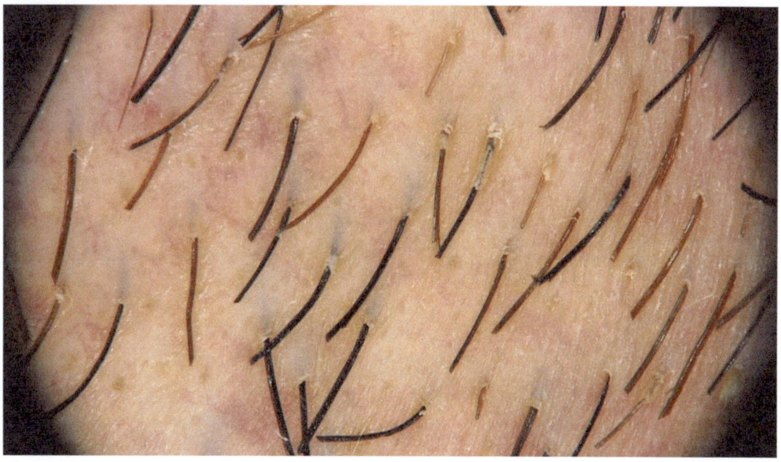

Fig. 9.25 Follicular mucinosis. White rims around follicular ostia and mucinous beard cast

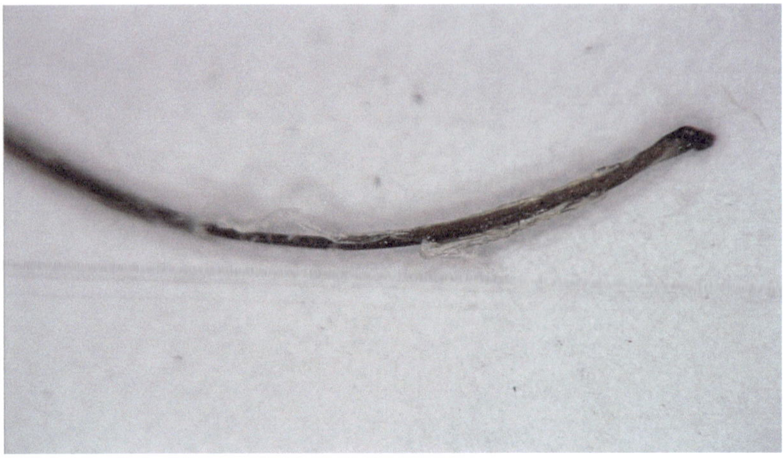

Fig. 9.26 Follicular mucinosis. Accumulation of mucin on the outer root sheath

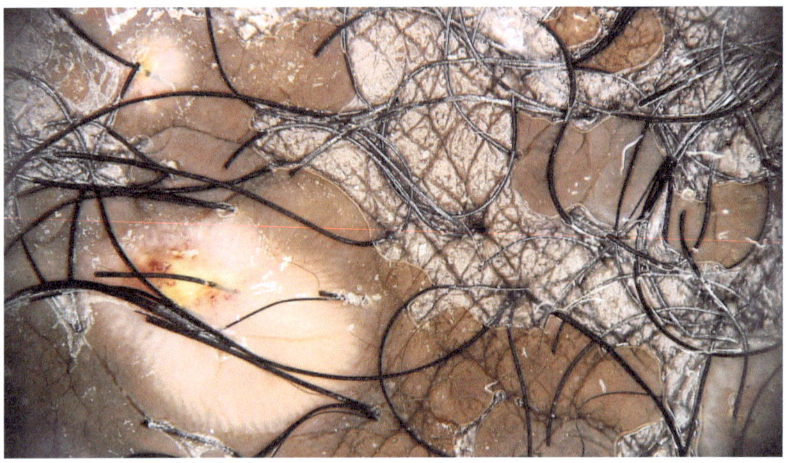

Fig. 9.27 Acne keloidalis nuchae. Perifollicular scales and hemorrhagic and honey-colored crust

Trichoscopy examination of Acne keloidalis nuchae (Fig. 9.27) may reveal follicular papules, pustules, scales around the follicles, and crusts that are either hemorrhagic or honey-colored in early stages. Another feature commonly seen is white rings around the hair follicles, which suggests perifollicular fibrosis. In advanced stages, tufted hair and enlarged follicular ostia can be seen.

Trichoscopy of Scalp Infestation and Infection

The indicators of pediculosis capitis (Figs. 9.28 and 9.29) include visible nits. These can sometimes be incorrectly identified as pseudo-nits or scales from other conditions such as seborrheic dermatitis, debris, or hair casts. Videodermoscopy for head lice reveals nits. Additionally, trichoscopy aids in diagnosing phthiriasis pubis (crab lice), which can infest the scalp hair or eyelashes (phthiriasis palpebrarum).

Comma hairs, corkscrew hair, and zigzag hairs (Fig. 9.30) are bent or twisted hairshaft features often seen in tinea capitis. Another tricoscopic findings of tinea capitis include Morse code-like hairs, bent hairs, block hairs, and i-hairs. Other common but nonspecific findings may include broken hairs, black dots, perifollicular scaling, and diffuse scaling [13].

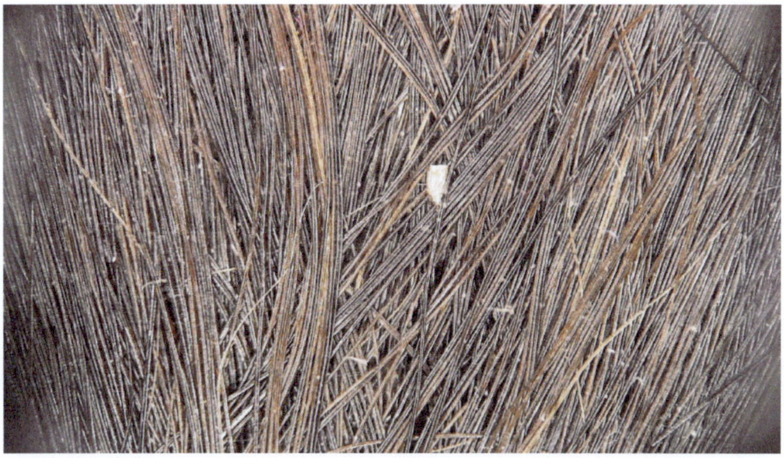

Fig. 9.28 Pediculosis capitis (a nit), 20×

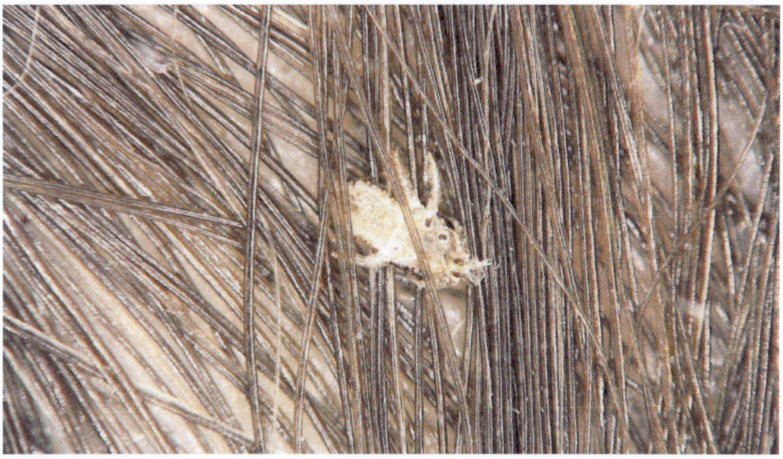

Fig. 9.29 Pediculosis capitis (Videodermoscopic observation), 50×

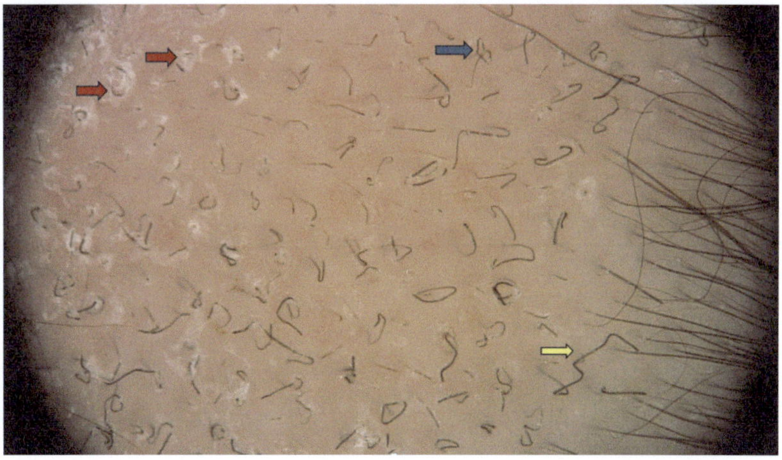

Fig. 9.30 Tinea capitus. Comma hairs (red arrows), zigzag hairs (yellow arrow), and corkscrew hairs (blue arrow)

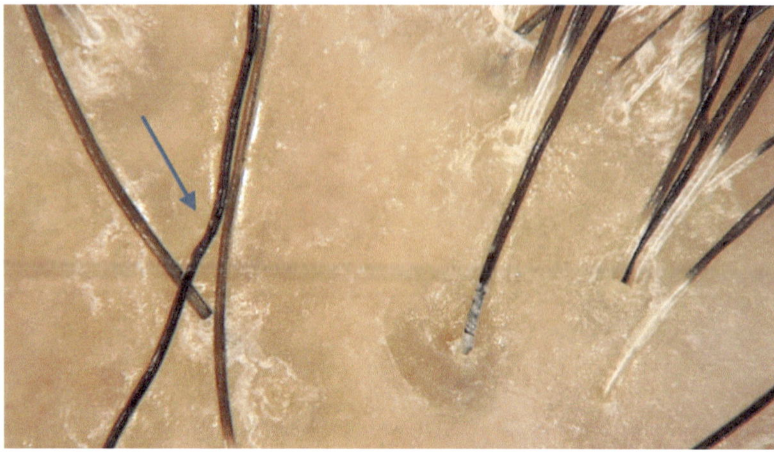

Fig. 9.31 Pili torti (blue arrow)

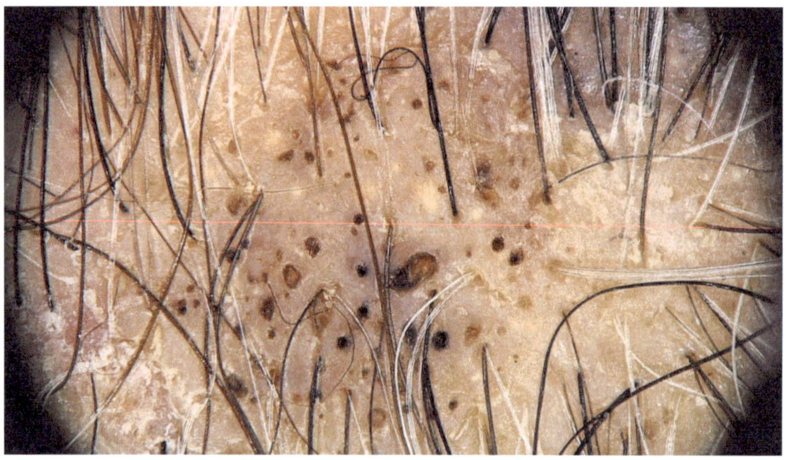

Fig. 9.32 Nevus comedonicus

Trichoscopy of Hair Shaft Disorders

Pili torti (Fig. 9.31) is characterized by the presence of the hair shaft flattened and twisted 180 degrees along its longitudinal axis. This can manifest in a variety of inherited and acquired hair disorders [14].

Other: Follicular Disorders

Trichoscopy findings of nevus comedonicus (Fig. 9.32) demonstrate multiple well-defined homogenous brown circles surrounding keratin plugs in the hair follicles.

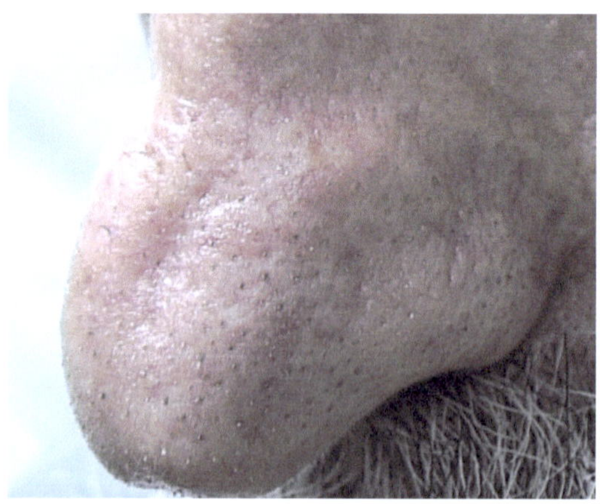

Fig. 9.33 Trichostasis Spinulosa

Trichosis spinulosa (Fig. 9.33) has a main trichoscopic characteristic feature of black dots, indicative of comedo-like cadaverized hairs, resulting from the retention of hairs within a keratinous sheath in dilated follicles (Fig. 9.34). Other common findings include keratotic plugs and the retention of fine, vellus hairs (Fig. 9.35) [15].

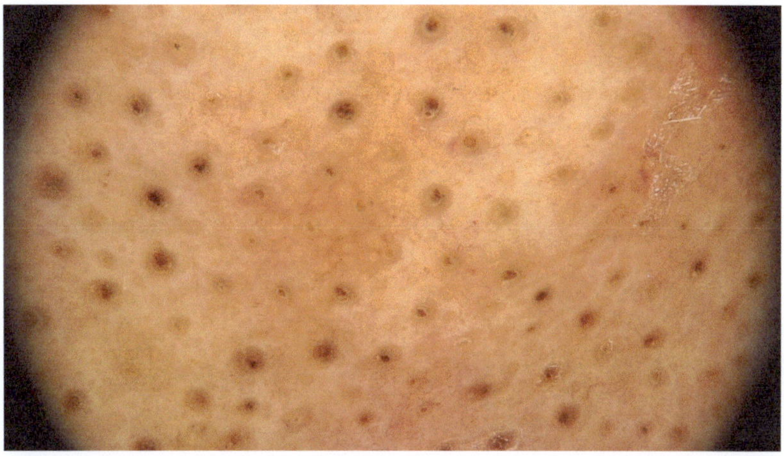

Fig. 9.34 Trichostasis Spinulosa. Black dots

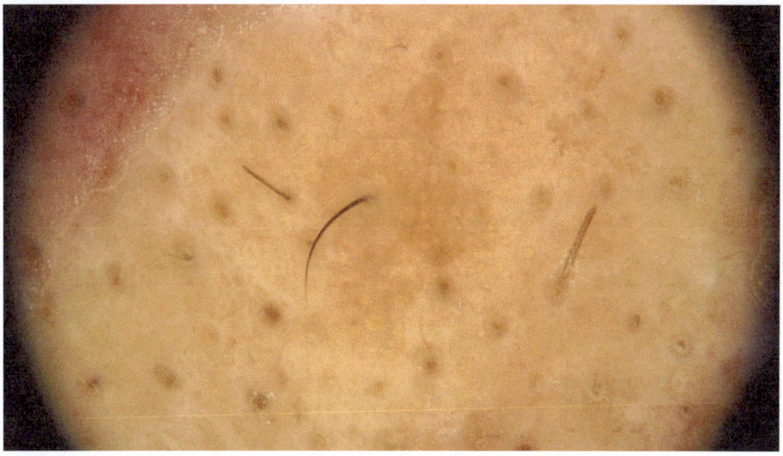

Fig. 9.35 Trichostasis Spinulosa. retention of vellus hairs

Acknowledgement Authors extend our sincere gratitude to Agnes Canazza for her generous time and effort in assisting us with the retrieval of valuable images.

References

1. Miteva M, Tosti A. Hair and scalp dermatoscopy. J Am Acad Dermatol. 2012;67(5):1040–8. https://doi.org/10.1016/j.jaad.2012.02.013.
2. Jain N, Doshi B, Khopkar U. Trichoscopy in alopecias: diagnosis simplified. Int J Trichology. 2013;5(4):170–8.
3. Ross EK, Vincenzi C, Tosti A. Videodermoscopy in the evaluation of hair and scalp disorders. J Am Acad Dermatol. 2006;55:799–806.
4. Lacarrubba F, Dall'Oglio F, Rita Nasca M, Micali G. Videodermatoscopy enhances diagnostic capability in some forms of hair loss. Am J Clin Dermatol. 2004;5(3):205–8.
5. Vincenzi C, Tosti A. Trichoscopy patterns. In: Tosti A, editor. Dermoscopy of the hair and nails. 2nd ed. Boca Raton: CRC Press; 2016. p. 1–20.
6. Pirmez R. The dermatoscope in the hair clinic: trichoscopy of scarring and nonscarring alopecia. J Am Acad Dermatol. 2023;89(2S):S9–S15.
7. Miteva M. Hair and scalp dermoscopy (Trichoscopy). In: Miteva M, editor. Hair pathology with trichoscopic correlations. Boca Raton: CRC Press; 2022. p. 1–9.
8. Rudnicka L, Oszewska M, Rakowska A, editors. Atlas of trichoscopy-dermoscopy in hair and scalp disease. 1st ed. London: Springer-Verlag; 2012.
9. Ummiti A, Priya P, Chandravathi PL, Kumar C. Correlation of trichoscopic findings in androgenetic alopecia and the disease severity. Int J Trichology. 2019;11:118–22.
10. Polat M. Evaluation of clinical signs and early and late trichoscopy findings in traction alopecia patients with Fitzpatrick skin type II and III: a single-center, clinical study. Int J Dermatol. 2017;56(8):850–5. https://doi.org/10.1111/ijd.13599.

11. Żychowska M, Reich A. Dermoscopy and trichoscopy in dermatomyositis—a cross-sectional study. J Clin Med. 2022;11(2):375.
12. Yamagishi H, Ota M, Nobeyama Y, Asahina A. Case of follicular mucinosis showing brownish yellow and red dots via dermoscopy. Clin Case Rep. 2022;10(5):e05815.
13. Waśkiel-Burnat A, Rakowska A, Sikora M, Ciechanowicz P, Olszewska M, Rudnicka L. Trichoscopy of tinea capitis: a systematic review. Dermatol Ther (Heidelb). 2020;10(1):43–52. https://doi.org/10.1007/s13555-019-00350-1.
14. Rudnicka L, Olszewska M, Waśkiel A, Rakowska A. Trichoscopy in hair shaft disorders. Dermatol Clin. 2018;36(4):421–30.
15. Panchaprateep R, Tanus A, Tosti A. Clinical, dermoscopic, and histopathologic features of body hair disorders. J Am Acad Dermatol. 2015;72(5):890–900.

The Transcriptomics and Epigenomics of Hair Follicles

10

Raquel Cuevas-Diaz Duran,
Emmanuel Martinez-Ledesma,
Melissa Garcia-Garcia, Andrea Sarro-Ramírez,
Carolina Gonzalez-Carrillo,
Denise Rodríguez-Sardin,
and Alejandro Cardenas-Lopez

Introduction

The skin is the largest organ of the human body, and it is also one of the most complex ones. Skin consists of a diverse variety of epithelial and mesenchymal cell types that perform coordinated functions underlying homeostasis. The skin appendages include sebaceous glands, apocrine and eccrine sweat glands, hair follicles (HF), and nails. HFs not only play an important role as a protein fiber factory and sensory organ, but they are also important for skin regeneration after injury. HFs are mini organs of the skin that are formed at an early embryonic stage through interactions between neuroectodermal and mesodermal stem cells, namely, epithelial, neural crest, and mesenchymal [1, 2]. Each of these stem cells gives rise to different populations of HF cells, highlighting their diversity. Furthermore, the HF is the only mammalian organ that undergoes cyclic transformations throughout its entire adult life, recapitulating embryonic growth. HFs cycle through periods of regeneration and rapid growth (anagen), apoptosis-driven regression (catagen), and relative quiescence (telogen) [3, 4]. This hair cycling is controlled by autocrine and paracrine signals that trigger changes in both cell state and cell identities.

HFs are characterized by highly heterogeneous cell subpopulations that work coordinately to periodically regenerate the hair shaft. Previous studies have tried to describe the heterogeneity of HFs, but they have been biased because of the use of *a priori* defined markers for cell enrichment [5–9]. These studies have also been limited by low sensitivity or small numbers of analyzed genes. Even so, these studies have uncovered more than 20 keratinocyte cell subpopulations and states, numerous fibroblasts and immune cell subtypes, melanocytes, and dermal papilla cells. Fortunately, advances in high throughput next generation sequencing technologies are changing

R. Cuevas-Diaz Duran (✉)
Tecnologico de Monterrey, Escuela de Medicina y Ciencias de la Salud, Monterrey, NL, Mexico

CapilarFix®, Monterrey, NL, Mexico
e-mail: raquel.cuevas.dd@tec.mx

E. Martinez-Ledesma
Tecnologico de Monterrey, Escuela de Medicina y Ciencias de la Salud, Monterrey, NL, Mexico

Institute for Obesity Research, Tecnologico de Monterrey, Monterrey, NL, Mexico
e-mail: juanemmanuel@tec.mx

M. Garcia-Garcia · A. Sarro-Ramírez · C. Gonzalez-Carrillo
CapilarFix®, Monterrey, NL, Mexico
e-mail: dra.melissa@capilarfix.com

D. Rodríguez-Sardin · A. Cardenas-Lopez (✉)
CapilarFix®, Monterrey, NL, Mexico

NeoMedics®, Monterrey, NL, Mexico
e-mail: dra.denise@capilarfix.com; dr.cardenas@capilarfix.com

P. J. Panagotacos, H. Maibach (eds.), *Hair Loss*, Updates in Clinical Dermatology,
https://doi.org/10.1007/978-3-031-74314-6_10

the way scientists are studying hair follicle (HF) functions at a molecular level with single-cell resolution. Recent studies are now allowing a better understanding of the diverse cell subpopulations residing in the HF, their transcriptional profiles at different stages of the hair cycle, and the potential interactions between them. Moreover, clues are emerging as to how specific cell subpopulations in the HF are replenished, as well as the molecular mechanisms allowing their fate selection and terminal differentiation. Elucidating the complex intercellular communication underlying the hair cycle will help us understand common hair pathologies and the cell subpopulations involved.

Herein, we briefly describe the functional anatomy of HFs and the major cell subpopulations that have been identified through conventional methods. We demonstrate through analyzing the number of papers published per year, that there is a growing interest in studying HF transcriptomics. We also discuss the technologies used to elucidate the transcriptomic profiles of HFs in bulk and with single-cell resolution. Furthermore, and given the relevance of single-cell transcriptomic studies, we describe prominent studies that have recently been published with the aim of understanding HF heterogeneity. We also introduce the use of sequencing technologies for querying epigenetic modifications and their use for elucidating cell subpopulations. Finally, we discuss the origin and the use of exosomes for hair regeneration.

Functional Anatomy of HFs and Major Cell Populations

The HF is a cylindrical structure consisting of eight concentric epithelial layers formed by subpopulations of cells organized into well-defined compartments [10]. The cells from each layer depict specific keratin expression profiles [11]. In a cross-section of the HF, the outermost layer is the outer root sheat (ORS), followed by the companion layer, the inner root sheat (IRS), and the hair shaft. The IRS is subdivided into Henle's layer, Huxley's layer, and IRS cuticle whereas the hair shaft consists of medulla, cortex, and hair cuticle. The whole epithelial concentric structure is surrounded by a mesoderm-derived connective tissue sheath. The hair shaft, located at the center of the HF is an outward-moving layer that originates proximally from an oval hair structure called the bulb. The bulb becomes an active hair shaft factory in the anagen phase, and it contains differentiated epithelial cells, undifferentiated keratinocytes of the hair matrix, melanocytes, and dermal papilla (DP) cells [12]. Matrix keratinocytes lie in the upper and lateral sides of the DP, the lowermost onion-like structure. Interestingly, matrix keratinocytes have a high proliferation rate, and they can be induced to differentiate into cells of the IRS and hair shaft medulla through interactions with DP cells [5]. The DP consists of a small cluster of mesoderm-derived densely packed fibroblasts. Interactions between DP cells and matrix keratinocytes regulate anagen duration, hair shaft diameter and length, and hair bulb size [13, 14].

Anatomically, the HF can be divided into four regions: infundibulum, isthmus, suprabulbar region, and the bulb. By the end of the anagen stage, the HF has an upper permanent segment (isthmus and infundibulum) and a cycling lower segment (suprabulbar region + bulb) subject to regeneration [12]. The infundibulum is the uppermost section of the HF and it extends towards the sebaceous duct. The isthmus lies between the sebaceous duct and the insertion of the arrector pili muscle (APM). A region of great scientific interest is the bulge, located in the lowermost isthmus. The bulge is a niche for multipotent hair follicle stem cells (HFSC) which are involved in hair regrowth [15]. During hair growth, DP cells secrete various paracrine factors that induce migration of HFSC downwards along the (ORS) to the hair bulb matrix, where they proliferate to form the secondary hair germ (SHG) [16, 17]. The SHG is a transitory structure that forms in the telogen phase. Cells from the SHG are in direct contact with DP cells and they transition to matrix progenitors (also known as matrix transient amplifying cell) [18]. Bulge HFSC not only contribute to SHG, but they can also be induced to differentiate into an interfollicular epidermis

(IFE)-like cell and migrate to act in wound healing [19]. Mounting studies have demonstrated that upon skin injury numerous cells including keratinocytes from the IFE, junctional zone, isthmus, and bulge regions are recruited for wound re-epithelialization [20–23]. Moreover, stem cell derived progenitors from any niche can rapidly contribute to wound healing demonstrating a high degree of plasticity.

Transcriptomic Profiling of HF Cells

Through transcriptomic profiling, scientists attempt to identify and quantify the set of messenger RNA molecules expressed in a cell or a group of cells under certain conditions. To address the importance of HF transcriptomics, we searched the PubMed NCBI database [ref] using the following query: *"hair follicle" AND ("single-cell" OR "single cell" OR ""RNA-seq""OR "transcriptome" OR "transcriptomics" OR "ChiP-seq" OR "ATAC-seq") AND human*. Selecting only papers published since 2010, we found a total of 156 manuscripts. Figure 10.1 shows that the number of papers published per year follows an exponential growth curve up to 2020 where it reaches a peak of 27 papers. The exponential model has a good adjusted R-squared of approximately 0.8. However, after 2020, the number of papers seems to stagnate around 20. Nonetheless, these numbers show an increasing interest in studying HF transcriptomics.

Almost 8% (12/156) of the papers involved the study HFs using single-cell, and from these, only 2 used single-cell multi-omics techniques. On the other hand, 14/156 (9%) of these articles researched alopecia, dividing the disease into androgenetic alopecia (8/14), alopecia areata (5/14), and scarring (cicatricial) alopecia (1/14). Surprisingly, ten papers (6%) analyzed HFs or elements of HFs related to cancer, in particular, five papers investigated skin tumors, two Merkel

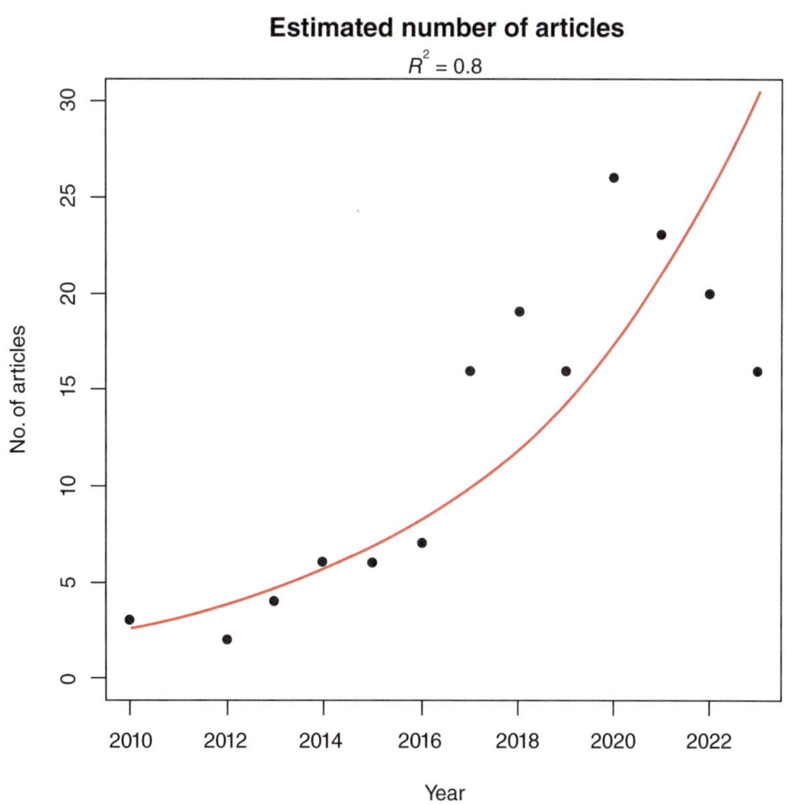

Fig. 10.1 Number of articles related to HF transcriptomics published per year since 2010. The red line represents the exponential growth in the number of articles with an adjusted R^2 of 0.8

cell carcinomas, two basal cell carcinomas, and one explored cancer and its relation to the skin's circadian clock. In addition to these interesting HF studies, we found the use of HF transcriptomic profiles as biomarkers to detect disorders of methamphetamine use [24].

Different technologies have been used to comprehensively profile transcripts, for example microarrays and next-generation RNA-sequencing (RNA-seq). However, RNA-seq has been well established as a higher resolution method that allows the identification of known and novel splice variants, non-coding transcripts, and genes not included in microarrays [25]. Thus, RNA-seq has been used in numerous studies in mouse and human to describe changes in gene expression in HFs at different stages of the growth cycle and under distinct biological conditions. In this section we will discuss relevant studies performed using RNA-seq technologies to describe the transcriptomics of hair follicles as a whole (bulk) and with single cell resolution.

Bulk RNA-Sequencing

Bulk RNA-seq comprises the sequencing of pooled cell populations, tissue sections, or biopsies to address gene expression. Due to the pooled origin of the samples, this method measures the average gene expression of individual genes across numerous (thousands to millions) input cells, limiting its scope to finding differences between conditions, disregarding cell subpopulations. Studies using bulk RNA-seq have mainly focused on finding transcriptional variations comparing HFs at different hair cycle stages, HFs from balding against non-balding regions, and HFs from healthy controls compared to specific hair diseases. Samples for bulk RNA-seq can be obtained through hair plucking, follicular unit extraction (FUE), and skin biopsies. Hair grafts obtained from patients undergoing hair transplantation and skin biopsies are generally composed of several HFs, hair bulbs, surrounding tissue including IFE, dermis, sebaceous and apocrine glands, vascular tissue, and immune cells [26]. In some cases, HFs are microdissected to enrich the bulge and the DP-containing bulb regions. The quality assessment of samples consists of determining their concentration and evaluating their integrity, defined as RNA integrity number (RIN). Samples passing quality control are then subjected to library preparation and then sequencing.

Single-Cell RNA-Sequencing

Single-cell sequencing (scRNA-seq) is a genomic approach that aims at identifying and quantifying transcripts with individual cell resolution. This technology has allowed the profiling of large numbers of cells or nuclei in parallel to systematically dissect the cellular composition of tissues and organs at unprecedented resolution [27–29]. Moreover, scRNA-seq has been successfully used to identify new cell types [30, 31] and to describe cell plasticity and lineage progression in dynamic systems [32–34]. One of the biggest ongoing research projects using scRNA-seq is the Human Cell Atlas, a large-scale effort whose main objective is to create cellular maps describing the position, function, and transcriptional profiles of all the cells in the human body [35]. This cellular reference map is to be used as a basis for understand human health, and as a tool for diagnosing, monitoring, and treating disease. A study describing the transcriptional signatures of human anagen hair follicle has recently been published as part of the Human Cell Atlas project [36]. This, and other prominent studies will be described herein after briefly discussing the experimental methodology used for scRNA-seq.

The first step in scRNA-seq is the preparation of high-quality single-cell or single-nuclei suspensions. Jaks and colleagues described a method for harvesting keratinocytes from mice [37]. The process starts by washing clipped and disinfected dorsal skin with Hank's Balanced Salt Solution (HBSS) and incubating skin strips in a 0.25% trypsin solution to detach the dermis from the epidermis. Next, epidermal tissue is scraped into S-MEM and single-cells are isolated through magnetic stirring. The suspension is filtered, and cells are separated using Anti-SCA-1-FITC magnetic beads to isolate SCA-1+ and SCA-1− cells. Cells within the suspension are then isolated or captured to obtain individual reaction volumes. Approaches for single cell capturing include fluorescence activated cell sorting (FACS) and microfluidic systems [38]. However, higher yields are obtained through microfluidics devices and droplets/nanowells. In sequential processing steps, cells are individually lysed, and their RNA is captured by poly(T) oligonucleotides. These mRNA molecules, complemented with single-cell-specific barcodes, are reverse transcribed into complementary DNA, amplified and processed to sequencing-ready libraries [29]. It should be noted that the unique extracellular composition of DP renders human HFs indigestible to a single cell suspension with common enzymes such as trypsin and collagenase [39, 40]. Instead, other protocols using dispase, microdissection, or explant cultures have been proposed [36, 41–43].

A pioneering study performed by Joost, and colleagues was the first to comprehensively address murine telogen epidermis and HF cellular heterogeneity [44]. Through sequencing 1422 single-cell transcriptomes, authors were able to identify 25 different subpopulations of interfollicular and follicular epidermal cells. Unsupervised clustering and affinity propagation using high variance genes confirmed the existence of 13 previously known epidermal subpopulations: sebaceous gland (SG cells), outer bulge and inner bulge keratinocytes, IFE basal cells, two stages of IFE differentiated cells, two terminally differentiated IFE keratinized layer cells, three distinct groups of upper HF cells, and two immune cell populations (Langerhans and resident T cells). Interestingly, subclustering of outer bulge, inner bulge, upper HF, and basal IFE populations derived in novel subpopulations which were confirmed by immunohistochemistry and single-molecule mRNA fluorescence in situ hybridization (smRNA-FISH). Analysis of each subpopulation's gene profiles led to the observation that most heterogeneity in the HF was a result of a combination of recurring gene signatures. Thus, authors performed pseudotemporal ordering of IFE cells and identified 1627 genes with significant expression level variation along a differentiation trajectory which robustly recapitulated epidermal stratification. Researchers further analyzed HF heterogeneity by separating basal IFE, upper HF, outer bulb and inner bulb gene signatures and found that cells were positioned along a path which reproduced their spatial localization along the proximal-distal axis of the HF. A total of 547 genes were differentially expressed along this pseudospace. Overall, these results demonstrate that the transcriptional heterogeneity of the telogen epidermis and HF subpopulations in homeostasis can be described by a differentiation trajectory and a proximal-distal axis [44].

Another prominent study combined single-cell transcriptomics and *in vivo* lineage tracing to elucidate the transcriptional changes that take place in epidermal and bulge stem cells in response to wounding [19]. Using transgenic mice, authors genetically labeled Lgr5 and Lrg6-expressing cells which in homeostatic conditions are found in the HF bulge region and in the IFE respectively. Tomato lineage tracing was induced by tamoxifen and dorsal wounds were performed. Skin surrounding wounded sites was excised and tomato-traced cells were sorted and sequenced. A total number of 1873 cells were captured from samples obtained at different time-points after wounding as well as from unwounded skin. The comparison of transcriptomic profiles of Lrg6^{TOM} and Lrg5^{TOM} cells to those from a previous study (the single-cell atlas of telogen skin [44]) demonstrated that these stem cells undergo transcriptional modifications in response to wounding. Most interestingly, Lrg5^{TOM} cells in the bulge rapidly increase the number of receptors enabling a response to signals from the wound environment, suggesting an initial priming before migration. In contrast, Lrg6^{TOM} cells in the IFE are primed in homeostatic conditions and respond to wounding. Results demonstrate how stem cells from different niches (IFE and HF bulge) undergo priming, proliferation, and migration and molecularly converge in wound healing [19].

A few years after the transcriptomic description of murine telogen epidermis, researchers from the same laboratory performed another unbiased systematic assessment of gene expression profiles and spatial location of all cell subpopulations, now using murine full-thickness skin during growth and rest [45]. Samples obtained from dorsal mouse skin during anagen and telogen were processed and 5767 and 7601 single cells were sequenced consisting of testing and validation datasets respectively. According to their expression profiles, cells were grouped into 7 main clusters: keratinocytes from the permanent epidermis (IFE, SG, non-cycling HF), keratinocytes from the anagen HF, fibroblast-like cells, immune cells (T-cells, macrophages, dendritic cells, Langerhans cells), vascular cells, neural crest-derived cells (melanocytes and Schwann cells), and others (skeletal muscle and red blood cells). These clusters were further stratified into 56 transcriptionally distinct cell types and cell states and were validated through smRNA-FISH. Interestingly, anagen-specific HF cells comprised 20 different subpopulations, suggesting that hair shaft growth is the result of a complex interplay between numerous subpopulations with multiple cell states. Given that anagen HF keratinocytes and fibroblast-like subpopulations undergo substantial remodeling through the hair cycle, authors focused on them to perform a more in-depth analysis. Interestingly, authors uncovered six distinct subpopulations of keratinocytes in the outer layer (OL) which were broadly classified into basal and suprabasal. The basal OL was composed of two different basal ORS populations (ORS B1 and ORS B2) and a lower proximal cup (LPC) group. Likewise, the suprabasal OL cluster was subdivided into a suprabasal ORS (ORS SB), a mid-part companion layer (mCP), and an upper companion layer (uCP) subpopulation. Basal and suprabasal OL cells were found to be intermingling even though they are transcriptionally distinct and depict no evidence of transitions between them. Moreover, authors revealed a trajectory from mCP to uCP cells, confirming that the companion layer is formed through upward dynamics from the hair bulb to the bulge [45–47]. Keratinocytes of the matrix and inner layers of the HF were grouped in a cluster that displayed a peculiar branching topology. RNA velocity analysis and an unsupervised Markov model predicted that uncommitted germinative layer cells reside at the starting point of this multi-branching topology. Pseudotemporal ordering showed that the three main branches corresponded to cells of the IRS, cortex/cuticle, and medulla, which passed through distinct intermediate states.

Table 10.1 lists the 56 cell subpopulations found by Joost and colleagues [45]. For each subpopulation, we included the top 10 most enriched genes with highest mean expression and lowest Benjamini-Hochberg adjusted *p-value* according to metrics reported by Joost et al. [45].

The human counterpart to the prominent research described elucidating murine HF heterogeneity, was published by Takahashi and collaborators [36]. The main challenge faced when studying the transcriptomics of human HFs is the scarcity of these appendages within the skin, as compared to murine models. Takahashi et al. used human skin samples discarded from hair transplant procedures to isolate and sequence 22,000 cells to obtain their transcriptomic profiles. Anagen HFs from five patients were used and cells were clustered into 23 groups. The identity of the clusters was determined according to differentially expressed genes, expression levels of keratin genes, and the expression of MKI-67, a marker of proliferation which has been used as a marker of the innermost layer of the ORS. The clusters found included bulge and lower bulge, IFE (spinous 1–3, granular, basal 1–2, mitotic), ORS (basal, suprabasal, companion layer), IRS (cuticle, Huxley's + Henley's layers), matrix/cortex/medulla, isthmus, infundibulum, melanocytes, mesenchymal, sebaceous/apocrine, immune, Langerhans, and endothelial. Furthermore, through pseudotemporal ordering, authors demonstrated that cells of the basal IFE differentiated into spinous and granular layers, consistent with previous knowledge of both mouse and human models. Authors also showed that cells belonging to the cortex/medulla/matrix cluster branch giving rise to ORS companion layer cells and to the IRS (Huxley's + Henley's layer) cells [36]. Overall, the work by Takahashi et al. [36] provides a landscape of the heterogeneity of human HF cells, however, their main limi-

Table 10.1 Cell subpopulations and states found in dorsal mouse skin samples during anagen and telogen phases of hair growth

Mayor cell class	Subpopulations identified	Top 10 enriched genes
Permanent epidermis keratinocytes	IFE cycling	B2m, Calm2, Fth1, H2-D1, H3f3b, Krt14, Krt5, Mt2, Ptma, Stmn1
	IFE basal	Ccl27a, Fos, H3f3b, Junb, Krt14, Krt15, Malat1, Rpl3, Rplp0, Sfn
	IFE suprabasal 1	Dmkn, Itm2b, Krt10, Krtdap, Lgals7, Ly6d, Rpl18a, Rplp0, Rps18, Sfn
	IFE suprabasal 2	Calm4, Dmkn, Itm2b, Krt10, Krt77, Krtdap, Lgals3, Lgals7, Ly6g6c, Sbsn
	Upper basal HF	Apoe, B2m, Ccl27a, Ftl1, Fxyd3, Krt17, mt-Cytb, mt-Nd4, Slc25a5, Sostdc1
	Upper suprabasal HF	Cst6, Cstb, Dapl1, Krt17, Krt79, Lgals7, Ly6d, Ly6g6c, Perp, Sprr1a
	Sebaceous gland	Akr1c18, Apoc1, Cidea, Dhcr24, Elovl6, Fabp5, Mgst1, Scd1, Scd3, Tecr
	Outer bulge	Apoe, Cxcl14, Dmkn, Ftl1, Krt15, Krt17, Ptn, S100a6, Tmsb4x, Ubb
	Hair germ	Ftl1, Rpl13, Rpl3, Rpl35, Rpl37a, Rps14, Rps19, Rps27, Rps4x, Rps5
Anagen HF keratinocytes	Basal ORS 1	Apoe, Cxcl14, Ftl1, Krt14, Krt17, Lgals7, Malat1, Tmsb10, Ubb, Ucp2
	Basal ORS 2	Apoe, Cd9, Cxcl14, Ftl1, Gjb2, Krt14, Krt15, Krt17, Malat1, Myl6
	Suprabasal ORS	Apoe, Dbi, Gja1, Krt14, Krt17, Krt5, Lgals7, S100a6, Sdc1, Tmsb4x
	Lower proximal cup	Cxcl14, Fgfbp1, Gclm, Igfbp7, Il11ra1, Krt15, Serpinh1, Slc39a10, Timp3, Tpm1
	Middle companion layer	Apoe, Dbi, Krt14, Krt17, Krt5, Lgals7, S100a6, Sbsn, Sdc1, Tmsb4x
	Upper companion layer	Apoe, Cst6, Cstb, Gsn, Krt14, Krt17, Lgals7, S100a6, Sbsn, Tmsb4x
	Germinative layer 1	Dcn, Fos, Ftl1, Id3, Ier2, Jun, Junb, Mt1, Mt2, Nfkbia
	Germinative layer 2	Dcn, Eif5a, H3f3b, Mt1, Mt2, Ppia, Ptma, Slc25a5, Stmn1, Ubb
	Germinative layer 3	Dcn, H2afz, Mt1, Mt2, Npm1, Ppia, Ptma, Slc25a5, Stmn1, Ybx1
	Germinative layer 4	Eif4a1, Eif5a, Hspa8, Mt1, Mt2, Npm1, Ppia, Ptma, Stmn1, Ybx1
	IRS 1	Fabp5, H2afz, H3f3b, Krt28, Krt71, Mgst1, Perp, Ptma, Stmn1, Tubb5
	IRS 2	Apoe, Fth1, Ftl1, H3f3b, Ifitm2, Jun, Junb, Mgst1, Ptma, Ybx1
	IRS 3	A430005L14Rik, Armcx3, C1qbp, Ctsc, Gsta2, Kat5, L2hgdh, Nolc1, Plxna2, Timm21
	IRS 4	Anxa1, Dmkn, Dynll1, Krt25, Krt27, Krt71, Ly6d, Prss53, Slc39a8, Tchh
	IRS 5	Crym, G6pdx, Lhfp, Pak1, Pdcd11, Pygl, Srf, Unk, Wnt10b, Zfp503
	IRS 6	2310007B03Rik, Avp, Cryba4, Crym, Ctps, Fam25c, Fbp1, Krt72, Prr9, Sp6
	Cortex cuticle 1	Chil1, Id1, Jun, Nfkbia, Nxpe2, Phlda2, Ptn, Rexo2, Sat1, Tnf
	Cortex cuticle 2	Calm2, Cdc20, Dapl1, Hmgb2, Krt35, Rexo2, Rnaset2a, Rnaset2b, Selenbp1, Ube2c
	Cortex cuticle 3	Dapl1, Gadd45g, Itm2b, Krt35, Mt4, Rexo2, Rnaset2a, Rnaset2b, Rps18, Sat1
	Cortex cuticle 4	Dapl1, Itm2b, Krt35, mt-Nd1, Mt4, Rnaset2a, Rnaset2b, Rpl37a, S100a3, Sfn
	Cortex cuticle 5	Dapl1, Krt31, Krt33a, Krt35, Krtap11–1, Krtap7–1, Krtap8–1, Mt4, S100a3, Sfn
	Medulla 1	Hmgb2, Mt1, Mt2, Ptma, Rexo2, Sat1, Stmn1, Tmsb10, Tuba1b, Tubb5
	Medulla 2	Fabp4, Gpnmb, Krt17, S100a10, S100a14, S100a3, S100a6, Sat1, Tmsb10, Txndc17
	Medulla 3	Atp6v1g1, Gpnmb, H3f3a, Malat1, Rplp0, Rps27, S100a3, S100a6, Sat1, Tmsb10

(continued)

Table 10.1 (continued)

Mayor cell class	Subpopulations identified	Top 10 enriched genes
Fibroblast-like cells	Skin fibroblasts 1	Cldn10, Col1a1, Col1a2, Col3a1, Cpz, Ndufa4l2, Nupr1, Ppic, Sparc, Tgfbi
	Skin fibroblasts 2	Aebp1, Ccl19, Cd63, Cyp2f2, Dcn, Fth1, Igfbp7, Lum, Mfap4, Mt1
	Skin fibroblasts 3	Cxcl12, Cygb, Dpt, F3, Gpx3, Gsn, Hmcn2, Mgst1, Myoc, Tmeff2
	Skin fibroblasts 4	Adm, Akr1c18, Anxa1, Anxa3, Ifi27l2a, Igfbp6, Mfap5, Pi16, Plac8, Prss23
	Dermal sheath 1	Abi3bp, Cd34, Col1a1, Col1a2, Col6a1, Cpxm2, Dcn, Lum, Mylk, Postn
	Dermal sheath 1	Cdc42ep3, Cryab, Dpep1, Galr2, Grem2, Igfbp7, Mfap5, Mgp, Prss12, Wnt11
	Anagen dermal papilla	Chodl, Cntn1, Crym, Emb, F5, Nrg2, Ptprz1, Rgs2, Rspo4, Sfrp1
	Telogen dermal papilla	Bcl2, Bmp4, Crabp1, Dkk2, Igfbp3, Malat1, Notum, Nrn1, Pappa2, Slc26a7
Immune cells	T-cells	Cd3d, Cd3e, Cd3g, Cd7, Ctla2a, Ctsw, Gem, Gzmc, Nkg7, Xcl1
	Macrophages 1	Apoe, C1qa, C1qb, C1qc, Ccl7, Ccl8, Ftl1, Itm2b, Pf4, Sepp1
	Macrophages 2	Ccl6, Clec4b1, Crip1, Ear2, Fn1, Gpx1, Lgals3, Lyz1, Lyz2, Retnla
	Macrophages 3	Abi3, Chil3, Emilin2, Gm9733, Gypc, Hp, Ly6c2, Serpinb10, Slpi, Vcl
	Dendritic cells	Cd209a, Cd74, H2-Aa, H2-Ab1, Il1b, Lsp1, Napsa, Plbd1, Pmaip1, Tspan13
	Langerhans cells	Cd207, Cd9, Dpep2, Grasp, H2-M2, Il1r2, Ltc4s, Mfge8, Pxdc1, Tnfaip2
Vascular cells	Endothelial cells 1	Cd36, Fabp4, Gpihbp1, Ly6a, Ly6c1, Rgcc, Tcf15, Tmsb4x, Tspan13, Ybx1
	Endothelial cells 2	Ackr1, Clu, Dbi, Plvap, Rps4x, Selp, Stom, Tmem252, Tmem255b, Vamp5
	Vascular smooth muscle	Acta2, Crispld2, Hspb6, Myh11, Myl9, Mylk, Rarres2, Tagln, Tpm1, Tpm2
	Lymph vessel cells	Arl4a, Fgl2, Fxyd6, Gm14964, Lbp, Lcn2, Mmrn1, Pard6g, Pdlim4, Thy1
Neural crest-derived cells	Melanocytes 1	Atp1a1, Ctsd, Dct, mt-Cytb, mt-Nd1, mt-Nd4, Pmel, Slc24a5, Tyr, Tyrp1
	Melanocytes 2	Atp6v1g1, Cdk4, Ftl1, Gstp1, Mgll, Rpl41, Rps3, Rps7, S100a1, Txn1
	Schwann cells	Cd9, Cnp, Cryab, Gatm, Mbp, Mfap5, Mpz, Pmp22, Rgcc, S100a6
Miscellaneous	Skeletal muscle	Rpl13, Rpl21, Rpl26, Rpl36, Rpl37, Rpl37a, Rps18, Rps19, Rps2, Rps27
	Red blood cells	Alas2, Bpgm, Fam220a, Ftl1, Hba-a1, Hba-a2, Hbb-bs, Hbb-bt, Mkrn1, Ube2l6

Top 10 enriched genes (highest mean expression and most significant adjusted p-value) are listed for each subpopulation. Data obtained from Joost et al. [45]

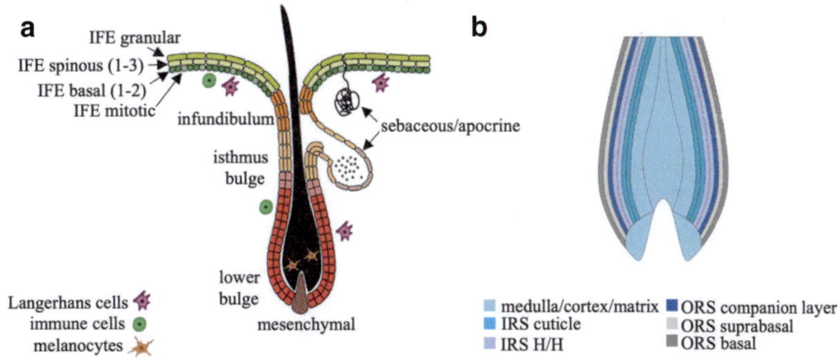

c

Cell subpopulation	Top 10 enriched genes
IFE granular	CALML3, KRT6B, KRT6A, LYPD3, FABP5, TACSTD2, SBSN, PKP1, S100A16, S100A11
IFE spinous 1	KRT10, LY6D, LGALS7B, DMKN, B2M, AQP3, KRT1, NEAT1, RHOV, LGALS7
IFE spinous 2	CHCHD10, SLC25A5, CSTB, LGALS7B, APOE, S100A16, TMEM45A, CALML3, S100A11, ATP5B
IFE spinous 3	LGALS7B, DMKN, KRT10, LY6D, KRTDAP, FABP5, KRT1, DBI, S100A7, CRABP2
IFE basal 1	KRT15, HLA-B, B2M, KRT14, KLF4, MT-ND1, PMAIP1, DUSP1, IFITM3, FTL
IFE basal 2	SAA1, CHI3L1, LY6E, MT-ND1, CYP27A1, C9orf16, MGST1, PTN, CTSB, CHCHD10
IFE mitotic	H2AFZ, STMN1, TUBA1B, HMGB1, TUBB, TK1, HMGB2, SMC2, TYMS, HMGN2
infundibulum	CCNL1, CYR61, HLA-B, PNRC1, SOCS3, NFKBIA, KRT15, SAT1, KLF10, MT-ND1
isthmus	KRT5, DST, KRT15, S100A6, TMSB4X, COL17A1, AQP3, RCAN1, CAV1, CYP1B1
bulge	CXCL14, KRT15, SFRP1, ITM2A, CAV1, DST, LGALS1, FTH1, S100A6, LMCD1
lower bulge	CXCL14, LGALS1, KRT14, IGFBP7, KRT15, RARRES2, SFRP1, FTH1, FGL2, MYL9
immune	B2M, MALAT1, HLA-B, VIM, S100A4, SRGN, CD52, CD69, TMSB4X, ARHGDIB
melanocytes	VIM, FTH1, MLANA, FTL, LGALS1, DCT, PMEL, GPM6B, MITF, NSG1
mesenchymal	VIM, SPARC, CALD1, FTL, S100A6, MALAT1, S100A4, SPARCL1, DCN, LGALS1
sebaceous/apocrine	PIP, AZGP1, DCD, SCGB2A2, SCGB1B2P, SCGB1D2, KRT19, KRT18, MUCL1, MAFF
langerhans	CD74, HLA-DRA, HLA-DPB1, HLA-DRB1, HLA-DPA1, TMSB4X, HLA-DRB5, CST3, RGS1, HLA-DMA
matrix/cortex/medulla	ALDH2, ID3, KRT85, LDHB, NME1, KRT35, DBI, ASS1, GJA1, ODC1
ORS SB	KRT5, S100A2, KRT14, APOE, FABP5, S100A14, KRT16, SDC1, LGALS7B, GJA1
ORS B	S100A2, FABP5, KRT14, KRT16, KRT5, TMSB4X, KRT6B, CALML3, APOE, GJB6
IRS H/H	PRR9, KRT25, FABP9, TCHH, KRT1, FABP5, KRT71, S100A9, S100A8, KRT74
IRS/cuticle	KRT28, DBI, GATA3, ARHGAP29, ID3, TACSTD2, KRT71, KRT25, SCEL, FABP5
endothelial	VIM, B2M, CD74, HLA-B, TMSB4X, SPARCL1, IFITM3, TMSB10, IFI27, GNG11

Fig. 10.2 Cell clusters identified through scRNA-seq in human anagen HFs and the top enriched genes (mena expression and adjusted *p-value*) found in each subpopulation. (**a**) Schematic diagram depicting the cell subpopulations identified in a longitudinal section of the human anagen HF and (**b**) concentric layers of the ORS, IRS, and shaft. Figure adapted from [36] with data obtained from [36]

tation was the depth of coverage, and this is potentially why the number of identified clusters was lower than the similar study performed by Joost et al. [45] in mouse. An overview of the cell subpopulations and the top 10 enriched genes found in human anagen HFs is depicted in Fig. 10.2.

Spatial Transcriptomics

Undoubtedly, scRNA-seq is the gold standard for defining cell states and phenotypes, however, a crucial practical obstacle remains: the need to isolate single cells from tissues without inducing stress, cell aggregation and/or apoptosis. Furthermore, tissue dissociation protocols suffer from losing the position of a given cell within a tissue and relative to its neighbors. Knowing a cell's location is important because it can determine the signals to which cells are exposed to as well as cell-cell interactions. Thus, emerging spatial transcriptomics techniques aim at simultaneously profiling hundreds to thousands of genes at subcellular resolution. In 2021, the spatially resolved transcriptomics (SRT) technology was named the "Method of the Year 2020" by *Nature Methods* [48]. Commercially available spatial transcriptomics technologies include Visium [49], by 10X Genomics, GeoMX [50] by Nanostring, and Slide-seq [51] by Curio Bioscience. At a broad level, this technology provides high quality transcriptomic data as well as a two-dimensional location information. Location information is possible by locating fresh or frozen tissue sections on special carrier chips with immobilized reverse transcription primers and spatial barcode. This technique, Spatial Transcriptomics (ST) [49] is the first in situ spatial barcoding-based technique. Mounting research using SRT and ST technologies have helped scientists to develop atlases of critical biological processes, for example during development [52, 53], brain plasticity [54], and human disease [55, 56]. Recently Shim and colleagues integrated spatial transcriptomics and scRNA-seq to compare nails and HFs obtained from human samples [57]. Authors concluded that nails and HFs share molecular similarities enriched by Wnt and BMP signaling pathways.

Currently, the pathogenesis of hair pathologies, for example, androgenetic alopecia are still unclear. Using scRNA-seq and spatial transcriptomics will provide means for cell subpopulation identification, pseudo-time analysis, cell-cell ligand-receptor interactions, and gene regulatory network reconstruction, tools which will allow a better understanding of hair pathologies and derivation of novel therapeutic targets.

Epigenetics of HF Cells

Epigenetics is an exciting field of research because it offers new insights into the underlying disease mechanisms. To do so, epigenetics studies the mechanisms that alter gene expression without modifying DNA sequence. These regulatory mechanisms include DNA methylation, histone post-transcriptional modifications, chromatin remodeling, noncoding RNA, and noncoding DNA [58, 59]. Mounting evidence has demonstrated that prominent transcriptional regulation is achieved through noncoding regions of the DNA, for example enhancers. Enhancers are important epigenetic mechanisms that orchestrate precise space and time gene expression patterns [60]. Enhancers serve as docking platforms for transcription factor binding, increasing the likelihood of transcription of one or more distal genes [61]. Chromatin accessibility assays, for example, single-cell assay for transposase-accessible chromatin using sequencing (scATAC-seq), have been used to investigate the dynamics of chromatin landscapes and to uncover putative enhancers. Changes in chromatin accessibility have been linked to the regulation of cell fate [62, 63]. Moreover, overlaying lineage-specific transcriptomes with chromatin accessibility landscapes has revealed potential master transcription factors and enhancer regions that participate in fate determination and differentiation of cells during the HF growth cycle [64].

A compelling study addressing chromatin accessibility and transcriptomic profiles with single-cell resolution was recently published by Ober-Reynolds and colleagues [65]. Authors collected samples from healthy human scalp punch biopsies, patients with alopecia areata, and discarded normal peripheral surgical tissue. Single-cells were isolated from digested tissue and libraries were prepared for paired scRNA-seq and scATAC-seq. In both single-cell chromatin profiles and transcriptomes, authors identified 22 cell clusters including keratinocytes, T lymphocytes, myeloid lineage cells, fibroblasts, and endothelial cells. Interestingly, authors demonstrated that GWAS variants associated to androgenetic alopecia (AGA) are strongly enriched in DP open chromatin regulatory regions, confirming that these cells are drivers of the pathogenesis. Moreover, these enhancer regions are linked to target genes enriched in WNT signaling. Results also indicated that HFSC subpopulations in alopecia areata samples are preserved whereas there is a significant depletion of sheath subpopulations of the bulb, suggesting that these cells are affected by the infiltration of immune cells [65]

Exosomes

Exosomes are a class of nanoscale extracellular vesicles that mediate intercellular communications. These extracellular vesicles are produced by inward budding of cells' endosomal membrane, and they are generally between 30 and 150 nm in size [66]. The phospholipid bilayer of exosomes integrates into the recipient cell's membrane transferring their cargoes into the cytosol. Therefore, exosomes are considered reliable messengers carrying various amounts of molecules such as DNA, mRNA, miRNA, long non-coding RNA, lipids, metabolites, and proteins, influencing physiological and pathological processes [67]. Furthermore, exosomes can move through the extracellular matrix and thus, they can be exchanged in an autocrine, paracrine, or endocrine form mediating communication between cells. Exosomes are found in every body fluid, and they can potentially reflect cells' physiological condition. Moreover, studies have shown that exosomes can induce cell proliferation, migration and angiogenesis and promote tissue repair.

One of the first contributions of exosomes to the field of regenerative medicine was through mesenchymal stem cells (MSC). MSC are multipotent stem cells with self-renewal abilities; they have been found mainly in bone marrow, adipose tissue, muscle, and umbilical cord [68]. Numerous researchers have demonstrated that MSC contribute to tissue repair not only through tissue replacement, but also through the delivery of wound healing promoting cytokines and growth factors inside exosomes [69, 70]. These factors include vascular endothelial growth factor (VEGF), transforming growth factor-β1 (TGF-β1), interleukin-6 (IL-6), interleukin-10 (IL-10), and hepatocyte growth factor (HGF) [69, 71]. Overall, these factors are able promote neovascularization, cell proliferation, and modulate immune responses. Thus, exosomes have been proposed as treatments for hair restoration and are currently being tested in clinical trials, as recently reviewed by Gupta et al. [72].

Research has shown that exosomes obtained from adipose-derived stem cells (ADSC) can promote hair follicle regeneration. For example, Wu et al. purified exosomes from murine ADSC using CD63, ALX1, and CD9 membrane markers [73]. Then, a mixture of dermal cells, epidermal cells, and ADSC exosomes were grafted into nude mice. Three weeks after transplantation the number of regenerated hairs was statistically higher in the group with ADSC exosomes compared to controls in which only dermal cells and epidermal cells were grafted [73]. A case series involving 39 androgenetic alopecia patients with mild to moderate hair loss, reported a significant improvement in hair thickness and hair density in the group that received ADSC exosome treatment [74]. Patients received a weekly application for 12 weeks of more than 6×10^{10} particles/vial of an ADSC exosome solution which was applied on the scalp area with a micro-needle roller [74]. Research has also demonstrated that exosomes secreted by 3D cultures of DP cells promoted the proliferation of human DP and ORS cells and increased hair shaft elongation and hair regeneration [75]. In a similar study, DP-derived mice exosomes were subcutaneously injected and the initiation of the HF anagen phase was stimulated, promoting the proliferation and migration of ORS cells [76]. Exosomes released from human ORS [77], DP cells [78], and myeloid-derived suppressor cells [79] have also been reported to regulate HF growth and development.

Exosomes present in platelet-rich plasma (PRP) have also been proposed, however, a recent study suggests that ADSC derived exosomes are more effective inducing hair proliferation *in vitro* [80]. Nonetheless, more studies are needed addressing hair regeneration abilities of exosomes from PRP. Other studies have focused on identifying the exosomal molecules that influence hair regeneration, for example, miRNAs. miRNAs are small non-coding RNA molecules (~22 nucleotides) that have a role in the regulation of gene expression by directly binding mRNAs in a sequence-specific manner [81]. Exosomal miRNAs that enhance HF growth and regeneration have been described, for example miR-218-5p [82], miR-181a-3p [83].

Overall, there is scarce information regarding the safety of exosome treatment in patients with hair disorders. Several preclinical studies examining the use of exosomes for hair growth have shown favorable outcomes. However, exosomes are currently not approved by the U.S. Food and Drug Administration (FDA) for treating hair disorders. Exosomes are also being studied for drug delivery and as novel biomarkers of disease. However, a better understanding of how they are released into circulation, how they transit body fluids and how their cargoes change in various physiological contexts is still under research.

Conclusions

The HF is a dynamic organ in which cells are replenished cyclically through controlled regulation of stem cell proliferation, migration, lineage commitment, and terminal differentiation. The cell subpopulations of the HF are highly diverse, and they undergo changes in cell states as they progress from stem cells to progenitors and finally to specialized keratinocytes. These states are tightly regulated by intrinsic mechanisms as well as by signals from the extracellular environment, for example, communication with other cells. Transcriptomic profiling with single-cell resolution has allowed the identification of numerous cell subpopulations and states in the anagen and telogen phases of the hair cycle both in mouse and human. Furthermore, researchers have found genes enriched for each cell subpopulation, allowing the development of molecular atlases containing expression profiles and spatial locations. A bigger number of cell subpopulations was discovered in the mouse HF model, compared to human, potentially due to a lower depth of coverage. Therefore, more scRNA-seq studies of human HFs are needed. Furthermore, studies integrating other omics with single cell resolution will also become important.

Research demonstrates that cells in the anagen HF undergo multistep differentiation programs and they exit the cell cycle upon an induction to intermediate progenitors. Similarly, in the telogen phase, HF cells transition along a differentiation trajectory and a proximal-distal axis. Overall, scRNA-seq HF studies are confirming that the hair cycle is a result of a complex interplay between cellular types and states. Understanding this diversity will help us understand the cell subpopulations involved in hair disorders as well as the interplay between them, allowing the emergence of novel therapeutic targets. These findings will help us understand dysregulated pathways in hair and skin disorders as well as in aging.

References

1. Sieber-Blum M, Grim M, Hu YF, Szeder V. Pluripotent neural crest stem cells in the adult hair follicle. Dev Dyn. 2004;231(2):258–69.
2. Christiano AM. Epithelial stem cells: stepping out of their niche. Cell. 2004;118(5):530–2.
3. Schmidt-Ullrich R, Paus R. Molecular principles of hair follicle induction and morphogenesis. BioEssays. 2005;27(3):247–61.
4. Alonso L, Fuchs E. The hair cycle. J Cell Sci. 2006;119(Pt 3):391–3.
5. Yang H, Adam RC, Ge Y, Hua ZL, Fuchs E. Epithelial-mesenchymal micro-niches govern stem cell lineage choices. Cell. 2017;169(3):483–496.e13.
6. Salzer MC, Lafzi A, Berenguer-Llergo A, Youssif C, Castellanos A, Solanas G, et al. Identity noise and adipogenic traits characterize dermal fibroblast aging. Cell. 2018;175(6):1575–1590.e22.
7. Philippeos C, Telerman SB, Oulès B, Pisco AO, Shaw TJ, Elgueta R, et al. Spatial and single-cell transcriptional profiling identifies functionally distinct human dermal fibroblast subpopulations. J Invest Dermatol. 2018;138(4):811–25.
8. Ghahramani A, Donati G, Luscombe NM, Watt FM. Epidermal Wnt signalling regulates transcriptome heterogeneity and proliferative fate in neighbouring cells. Genome Biol. 2018;19(1):3.
9. Cheng JB, Sedgewick AJ, Finnegan AI, Harirchian P, Lee J, Kwon S, et al. Transcriptional programming of normal and inflamed human epidermis at single-cell resolution. Cell Rep. 2018;25(4):871–83.
10. Schneider MR, Schmidt-Ullrich R, Paus R. The hair follicle as a dynamic miniorgan. Curr Biol. 2009;19(3):R132–42.
11. Kalabusheva EP, Shtompel AS, Rippa AL, Ulianov SV, Razin SV, Vorotelyak EA. A kaleidoscope of keratin gene expression and the mosaic of its regulatory mechanisms. Int J Mol Sci. 2023;24(6):5603.
12. Krause K, Foitzik K. Biology of the hair follicle: the basics. Semin Cutan Med Surg. 2006;25(1):2–10.
13. Paus R, Foitzik K. In search of the 'hair cycle clock': a guided tour. Differentiation. 2004;72(9–10):489–511.
14. Stenn KS, Paus R. Controls of hair follicle cycling. Physiol Rev. 2001;81(1):449–94.
15. Cotsarelis G, Sun TT, Lavker RM. Label-retaining cells reside in the bulge area of pilosebaceous unit: implications for follicular stem cells, hair cycle, and skin carcinogenesis. Cell. 1990;61(7):1329–37.
16. Wilson C, Cotsarelis G, Wei ZG, Fryer E, Margolis-Fryer J, Ostead M, et al. Cells within the bulge region of mouse hair follicle transiently proliferate during early anagen: heterogeneity and functional differences of various hair cycles. Differentiation. 1994;55(2):127–36.
17. Ito M, Kizawa K, Hamada K, Cotsarelis G. Hair follicle stem cells in the lower bulge form the secondary germ, a biochemically distinct but functionally equivalent progenitor cell population, at the termination of catagen. Differentiation. 2004;72(9–10):548–57.
18. Panteleyev AA, Jahoda CA, Christiano AM. Hair follicle predetermination. J Cell Sci. 2001;114(Pt 19):3419–31.
19. Joost S, Jacob T, Sun X, Annusver K, La Manno G, Sur I, et al. Single-cell transcriptomics of traced epidermal and hair follicle stem cells reveals rapid adaptations during wound healing. Cell Rep. 2018;25(3):585–597.e7.
20. Page ME, Lombard P, Ng F, Göttgens B, Jensen KB. The epidermis comprises autonomous compartments maintained by distinct stem cell populations. Cell Stem Cell. 2013;13(4):471–82.

21. Füllgrabe A, Joost S, Are A, Jacob T, Sivan U, Haegebarth A, et al. Dynamics of Lgr6[+] progenitor cells in the hair follicle, sebaceous gland, and interfollicular epidermis. Stem Cell Rep. 2015;5(5):843–55.
22. Brownell I, Guevara E, Bai CB, Loomis CA, Joyner AL. Nerve-derived sonic hedgehog defines a niche for hair follicle stem cells capable of becoming epidermal stem cells. Cell Stem Cell. 2011;8(5):552–65.
23. Ito M, Liu Y, Yang Z, Nguyen J, Liang F, Morris RJ, et al. Stem cells in the hair follicle bulge contribute to wound repair but not to homeostasis of the epidermis. Nat Med. 2005;11(12):1351–4.
24. Jang WJ, Song SH, Son T, Bae JW, Lee S, Jeong CH. Identification of potential biomarkers for diagnosis of patients with methamphetamine use disorder. Int J Mol Sci. 2023;24(10):8672.
25. Mortazavi A, Williams BA, McCue K, Schaeffer L, Wold B. Mapping and quantifying mammalian transcriptomes by RNA-Seq. Nat Methods. 2008;5(7):621–8.
26. Kiani MT, Higgins CA, Almquist BD. The hair follicle: an underutilized source of cells and materials for regenerative medicine. ACS Biomater Sci Eng. 2018;4(4):1193–207.
27. Cuevas-Diaz Duran R, Wei H, Wu JQ. Single-cell RNA-sequencing of the brain. Clin Transl Med. 2017;6(1):20.
28. Wei H, Wu X, Withrow J, Cuevas-Diaz Duran R, Singh S, Chaboub LS, et al. Glial progenitor heterogeneity and key regulators revealed by single-cell RNA sequencing provide insight to regeneration in spinal cord injury. Cell Rep. 2023;42(5):112486.
29. Mereu E, Lafzi A, Moutinho C, Ziegenhain C, McCarthy DJ, Álvarez-Varela A, et al. Benchmarking single-cell RNA-sequencing protocols for cell atlas projects. Nat Biotechnol. 2020;38(6):747–55.
30. Aizarani N, Saviano A, Sagar, Mailly L, Durand S, Herman JS, et al. A human liver cell atlas reveals heterogeneity and epithelial progenitors. Nature. 2019;572(7768):199–204.
31. Montoro DT, Haber AL, Biton M, Vinarsky V, Lin B, Birket SE, et al. A revised airway epithelial hierarchy includes CFTR-expressing ionocytes. Nature. 2018;560(7718):319–24.
32. Tanay A, Regev A. Scaling single-cell genomics from phenomenology to mechanism. Nature. 2017;541(7637):331–8.
33. Sandberg R. Entering the era of single-cell transcriptomics in biology and medicine. Nat Methods. 2014;11(1):22–4.
34. Camp JG, Treutlein B. Human organomics: a fresh approach to understanding human development using single-cell transcriptomics. Development. 2017;144(9):1584–7.
35. Regev A, Teichmann SA, Lander ES, Amit I, Benoist C, Birney E, et al. The human cell atlas. elife. 2017;5:6.
36. Takahashi R, Grzenda A, Allison TF, Rawnsley J, Balin SJ, Sabri S, et al. Defining transcriptional signatures of human hair follicle cell states. J Invest Dermatol. 2020;140(4):764–773.e4.
37. Jaks V, Barker N, Kasper M, van Es JH, Snippert HJ, Clevers H, et al. Lgr5 marks cycling, yet long-lived, hair follicle stem cells. Nat Genet. 2008;40(11):1291–9.
38. Lafzi A, Moutinho C, Picelli S, Heyn H. Tutorial: guidelines for the experimental design of single-cell RNA sequencing studies. Nat Protoc. 2018;13(12):2742–57.
39. Messenger AG, Elliott K, Westgate GE, Gibson WT. Distribution of extracellular matrix molecules in human hair follicles. Ann N Y Acad Sci. 1991;642:253–62.
40. Topouzi H, Logan NJ, Williams G, Higgins CA. Methods for the isolation and 3D culture of dermal papilla cells from human hair follicles. Exp Dermatol. 2017;26(6):491–6.
41. Gledhill K, Gardner A, Jahoda CAB. Isolation and establishment of hair follicle dermal papilla cell cultures. Methods Mol Biol. 2013;989:285–92.
42. Magerl M, Kauser S, Paus R, Tobin DJ. Simple and rapid method to isolate and culture follicular papillae from human scalp hair follicles. Exp Dermatol. 2002;11(4):381–5.
43. Wu JJ, Liu RQ, Lu YG, Zhu TY, Cheng B, Men X. Enzyme digestion to isolate and culture human scalp dermal papilla cells: a more efficient method. Arch Dermatol Res. 2005;297(2):60–7.
44. Joost S, Zeisel A, Jacob T, Sun X, La Manno G, Lönnerberg P, et al. Single-cell transcriptomics reveals that differentiation and spatial signatures shape epidermal and hair follicle heterogeneity. Cell Syst. 2016;3(3):221–237.e9.
45. Joost S, Annusver K, Jacob T, Sun X, Dalessandri T, Sivan U, et al. The molecular anatomy of mouse skin during hair growth and rest. Cell Stem Cell. 2020;26(3):441–457.e7.
46. Sequeira I, Nicolas JF. Redefining the structure of the hair follicle by 3D clonal analysis. Development. 2012;139(20):3741–51.
47. Mesler AL, Veniaminova NA, Lull MV, Wong SY. Hair follicle terminal differentiation is orchestrated by distinct early and late matrix progenitors. Cell Rep. 2017;19(4):809–21.
48. Marx V. Method of the Year: spatially resolved transcriptomics. Nat Methods. 2021;18(1):9–14.
49. Ståhl PL, Salmén F, Vickovic S, Lundmark A, Navarro JF, Magnusson J, et al. Visualization and analysis of gene expression in tissue sections by spatial transcriptomics. Science. 2016;353(6294):78–82.
50. Merritt CR, Ong GT, Church SE, Barker K, Danaher P, Geiss G, et al. Multiplex digital spatial profiling of proteins and RNA in fixed tissue. Nat Biotechnol. 2020;38(5):586–99.
51. Stickels RR, Murray E, Kumar P, Li J, Marshall JL, Di Bella DJ, et al. Highly sensitive spatial transcriptomics at near-cellular resolution with Slide-seqV2. Nat Biotechnol. 2021;39(3):313–9.

52. Shi H, He Y, Zhou Y, Huang J, Maher K, Wang B, et al. Spatial atlas of the mouse central nervous system at molecular resolution. Nature. 2023;622(7983):552–61.
53. Lohoff T, Ghazanfar S, Missarova A, Koulena N, Pierson N, Griffiths JA, et al. Integration of spatial and single-cell transcriptomic data elucidates mouse organogenesis. Nat Biotechnol. 2022;40(1):74–85.
54. Vanrobaeys Y, Mukherjee U, Langmack L, Beyer SE, Bahl E, Lin LC, et al. Mapping the spatial transcriptomic signature of the hippocampus during memory consolidation. Nat Commun. 2023;14(1):6100.
55. Wang C, McNutt M, Ma A, Fu H, Ma Q. ssREAD: a single-cell and spatial RNA-seq database for Alzheimer's disease. bioRxiv. 2023.
56. Parigi SM, Larsson L, Das S, Ramirez Flores RO, Frede A, Tripathi KP, et al. The spatial transcriptomic landscape of the healing mouse intestine following damage. Nat Commun. 2022;13(1):828.
57. Shim J, Park J, Abudureyimu G, Kim MH, Shim JS, Jang KT, et al. Comparative spatial transcriptomic and single-cell analyses of human nail units and hair follicles show transcriptional similarities between the onychodermis and follicular dermal papilla. J Invest Dermatol. 2022;142(12):3146–3157.e12.
58. Allis CD, Jenuwein T. The molecular hallmarks of epigenetic control. Nat Rev Genet. 2016;17(8):487–500.
59. Virolainen SJ, VonHandorf A, Viel KCMF, Weirauch MT, Kottyan LC. Gene-environment interactions and their impact on human health. Genes Immun. 2023;24(1):1–11.
60. Giacoman-Lozano M, Meléndez-Ramírez C, Martinez-Ledesma E, Cuevas-Diaz Duran R, Velasco I. Epigenetics of neural differentiation: spotlight on enhancers. Front Cell Dev Biol. 2022;10:1001701.
61. Gasperini M, Tome JM, Shendure J. Towards a comprehensive catalogue of validated and target-linked human enhancers. Nat Rev Genet. 2020;21(5):292–310.
62. Buenrostro JD, Wu B, Litzenburger UM, Ruff D, Gonzales ML, Snyder MP, et al. Single-cell chromatin accessibility reveals principles of regulatory variation. Nature. 2015;523(7561):486–90.
63. Yadav T, Quivy JP, Almouzni G. Chromatin plasticity: a versatile landscape that underlies cell fate and identity. Science. 2018;361(6409):1332–6.
64. Adam RC, Yang H, Ge Y, Lien WH, Wang P, Zhao Y, et al. Temporal layering of signaling effectors drives chromatin remodeling during hair follicle stem cell lineage progression. Cell Stem Cell. 2018;22(3):398–413.e7.
65. Ober-Reynolds B, Wang C, Ko JM, Rios EJ, Aasi SZ, Davis MM, et al. Integrated single-cell chromatin and transcriptomic analyses of human scalp identify gene-regulatory programs and critical cell types for hair and skin diseases. Nat Genet. 2023;55(8):1288–300.
66. van Niel G, Carter DRF, Clayton A, Lambert DW, Raposo G, Vader P. Challenges and directions in studying cell-cell communication by extracellular vesicles. Nat Rev Mol Cell Biol. 2022;23(5):369–82.
67. Jiang X, You L, Zhang Z, Cui X, Zhong H, Sun X, et al. Biological properties of milk-derived extracellular vesicles and their physiological functions in infant. Front Cell Dev Biol. 2021;9:693534.
68. Pittenger MF, Discher DE, Péault BM, Phinney DG, Hare JM, Caplan AI. Mesenchymal stem cell perspective: cell biology to clinical progress. NPJ Regen Med. 2019;4:22.
69. An Y, Lin S, Tan X, Zhu S, Nie F, Zhen Y, et al. Exosomes from adipose-derived stem cells and application to skin wound healing. Cell Prolif. 2021;54(3):e12993.
70. Kim HJ, Kim G, Lee J, Lee Y, Kim JH. Secretome of stem cells: roles of extracellular vesicles in diseases, stemness, differentiation, and reprogramming. Tissue Eng Regen Med. 2022;19(1):19–33.
71. Zhou C, Zhang B, Yang Y, Jiang Q, Li T, Gong J, et al. Stem cell-derived exosomes: emerging therapeutic opportunities for wound healing. Stem Cell Res Ther. 2023;14(1):107.
72. Gupta AK, Wang T, Rapaport JA. Systematic review of exosome treatment in hair restoration: preliminary evidence, safety, and future directions. J Cosmet Dermatol. 2023;22(9):2424–33.
73. Wu J, Yang Q, Wu S, Yuan R, Zhao X, Li Y, et al. Adipose-derived stem cell exosomes promoted hair regeneration. Tissue Eng Regen Med. 2021;18(4):685–91.
74. Park BS, Choi HI, Huh G, Kim WS. Effects of exosome from adipose-derived stem cell on hair loss: a retrospective analysis of 39 patients. J Cosmet Dermatol. 2022;21(5):2282–4.
75. Kwack MH, Seo CH, Gangadaran P, Ahn BC, Kim MK, Kim JC, et al. Exosomes derived from human dermal papilla cells promote hair growth in cultured human hair follicles and augment the hair-inductive capacity of cultured dermal papilla spheres. Exp Dermatol. 2019;28(7):854–7.
76. Zhou L, Wang H, Jing J, Yu L, Wu X, Lu Z. Regulation of hair follicle development by exosomes derived from dermal papilla cells. Biochem Biophys Res Commun. 2018;500(2):325–32.
77. Nilforoushzadeh MA, Aghdami N, Taghiabadi E. Human hair outer root sheath cells and platelet-lysis exosomes promote hair inductivity of dermal papilla cell. Tissue Eng Regen Med. 2020;17(4):525–36.
78. le Riche A, Aberdam E, Marchand L, Frank E, Jahoda C, Petit I, et al. Extracellular vesicles from activated dermal fibroblasts stimulate hair follicle growth through dermal papilla-secreted norrin. Stem Cells. 2019;37(9):1166–75.
79. Zöller M, Zhao K, Kutlu N, Bauer N, Provaznik J, Hackert T, et al. Immunoregulatory effects of myeloid-derived suppressor cell exosomes in mouse model of autoimmune alopecia areata. Front Immunol. 2018;9:1279.

80. Nilforoushzadeh MA, Aghdami N, Taghiabadi E. Effects of adipose-derived stem cells and platelet-rich plasma exosomes on the inductivity of hair dermal papilla cells. Cell J. 2021;23(5):576–83.
81. Bartel DP. MicroRNAs: genomics, biogenesis, mechanism, and function. Cell. 2004;116(2):281–97.
82. Hu S, Li Z, Lutz H, Huang K, Su T, Cores J, et al. Dermal exosomes containing miR-218-5p promote hair regeneration by regulating β-catenin signaling. Sci Adv. 2020;6(30):eaba1685.
83. Zhao B, Li J, Zhang X, Dai Y, Yang N, Bao Z, et al. Exosomal miRNA-181a-5p from the cells of the hair follicle dermal papilla promotes the hair follicle growth and development via the Wnt/β-catenin signaling pathway. Int J Biol Macromol. 2022;207:110–20.

Hair Follicle Cloning and Stem Cells

11

Anastasakis Konstantinos

Basic Concepts

- The domain of Biomedical Engineering has witnessed significant advancements throughout the twenty-first century, notably following the discovery that adult body stem cells exhibit trans-differentiation capabilities, allowing them to differentiate into various cell types beyond their germline lineage or originating tissue.
- The utilization of human hair follicle cells to stimulate novel hair growth is termed hair follicle neogenesis, posited as the ultimate remedy for AGA/FPHL.
- Hair follicle (HF) neogenesis represents the third tier of complexity within Biomedical Engineering, necessitating intricate, three-dimensional organization to develop fully functional follicular constituents.
- While HF neogenesis has been realized in vivo solely within animal models, their reliability and predictability are compromised by formidable technical challenges. Conversely, employing stem cells to augment existing hair has yielded outcomes just comparable to topical Minoxidil.
- Regrettably, outcomes from hair growth cell cultures fail to mirror realistic scenarios of human application, and the neogenesis of human follicles derived from cultured HF dermal cells remains unattained.
- Presently, three therapeutic mechanisms concerning HF regeneration through stem cell utilization are identified: reversing the pathogenesis of hair loss (particularly in AGA/FPHL), regenerating HFs with "bulge" stem cells, and inducing HF neogenesis from stem cell cultures.
- The process of reversing the pathological mechanism of AGA/FPHL may predominantly rely on the secretion of bioactive factors, such as growth factors and cytokines, capable of inducing hair follicle stem cells (HFSCs) within their natural environment. Essentially, stem cells can secrete these factors to initiate repair cascades for host-site damage through paracrine effects. Considering that adipose-derived stem cells (ADSCs) represent one of the most accessible sources of MSCs, proteins derived from ADSCs could serve as viable clinical therapeutic agents for treating hair loss.
- Stem cell transplantation for the production of hair follicles, whether conducted in vitro or in vivo, presents several challenges. It is a costly procedure with uncertain safety implications, including concerns regarding potential tumorigenicity. Moreover, maintaining the induction properties of dermal papilla cells in culture is problematic, and the implantation process is exceptionally challenging. Addi-

A. Konstantinos (✉)
Anastasakis Hair Clinic, Athens, Attiki, Greece

P. J. Panagotacos, H. Maibach (eds.), *Hair Loss*, Updates in Clinical Dermatology,
https://doi.org/10.1007/978-3-031-74314-6_11

tionally, unresolved ethical issues further complicate matters.
- Despite recent advancements, the clinical application of tissue engineering strategies for treating hair loss remain elusive. Notably, the successful neogenesis of human follicles from cultured HF dermal cells has yet to be achieved.

Hair Cloning

Throughout the initial decades of the new millennium, there has been an unparalleled interest in the role of stem cells within the realms of Regenerative Medicine and Biomedical Engineering. Within the domain of hair follicle disorders, the concept of manipulating human hair follicle cells to stimulate hair growth is commonly referred to as "hair follicle neogenesis," "folliculo-neogenesis," or "hair cloning." Many regard it as the sole viable solution to address the constraints of limited donor supply in hair restoration surgery and to mitigate excessive scarring in donor areas resulting from harvesting procedures. Stem cells appear to be pivotal in unlocking the potential of hair follicle cloning, and since the early 1990's, the promise of hair cloning always seems to be 5 years away, into a never-reached horizon.

What Are the Stem Cells?

Prof. Cotsarelis argues that perhaps the simplest definition of an epithelial stem cell is based on lineage: a stem cell is the cell of origin for terminally differentiated cells in adult tissues [1].

However, the definition of stem cells must rely on functional, not on morphological attributes. Functionally, a stem cell represents an undifferentiated cell that is able to produce a progeny of other stem cells (self-renewal), or one that can divide asymmetrically into another stem cell (thereby retaining its undifferentiated status) and a transient amplifying cell, which has lost its capacity for unlimited self-renewal and differentiates down a specific pathway [2]. Tissues with self-renewal capacity, such as the epidermis and hair follicles, undergo continuous cell regeneration to replace the shedding squames and hairs relying on stem cells.

The most captivating aspect of stem cells lies in their remarkable plasticity. Stem cell "transdifferentiation," often synonymous with "plasticity," describes the phenomenon wherein stem cells can transition across germ lines and differentiate into a diverse array of cell types distinct from their germ lineage or originating tissue. Examples include adult bone marrow-derived mesenchymal stem cells (MSCs) differentiating into various skin cell types, adipose-derived stem cells (ADSCs) transforming into hepatocytes, and dermal stem cells giving rise to neurons, capable of migrating into the spinal cord following traumatic injury in rats [3].

Therefore, for a cell to be considered as a stem cell, three requirements must be met:

1. Self-renewal,
2. Ability to differentiate into multiple cell types,
3. Ability to restore tissues in vivo.

The exploration of stem cell applications initially focused on embryonic cells; however, due to legal and ethical considerations, researchers swiftly shifted their attention to alternative sources. Cutaneous MSCs emerged as a promising alternative, possessing multipotent capabilities unlike pluripotent embryonic stem cells, which can differentiate into all derivatives of the three primary germ layers: ectoderm, endoderm, and mesoderm. MSCs demonstrate the capacity to develop into various cell types, including smooth muscle cells, adipocytes, osteocytes, glial cells, and neurons, thus addressing previous limitations.

How Could We Use Stem Cells in Hair Follicle Disorders?

Cutaneous MSCs research traces back to a study by Toma et al., who isolated multipotent adult stem cells from the dermis [4] and showcased that the transplantation of MSCs derived from adipose tissue, bone marrow, and umbilical cord blood could facilitate hair follicle regeneration within the skin.

The concept of stem cell-based therapies to generate new hair follicles holds significant theoretical promise. The proposed model initially isolates hair follicles from the occipital scalp of patients with AGA/FPHL. Subsequently, folliculo-neogenesis could hypothetically be achieved through one or more of the following approaches:

1. Isolation, culture, and implantation of stem cells into the scalp, leading to their integration into existing miniaturized hair follicles, directing them towards a different morphology (morphogenic switch model). This process could potentially reverse the pathogenesis of hair loss resulting from disease, injury, or aging (Fig. 11.1)
2. Isolation, culture, and implantation of stem cells or follicular fragments into bald scalp areas, facilitating the generation of new hair follicles in situ (full-neogenesis model) (Fig. 11.1). This approach may involve harvesting a small portion of the non-balding scalp, micro-dissecting the stem cells, amplifying them in vitro, and implanting them into balding areas [6]
3. De novo formation of hair follicles in vitro for implantation into the scalp as fully functional organs (proto-hair model), either with or without external support, using established hair transplantation techniques (Fig. 11.2)

However, each of these ideas faces major obstacles. A primary challenge is the loss of hair follicle-inducing ability in cultured dermal papilla cells (DPCs). Additionally, concerns exist regarding the appearance of "cloned hairs," including their color, size, alignment, and curl. Moreover, follicles must be induced to grow in specific directions to ensure proper angulation, direction, and density for their position on the scalp [7]. Other critical considerations include long-term safety concerns related to the tumorigenic potential of stem cells and the financial feasibility of the method. Cloning hair follicles is an amazingly tough challenge, after all.

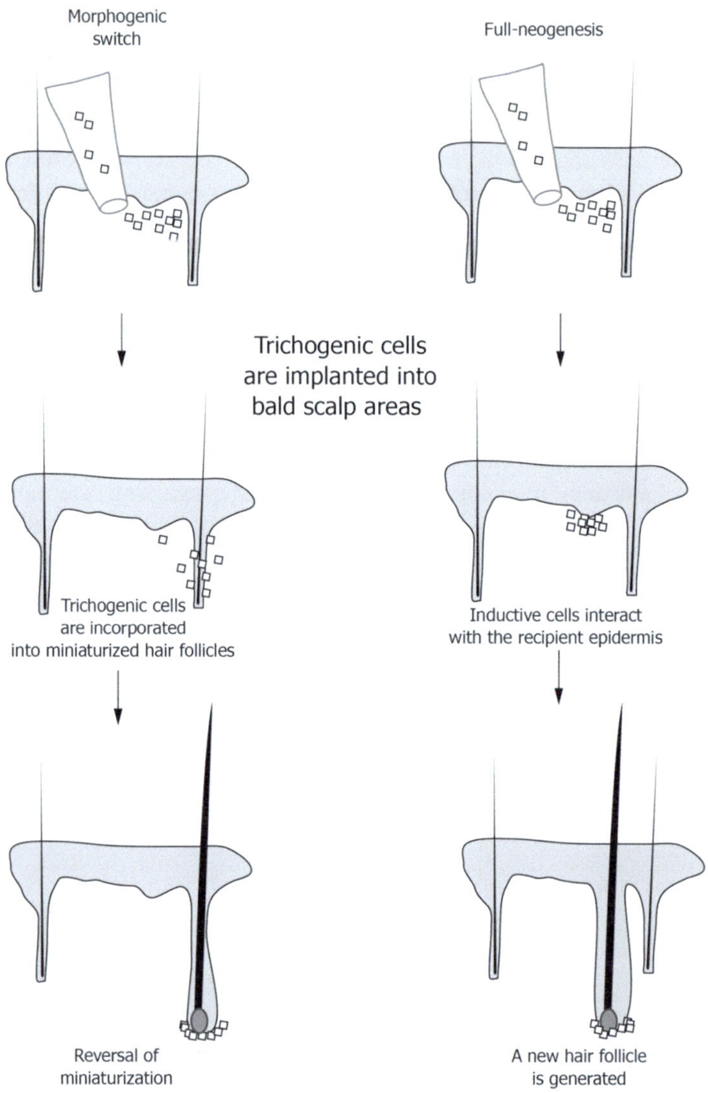

Fig. 11.1 Diagrammatic representation of the concept underlying full-neogenesis and morphogenic switch. (adapted from Stenn et al. [2]) (**a**) Trichogenic cells are implanted into bald areas of the scalp and assimilate into miniaturized hair follicles, prompting them to produce significant, terminal follicles (morphogenic switch), (**b**) Trichogenic cells are implanted into bald areas of the scalp; the inductive cells interact with the recipient epidermis to generate a follicle in a pattern similar to that observed in the fetus (full-neogenesis) (from [5], used with permission)

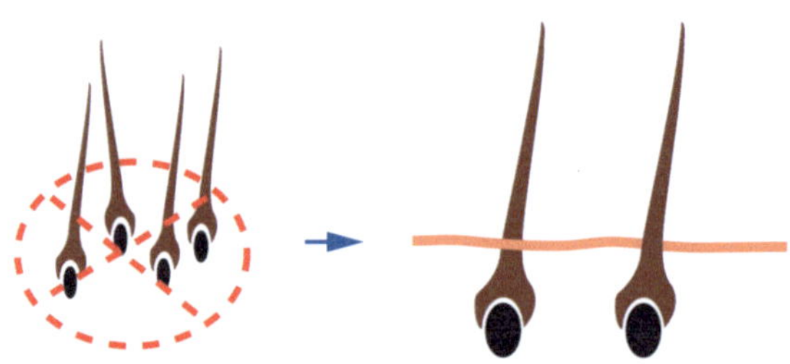

Fig. 11.2 Trichogenic cells are cultured, and hair follicles are produced in vitro (proto-hairs), with or without external support, which are subsequently implanted into bald areas of the scalp using established hair transplantation techniques (from [5], used with permission)

Basic Embryology and Anatomy of Hair Follicles

The development and regeneration of hair follicles are widely understood to arise from intricate molecular interactions between the follicular epithelium and the mesenchymal DPCs. A finely tuned series of reciprocal and sequential interactions between these two components is indispensable for hair follicle morphogenesis [8].

Generally, dermal cells are regarded as inducers, while epithelial cells act as responders in hair follicle formation. The signaling between these cell types is reciprocal and highly complex [9]. Interestingly, despite originating from mammalian species with a common ancestor older than 120 million years ago, how hair-forming cells generate a hair follicle organ exhibits remarkable similarity, earning it the descriptor "universal [10, 11].

Epithelial-mesenchymal interaction is a prerequisite for functional HF formation, regeneration, and cycling, mainly through paracrine mechanisms, and has become the theoretical basis of tissue engineering for HF regeneration. Current strategies to regenerate HF in vivo are aimed at simulating these interactions, mostly adopting the principle of combining epithelial and mesenchymal DPCs and skin-derived precursor components [12].

Understanding the steps of follicle morphogenesis, identifying signaling molecules, cultivating stem cells, and creating components of hair follicles in vitro represent significant accomplishments. However, orchestrating the intricate molecular interactions necessary for the development of a viable hair follicle presents a challenge of an entirely different magnitude.

Levels of Complexity

Recent progress in stem cell biology has enabled significant advancements in generating mature organs from dissociated cells, such as the intestine [13], mammary gland [14], and tooth [15]. These achievements suggest potential clinical applications in the near future [11]. However, transitioning stem cells into regenerative medicine products faces challenges due to the varying levels of morphological complexity and unique barriers to research [16]:

1. Bone marrow stem cells, already in clinical use, represent the first level of complexity, as blood cells do not require spatial organization and can function upon release into the bloodstream.
2. Tissues secreting molecules like insulin and dopamine represent the second level of complexity. While topological organization is not critical, strict regulation of molecule synthesis and secretion is essential.
3. Tissues where cell morphology, structure, and organization are critical, such as skin, cartilage, and bone, represent the third complexity level.
4. The most complex tissues/organs require proper architecture and functional integration, as seen in cardiac systems and neural circuits.

Normal skin regeneration involves various cell types derived from two germ layers giving rise to multiple cell types. However, these cells require additional tissue interaction and anatomical orientation to function properly, adding significant complexity [15] to the process. Hair follicle bioengineering is of the third order of complexity in organ regeneration because a complex three-dimensional organization is required to promote fully functional tissue appendages.

Tiny But Mighty

The hair follicle, despite its small size and non-essential function for life, has often been erroneously perceived as a simple structure. However, this simplicity is utterly deceptive. In reality, even though the hair follicle is readily accessible in the human body, it is a complex and multicellular mini-organ that shares biological complexities with larger and more significant organs. Consequently, the scientific inquiries and obstacles in engineering a hair follicle closely resemble those encountered when engineering other tissues and organs [1, 2]. In fact, some of the most noteworthy current research on epithelial-mesenchymal interactions and adult organ formation is being conducted using the hair follicle as a model [17–19].

What Kind of Hair Follicles Do We Need to Create?

Chuong and Cotsarelis [20] outlined the essential criteria for engineering hair follicles for human hair restoration:

1. Proximal end with follicle configuration, an epithelial filament coming out of the distal end of the follicle, and a DP sitting at the base of the follicle,
2. Proximal-distal growth mode with proliferating and differentiating cells positioned distally,
3. Concentric layers of outer and inner root sheaths, cuticle, cortex, and medulla,
4. Hair shaft with unique molecular constitution,
5. Association with a sebaceous gland,
6. Machinery for shedding old shaft while preserving stem cells and DPCs for the next hair cycle,
7. Inherent ability to regenerate a new hair organ through repeated cycles.

Meeting all these criteria is necessary for a bioengineered product to be rightfully named a "hair follicle." Failure of any of these events will lead to disrupted hair-follicle structures, resulting in various degrees of incomplete hair follicle formation.

Trichogenic Cell Assays: The Test Field of Folliculo-Neogenesis

Trichogenic cell assays have been used for decades to understand how dissociated cells interact to assemble a hair follicle. Trichogenic cell assays assess isolated cell populations' hair-inductive properties. Various in vivo tissue and cellular recombination assays, using same-species (allograft) or trans-species (xenograft) models, have been used to investigate hair follicle regeneration.

Despite the large variety of trichogenic cell assays reported in the literature, all assays are based on the same principle: combining responder epithelial cells with inducer mesenchymal cells, all placed into a permissive environment [21]. Epidermal stem or progenitor cells can originate from various sources, including embryonic stem cells, engineered embryonic stem cells or cell lines, interfollicular epidermal stem cells, bulge stem cells, ADSCs, or bone marrow stem cells.

As far back as the 1960s, researchers demonstrated that whole follicle bulbs and isolated whisker papillae remained viable and produced hair follicles in new sites [22]. The trichogenic capacity of DPCs in mature hair follicles was experimentally shown in seminal studies by Oliver et al. and Jahoda et al., using adult rat vibrissa or whisker follicles [23–25]. Several trichogenic assays have since been reported [26]:

- The "wound assay" involves inserting freshly prepared or cultured DPCs into a small incision in the skin to reconstitute hair follicles [27].
- The "chamber assay used suspensions of fresh or cultured DPCs and neonatal rat epidermal cells into a transparent chamber on the dorsal skin of nude mice [28, 29]. Because hair shaft growth is apparent upon visual inspection, the chamber assay has been widely used to examine the ability of epithelial and/or mesenchymal cells to induce hair growth [30–32].
- The "sandwich assay" prepares a complex by inserting DPCs between enzymatically-treated epidermis and dermis fragments, transplanted into subcutaneous tissue [33, 34] or under the kidney capsule [35, 36].
- The "flap assay" uses a sandwiched construct with an epidermis fragment and dermal side of a skin flap [37] to induce regenerated hair follicles [38].
- The "hair patch assay" involves injecting mixed epithelial cells and DPCs subcutaneously or under the kidney capsule [39, 40].

- Variation includes using freshly isolated bulge cells combined with neonatal dermal cells to form hair follicles after injection into immunodeficient mice1 [41, 42].

According to Prof. Cotsarelis, these studies provided proof of concept that isolated stem cells could be a part of tissue-engineering approaches for treating AGA/FPHL [1].

In addition to hDPCs and bulge cells, dermal stem cells (DSCs) also exhibit hair-inductive properties, particularly in adult hair follicles. Early studies by Oliver in the 1960s demonstrated that when the end-bulb or the DP alone was surgically removed from the follicular bulb, a new DP formed [23], suggesting that DSCs contributed to DP reconstitution [43, 44]. The hair inductive capacity of DSCs was further demonstrated by implanting micro-dissected DSCs into the upper half of rat vibrissa follicles [45], resulting in shaft elongation and DP regeneration from the implanted DSCs [23].

In a seminal study published in "Nature" by Reynolds et al. [46], DSCs from a male human scalp follicle implanted into the arm of a female co-worker led to the formation (or transformation) of a new hair follicle. These findings suggest that DSCs possess trichogenic activity akin to the DP. Moreover, the allotransplant experiment indicated that DSCs and the DP may evade immunological rejection, possibly due to a level of immune privilege, although they are unlikely to represent immune-privileged tissues themselves [47]. After all, follicular neogenesis might be more straightforward than initially considered.

Growth Factors and Stem Cells Might Be Enough

A goal of Biomedical Engineering approaches for treating AGA/FPHL involves augmenting the number of existing follicles. This can be achieved by amplifying keratinocyte and DPC numbers in vitro before transplantation. Stem cells can secrete growth factors and cytokines that can set forth vital signals for SC differentiation to keratinocytes that later secrete keratinocyte growth factor (KGF), an essential endogenous mediator of follicular growth, development, and differentiation.

Several other growth factors, such as Insulin Growth Factor-1 [48] and FGF-7 [49] have been reported to mediate the hair induction signaling pathways from DPCs to follicular epithelial cells. Wnt signaling is essential to embryonic morphogenesis and postnatal hair follicle neogenesis of hair follicles [50]. TGF-β2 is expressed in hair-inducing DPCs but not in dermal fibroblasts [51]. Alkaline phosphatase activity is highly maintained in hair-inducing DPCs [23], and both versican expression [27] and alkaline phosphatase activity [23] are gradually lost with culture expansion of DPCs. Bone morphogenetic protein (BMP)-6 [52] has been shown to enhance mouse hair folliculogenesis [53] among others.

Despite the progress made, there still needs to be a reliable biomarker for assessing the hair-inductive capacity of hDPCs. Animal models remain the primary method for evaluating this capacity. Throughout each morphogenetic stage, numerous elements serve as responsible molecules for the reciprocal signaling between the epithelial and dermal components of the hair follicle. However, in the context of follicular neogenesis, it remains unclear which signaling molecules among these pathways function in hair induction in transplanted DPCs [54]. Thus far, specific signaling molecules have been identified as candidates for hair-inducing activity through sophisticated transgenic approaches such as specific knockout or overexpression in vivo. Nevertheless, applying transgenic approaches in humans presents challenges, hindering studies on specific in vivo gene function [55].

Although various biomarkers specifically expressed in hDPCs have been reported [56, 57], their functions remain to be fully elucidated. Interestingly, ADSCs stimulate hair growth through the combined effects of diverse bioactive factors.

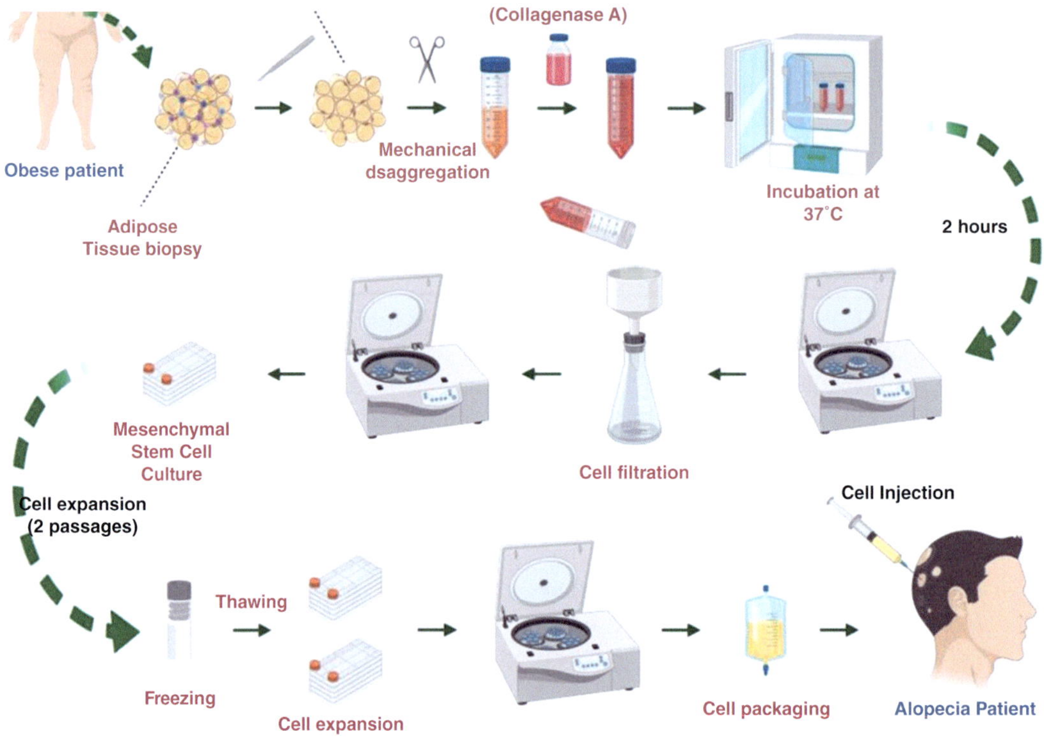

Fig. 11.3 Acquisition and generation of adipose tissue mesenchymal stem cells. Created with Biorender.com (from Martinez-Lopez et al. [58], used with permission)

Role of Mesenchymal Stem Cell Therapy and Adipose Tissue-Derived Stem Cells

Human mesenchymal stem cell (hMSC)-based therapies have been applied in regenerative medicine across various medical fields, including orthopedics, neurology, cardiology, and dermatology. Originating from the mesoderm (like the skin), hMSCs are well-suited for repairing and regenerating skin abnormalities due to their responsiveness to paracrine factors when implanted in damaged tissues [3, 58, 59] (Fig. 11.3).

Adipose-derived stem cells (ADSCs) [60], arising from multipotent stem cells within the adipose tissue, offer promising potential for regenerative medicine. They lack immunogenic properties, are easily obtained from subcutaneous fat [61], and demonstrate multi-lineage differentiation potential and angiogenic capabilities. ADSCs can display multi-lineage plasticity and share characteristics similar to those of bone marrow-derived MSCs [62]. Moreover, ADSCs have various cytokine-secreting properties and beneficial paracrine effects on surrounding cells or tissues [63]. The paracrine function is considered as one of the most important therapeutic benefits of therapy using MSCs [64–66], and more than 80% of the regenerative potential in transplanted stem cells is regulated through paracrine activities of paracrine factors.

ADSCs' paracrine action involves a complex interplay of secreted factors, collectively termed "secretomes," which include nucleic acids, extracellular vesicles (including exosomes), proteins, growth factors, and other molecules. These secreted factors, encoded by approximately 10% of the human genome, mediate inter-cellular communication [63, 67], and are released through various secretion mechanisms. When cultured stem cells' secretomes are present in a nutrient-rich medium, they form a stem cell-derived "conditioned medium" (CM), which has shown promising effects on human hair follicles in research studies.

Hair Growth-Stimulating Effects of ADSCs

Several studies have highlighted the ability of ADSCs to stimulate hair growth in both ex vivo and animal models by leveraging diverse bioactive factors [68, 69]. These factors work together to enhance the proliferation of DPCs through the activation of Erk and Akt signaling pathways, regulate the cell cycle of DPCs by increasing Cyclin D1 and CDK2 expression, and shield DPCs from damage caused by androgens and reactive oxygen species [70–72]. Additionally, secretory factors identified from ADSCs, including IGF binding protein precursors, PDGF, KGF, HGF, VEGF, and fibronectin [73, 74], have been shown to play crucial roles in stimulating hair growth [62].

Park et al. demonstrated that applying ADSCs in hair follicles can promote hair growth through a paracrine mechanism, further enhanced by hypoxia. Low oxygen concentrations (1–5%) have been found to increase the expression levels of various stem cell factors, including VEGF, basic FGF, IGF binding protein 1 (IGFBP-1), IGF binding protein 2 (IGFBP-2), macrophage colony-stimulating factor (M-CSF), M-CSF receptor (M-CSFR), and PDGF receptor β (PDGFR-β) [75].

All these exciting properties of ADSCs have allowed researchers to focus their efforts on this field and experiment with ADSCs in clinical practice. Actually, the field of ADSCs is the only one that has shown promising findings concerning hair growth in a fashion that is relevant to "traditional cloning" [67–72, 76–84].

The findings indicate that ADSCs enhance hair growth by boosting the proliferation of DPCs and potentially epithelial cells, thereby modulating the cell cycle and activating the anagen phase in hair cycles. Manipulating ADSCs holds promise for promoting hair growth; however, their efficacy has to surpass that of current FDA-approved drug therapies against hair loss to be considered a viable option. For a comprehensive understanding of the theory and practical applications of ADSCs in hair regrowth, interested readers can refer to recent extensive reviews on the subject by Owczarczyk-Saczonek et al. [85].

Research in Humans

Stem cell use for promoting hair growth in humans is currently restricted. Gentile et al. showcased the Rigeneracons® bioreactor's application in delivering autologous micrografts directly for clinical use [86]. Rigenera® technology retrieves mature autologous stem cells from patient biopsies through mechanical disintegration and tissue filtration.

The "Rigenera® procedure" complies with Regulation n.1394/2007 of the European Parliament (EC), which restricts extensively manipulated bioprocess engineering. Several studies [87–89] have explored this procedure, but they all suffer from severe methodological limitations. These include poor-quality before-and-after photos of patients with AGA, depicting minimum improvement, making it impossible to evaluate results properly. Additionally, the invasive nature of this procedure raises questions about its clinical applicability, given the controversial outcomes.

Studies comparing bone marrow-derived mononuclear cells (BMMCs) to follicular stem cells (FSCs) for treating resistant cases of Alopecia Areata (AA) and AGA [90], as well as ADSC-constituent extract (ADSC-CM) for AGA in men and FPHL [91], report optimistic findings. However, the full-text articles contain low-quality, small-size patient photos showing minimal improvement, casting doubt on the authors' claims.

ADSC-CM shows promise as a future hair regrowth modality, but it has limitations. The composition of factors in ADSC-CM can vary significantly, highlighting the need for standardization in its preparation to enhance clinical outcomes. Moreover, the rapid turnover and depletion of ADSC-CM factors in vivo may require large quantities and frequent application for efficacy.

According to the review by Egger et al. [60], more solid studies are encouraged for stem cell-based transplants and ADSC-CM in alopecias. Actually, several clinical trials are currently underway and are awaiting results (ClinicalTrials.gov Identifiers: NCT01673789, NCT02865421, NCT03078686, NCT02849470, NCT03676400, NCT03662854, NCT 01501617) [92–97].

Neogenesis of Hair Follicles by Tissue Engineering: The Holy Grail!

The trichogenic cell assays previously described have yielded valuable insights into the hair neogenesis process and the involved cells. However, challenges such as the high cell demand, the necessity for suitable animal models, and subpar results with human cellular sources currently hinder their clinical applicability.

New strategies focusing on tissue engineering-based follicle neogenesis have emerged to address these limitations. These innovative techniques, primarily centered on three-dimensional cell culture conditions facilitated by cells or biocompatible scaffolds [98, 99], have shown promise in various studies published in reputable journals. These studies demonstrate the potential of dissociated cells to form hair follicle germs or proto-hairs capable of generating mature hair follicles through ectopic and orthotopic implantation. Collectively, these findings support the feasibility of Follicular Cell Implantation for hair restoration in individuals with hair loss [100–105], with recent advancements involving the use of ADSCs and disaggregated cells.

However, the prospect of actual follicle bioengineering, often referred to as "hair cloning" in humans, remains a majestic topic of interest and exploration.

Folliculo-Neogenesis in Humans

No studies on folliculo-neogenesis have been conducted in humans. Success in de-novo hair regeneration has mainly relied on mouse models, particularly using cells from newborn or embryonic mice. Despite efforts, there is currently no established cell-based therapy for human hair follicle formation.

Testing cell-based treatments on human skin grafted to immunodeficient mice is an intermediate step, but regenerating human hair follicles remains elusive, requiring breakthroughs in several diverse scientific fields. The inability to manufacture pure human hair follicles suggests missing factors in the microenvironment, disrupting the differentiation process [106]. Before engineering new hair follicles, we must acknowledge the limitations of translating laboratory animal studies to humans.

Issues Remaining to Be Solved

Efforts focus on enhancing 3D microenvironments for culturing hair follicular cells in vitro. Tissue engineering seeks to regenerate tissues and organs using cells within a scaffold. Dermal cells, including DPCs and sheath cells, can induce hair growth when transplanted into intact recipient epithelium. Yet, challenges persist on the path to human hair follicle induction:

- Most research on HFSCs has been conducted on mouse or rat hair follicles, desperately needing validation in human systems. While these models are helpful for showcasing hair induction by DPCs, they lack efficiency in inducing hair on the human scalp.
- While rodent studies of folliculo-neogenesis have been impressive, success has primarily been with cells from newborn or fetal animals (hybrid or chimeric) [38]. Attempts with adult cells have been incomplete and disappointing, suggesting a notable challenge in forming new hair follicles from dissociated cells [107].
- Human hair regeneration has been achieved by grafting DPs onto immunodeficient mice, revealing the reprogramming ability of DPs compared to dermal fibroblasts [31, 108]. However, differences between rodent and human follicles, especially human scalp hair, pose challenges due to size and structural variations.

- Existing animal models for hair regeneration are unreliable and impractical for clinical use, often resulting in inconsistent outcomes or requiring invasive procedures unsuitable for non-life-threatening conditions like AGA/FPHL.
- Transplanting hDPCs into rat auricles [51, 109] or injecting them subcutaneously [36, 38] has yielded confusing results, with difficulties in distinguishing original hairs from regenerated ones, and have been unsuccessful in regenerating human hair follicles [1, 2].
- Until today, success has been hindered by issues still outside our understanding [31]:
- While immunodeficient mice have been utilized as hosts, they may not be ideal for xenografting human cells, as grafted human cells are progressively replaced by murine wound healing epidermis [31, 110].
- Mouse DPCs tend to spontaneously aggregate in vitro or upon subcutaneous injection, facilitating epithelial-mesenchymal interaction and hair follicle formation. Human DPCs do not possess this property and scatter in the dermis and subcutaneous tissue when injected [111].
- The loss of hair inductivity of hDPCs during culture poses a challenge, as the molecules and mechanisms responsible for their hair-inducing capacity remain incompletely understood [1, 2, 57].
- The epidermal component from human tissues, typically cultured keratinocytes, maintains adequate differentiation ability, potentially due to insufficient numbers of HFSCs. Discrepancies in characteristics, behaviors, and differentiation potentials of stem cells between humans and rodents have been noted in epidermal tissue research [31, 112]. However, clarifying how these factors contribute to hair follicle reconstitution in humans is challenging due to the interdependence of the hair inductivity of the mesenchymal source and the differentiation ability of the epidermal component [31].
- Obtaining sufficient numbers of inductive human DPCs and undifferentiated epidermal stem cell components presents further challenges, as the ratio of epithelial and dermal cells significantly influences hair follicle formation efficiency. Notably, approx. 5000 dermal cells and 2500 epidermal cells will produce a single follicle, making hair follicle engineering extremely expensive [39].
- Additionally, variability in the growth cycle of human scalp follicles complicates analysis, as follicles in different stages of anagen may yield disparate results in colony-forming efficiency [113].
- The inductive capability of hDPCs alone is insufficient for effective hair restoration, necessitating the development of methods for both producing and implanting hair-inductive DPCs efficiently. While methods for culturing hair-inductive DPCs exist [114], techniques for their effective implantation to induce hair growth efficiently are yet to be developed [95].

Where Can We Go from Here?

Early efforts in cell-based alopecia treatments may focus on using the patient's own tissue to engineer hair follicles, reducing the risk of immune rejection. Nonetheless, an intriguing prospect emerges: developing heterologous (allogeneic) hair follicle tissue for tissue transplantation. This proposition rests on the premise that the hair follicle is an immune-privileged organ devoid of MHC (major histocompatibility complex) class I antigens [115]. Nevertheless, the safety testing and regulatory hurdles for this approach would require enormous resources.

Recent advances have shed light on the process of new hair formation when dissociated cells are injected into the skin, especially in AGA patients with existing vellus hair follicles [95, 116]. However, it remains uncertain whether injected DPCs prompt the formation of a new follicle from adjacent epithelium (folliculoneogenesis) or integrate into a neighboring follicle to convert it into a larger follicle (vellus to terminal switch) [117].

Besides these technical issues, several challenges remain to be overcome for clinical success as well. Optimizing the cell preparation method is paramount, representing a significant challenge.

Both epithelial stem cells and adult DPCs must be prepared while preserving their original functions, given their crucial roles in interacting, forming hair follicles, and regulating the hair cycle. Due to limited donor tissue, culture expansion of DPCs becomes necessary, but maintaining their hair-inducing capacity poses a considerable challenge, as expanded DPCs tend to lose this ability. Strategies such as supplementation with keratinocyte-conditioned media [28], or basic FGF [30] have been explored to address this issue. It has been reported that a supplementary grafting of dermal sheath cells combined with DPCs might enhance experimental hair growth [118], but the results are still preliminary [119].

Additionally, improving the transplantation of DPCs is essential. Determining the optimal number of DPCs and the best preparation method (e.g., aggregates, spheres, sheets, or bio-scaffolds) is crucial, as it directly impacts DPC function. Studies using microencapsulated cultured human DPCs have shown promising results in producing hairs at high density [120], but further investigation is needed to ascertain their role in the neogenesis of hair follicles. Moreover, refining the grafting procedure to enhance hair growth efficiency and minimize invasiveness is essential for its acceptance as a viable aesthetic treatment. While significant progress has been made in achieving hair folliculogenesis, improving the quality of the hair shaft remains a priority for clinical applications [25].

Role of Bulge Stem Cells in Tumorigenesis [1, 2]

According to the theory that epithelial stem cells possess a lifespan equivalent to that of the organism, they are believed to be prone to accumulating genetic mutations, potentially leading to tumor formation [121]. This notion is supported by ample evidence from mouse models, indicating that numerous skin tumors originate from hair follicles and their associated stem cells [122, 123]. Keratinocyte stem cells, being the slowest cycling cells in the vicinity, appear to be particularly vulnerable to cutaneous carcinogens. Their prolonged retention of carcinogens increases their susceptibility to tumor promotion [124].

Significant evidence suggests that basal cell carcinomas (BCCs) may originate from hair follicle stem cells (HFSCs) [125]. BCCs express Bcl-2 [126], a marker found in the permanent parts of hair follicles, notably the bulge area [127]. Furthermore, over-expression of sonic hedgehog (Shh) in mouse epidermis is causing BCC-like tumors from invaginating hair follicles but has little effect on interfollicular epidermis [128], which further supports the hypothesis of BCC's follicular origin [129].

Trichoepithelioma (TE), a benign tumor resembling BCC clinically and histologically, often coexists with BCCs in some patients. Both tumors are hypothesized to arise from a common precursor cell type within hair follicles [130]. Mutations in the PTC gene [131, 132] found in both sporadic TEs and BCCs provide compelling evidence for a shared tumorigenic mechanism linked to the hair follicle. Further exploration of TEs, BCCs, and other hair follicle tumors using additional markers on HFSCs will likely yield new insights into their pathogenesis. However, until then, the long-term safety of using stem cells for folliculo-neogenesis remains uncertain.

Where Are We Standing Right Now?

The main challenge in tissue engineering is assembling fully functional organ systems from dissociated cells grown under specific culture conditions [1, 31].

Many scientists believe that manufacturing human hair follicles in culture is within reach, with significant scientific effort and investment directed toward this objective. Balañá et al. reviewed numerous patents related to hair regeneration, indicating substantial interest in this area within the industry. They highlighted current technical advancements, preferred research approaches, and critical areas of focus [99]. Biotech companies, including Shiseido Co Ltd., Aderans Research Institute Inc., and Follica Inc., actively investigate methods to stimulate hair growth by converting stem cells into progenitor cells. Follica Inc., for instance, has explored disrupting the skin on balding scalps to create an "embryonic window" for epithelial stem cell differentiation towards hair follicular fate. Replicel Inc. has examined transferring healthy outer root sheath cells to bald areas to rejuvenate new follicles. Intercytex and Aderans Research Institute have investigated expanding hair follicular cells in vitro to create a reserve for transplantation [133]. Additionally, non-profit institutions such as Jilin University, the University of Pennsylvania, the University of Southern California, and the National Taiwan University actively engage in hair regeneration research, underscoring the productivity of academic institutions in this field [89].

Most experts agree that achieving folliculo-neogenesis through follicular cell implantation appears to be a more feasible goal. However, before stem cells can be effectively utilized to grow hair in animals and eventually in humans, two major challenges must be overcome:

1. Understanding the intricate molecular signaling that governs cellular fate specification, particularly in hair follicles, involves addressing cell types originating from two different germ layers.
2. Enhancing our understanding of tissue architecture construction, including the appropriate arrangement, ratio, and orientation of each cellular component. This entails deciphering the regulation of hair follicle number, size, and topological arrangement, ensuring consistency and repeatability across mammalian species.

   In order to by-pass these obstacles, deep understanding and appreciation of several biological functions are necessary, such as:
   - stem cell biology,
   - epithelial-mesenchymal interactions,
   - cell adhesion,
   - cytoskeleton and intermediate filament formation,
   - controls of cell lineage formation and differentiation,
   - cell attachments, formation, and breakage,
   - cell motility,
   - cell-cell communication,
   - cellular apoptosis,
   - hormone sensitivity,
   - neuro humoral immune interactions,
   - cell pigmentation.

Combining all these various disciplines has presented significant challenges. While nature took millions of years to evolve the intricate structure of the hair follicle, it remains uncertain how long it will take humans to master the engineering of fully functional hair follicles with organized architecture, proper differentiation, and cyclic regeneration. Moving forward, efforts should concentrate on creating more realistic and aesthetically pleasing models, facilitating the clinical translation of hair loss treatments. Through incremental progress, we will gradually move closer to the ultimate objective of engineered skin and hair follicles that function seamlessly [134].

However, Is Folliculo-Neogenesis the Answer?

The concept of manipulating, culturing, and re-implanting stem cells in bald areas has gained widespread acceptance, with many believing it to be a near-future breakthrough. Some researchers envision cultivating hair follicles in laboratories for surgical implantation into bald scalps. Consequently, biotech companies invest heavily in research, while concerns arise among hair restoration surgeons about the potential obsolescence of their surgical skills. Influenced by media narratives, patients question the delay in producing hair follicles in labs for easy transplantation. As pressure mounts, it prompts reflection on the underlying beliefs:

- What is the basis of these beliefs?
- Are stem cells and folliculo-neogenesis indispensable for effectively managing or curing AGA/FPHL?

Reality-Checking on Hair Loss

1. The most prevalent hair follicle disorders encountered in clinical practice are AGA/FPHL, telogen effluvium, and AA, collectively accounting for over 97% of hair loss cases in both genders. (Fig. 11.4)
2. AGA/FPHL are non-scarring alopecias characterized by the depletion of hair progenitor cells while HFSCs remain intact. This characteristic implies that AGA/FPHL are reversible conditions. Drug treatments, such as Minoxidil, Finasteride, and Dutasteride, likely act by re-converting vellus hair follicles into terminal ones, leveraging the viability and responsiveness of HFSCs.
3. There is no evidence of "organ deletion" in AGA/FPHL. Instead, large terminal hair follicles are gradually replaced by miniaturized vellus follicles that can still cycle. This potential for reconversion is evidenced by cases such as those undergoing male-to-female sex reassignment surgery [135]. (Fig. 11.5)
4. HFSCs in miniaturized hair follicles affected by AGA/FPHL show no damage or defects compared to adjacent terminal follicles. Vellus follicles maintain complete stem cell populations [15], explaining their impressive conversion to terminal follicles and maintenance of circularity.
5. Scarring alopecias are irreversible conditions where both vellus and terminal follicles lose their cycling ability due to irreversible damage to their epithelial stem cells.

Thus, the most prevalent causes of hair loss (>97%) are not related to stem cell disorders or to reduced numbers of hair follicles. Hair follicles, even though miniaturized, are still there.

Hence, the fundamental question emerges: What is the stem cell issue purportedly necessitating correction through stem cell "therapies"?

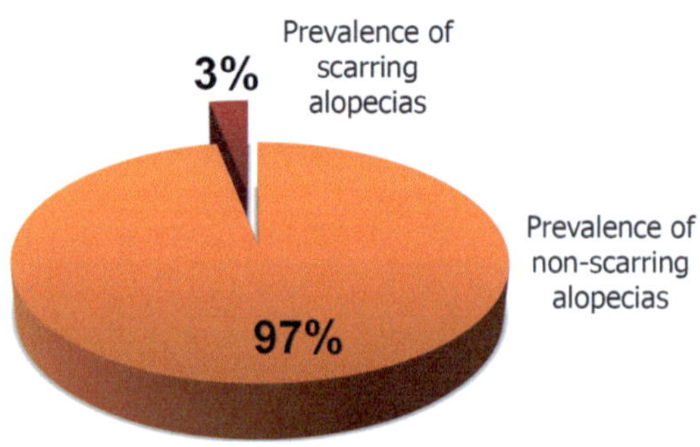

Fig. 11.4 The incidence of scarring alopecias stemming from the permanent damage to vital epithelial stem cells of the hair follicle is less than 3%. Non-scarring alopecias, characterized by intact, healthy stem cell populations, encompass over 97% of hair loss conditions (from [5], used with permission)

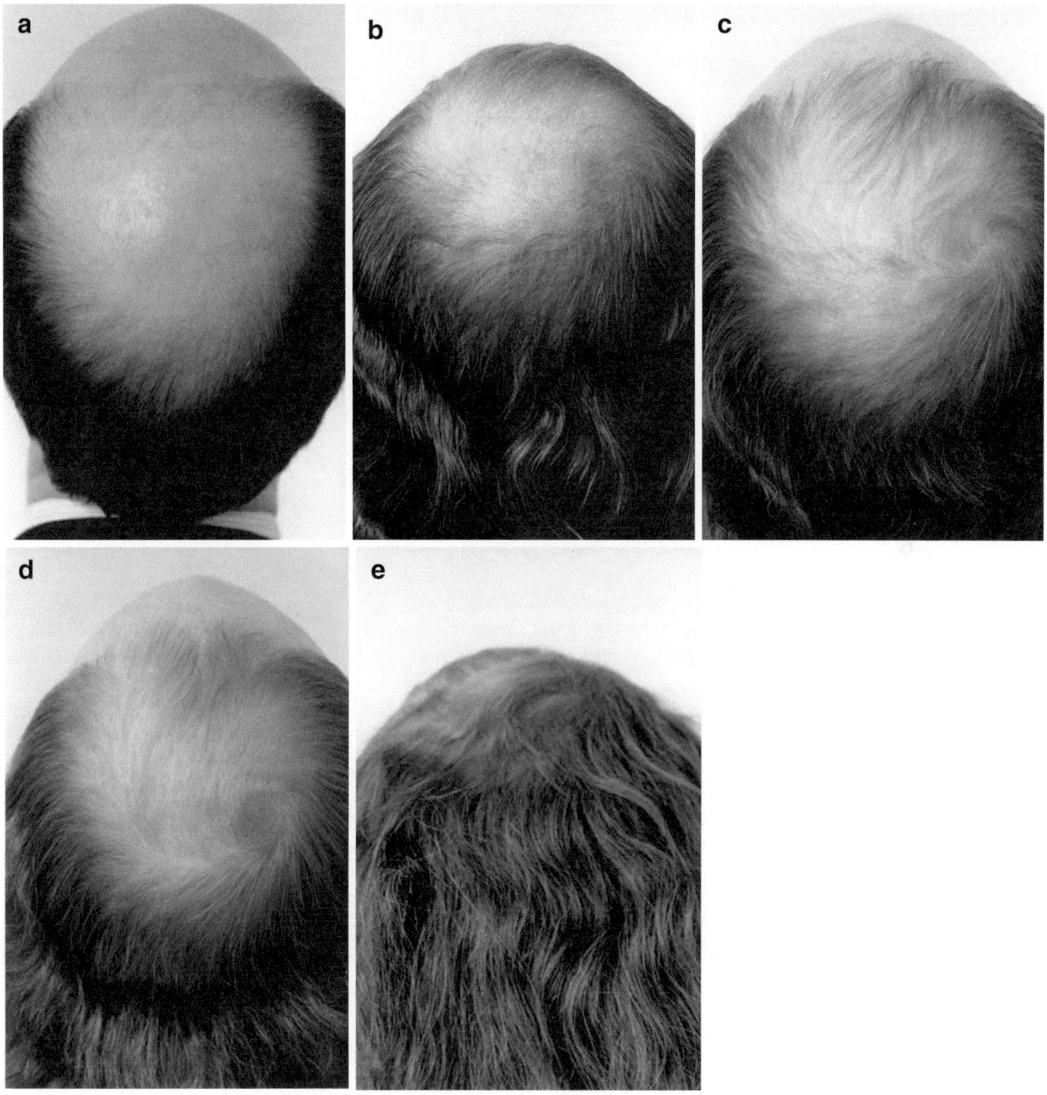

Fig. 11.5 In a case study of a transgender male-to-female patient, following a two-year regimen of oral and topical hair growth treatments (including estradiol, estrone solution, minoxidil, spironolactone, and tretinoin), significant regrowth of terminal scalp hair was observed. The patient progressed from Norwood-Hamilton stage VII to stage IIIv, with nearly complete restoration of hair coverage, albeit with some thinning at the vertex (adapted from Adenuga et al. [135], used with permission)

Should We Really Aim for Stem Cell "Therapies"?

With a clear head, one should honestly revisit the whole idea behind the "hair cloning" trend and promise, how necessary and feasible it might be:

Concept of De Novo Folliculo-Neogenesis

This argument may only find favor among those who advocate rebuilding an entire house instead of repairing a broken front door. In AGA/FPHL, despite the presence of

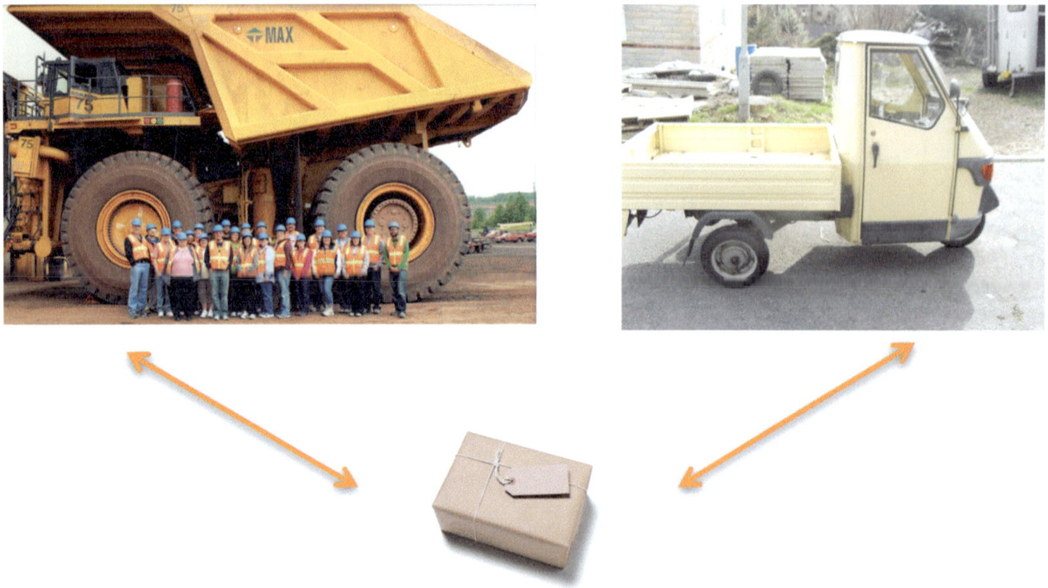

Fig. 11.6 When transporting this small package, it is essential to select a vehicle that matches the size and importance of the cargo. Opting for a heavy-duty truck might seem like overkill, echoing the caution against therapeutic overkill in hair loss treatment. Instead, a smaller, more precise vehicle, such as a compact delivery van or even a courier bike, could be a better choice. This mirrors the principle of selecting the most appropriate and targeted treatment for hair loss and avoiding excessive or unnecessary interventions (from [5], used with permission)

stem cells and existing hair follicles (albeit vellus), some insist on the need to start afresh. Besides being therapeutically excessive (Fig. 11.6), akin to seeking trouble, this approach raises concerns about potential complications such as malignant transformation, cyst formation, or painful granulomas instead of normal hair follicles and hair. If these concerns are not enough to provoke worry, the cosmetic outcome should certainly give pause for thought.

The true beauty of human hair is found in its luster, color, strength, uniformity, and the precise alignment of strands. However, current data from even the most successful attempts at folliculo-neogenesis indicate that patients are likely to have hair that is asymmetrical in thickness, curly, randomly distributed, and positioned at varied angles. This results in a texture resembling scrotum hairs rather than the desired straight, natural, thick, and glossy scalp hair. Not exactly what candidate for these therapies would hope for.

Concept of Follicular Cell Implantation to Vellus Hair Follicles

Once more, despite the presence of stem cells and existing hair follicles (albeit vellus), some proponents argue for the necessity of introducing additional stem cells to generate terminal hair follicles. However, the precise delivery of these stem cells to the specific regions of small, colorless, and thus difficult-to-identify vellus hair follicles poses considerable challenges. Even setting aside the ethical concerns associated with such an approach, the safety implications and potential cosmetic outcomes of this intervention remain largely uncertain.

Legal Framework and Caution in Stem Cell Therapies

The U.S. Food and Drug Administration (FDA) holds regulatory authority over stem cell products in the United States. Currently, only stem cell-based products derived from cord blood, specifically blood-forming stem cells (hematopoietic progenitor cells), are FDA-approved for use in the country [136].

In 2017, the FDA introduced a comprehensive regenerative medicine policy framework through four guidance documents. These guidelines were designed to support and accelerate the development of regenerative medicine products, including human cells, tissues, and cellular and tissue-based products (HCT/Ps). As part of this framework, the FDA implemented a 3-year period of risk-based enforcement discretion for specific HCT/Ps. This grace period allowed manufacturers to evaluate whether they needed to submit an investigational new drug application (IND) or marketing application to the FDA or if they met the regulatory criteria to continue marketing their products under sect. 361 of the Public Health Service Act (PHSA), which does not require pre-market review and approval [137].

Since 2019, the FDA has issued over 350 "Warning Letters" and "Untitled Letters" to manufacturers, clinics, and healthcare providers regarding unapproved regenerative medicine products. Recent actions taken by the FDA, including citations, warning letters, product seizures, and even criminal charges, underscore the government's heightened vigilance and commitment to regulating stem cell therapies [137].

In a JAMA article published in June 2020, then-FDA Commissioner Stephen Hahn, M.D., and Dr. Marks emphasized the risks associated with unproven and unapproved regenerative medicine products. They highlighted these products as uncontrolled experimental procedures that impose financial and physical costs on patients [138]. Due to the challenges posed by the COVID-19 pandemic, the FDA extended the grace period by an additional 6 months until May 31, 2021.

As of June 1, 2021, compliance with HCT/P regulations will require clinical trials or regulatory approvals for these products. This has already irreversibly impacted thoughtless promises and hopes as well as announced research efforts.

Conclusion

HFSCs are poised to play a pivotal role in the future of regenerative medicine, extending beyond the restoration of hair follicles alone. With a deep understanding of hair follicle morphogenesis and the cyclic regulation of regeneration, coupled with refined protocols for isolating and culturing HFs and/or HFSCs, there has been a surge in bioengineering innovations to address hair loss.

Undoubtedly, biomedical engineering holds hypothetical promise as a prospective therapy for hair regrowth. However, like any medical intervention, it comes with inherent limitations. Future endeavors must focus on overcoming these limitations and translating our knowledge into effective tissue engineering solutions for hair restoration.

Realistically, we need to target our systematic efforts in identifying effective, predictable, and lasting treatments for the:

1. control of follicular circularity,
2. protection of follicular stem cells,
3. restoration of the hair follicle's immune privilege,
4. inhibition of exogen stage,
5. re-conversion of vellus hair follicles to terminal ones.

In addition, the "hair cloning" concept raises numerous critical academic, safety, and ethical concerns that could dampen enthusiasm and optimism surrounding its potential. Moreover, a fundamental question persists: is stem cell therapy or folliculo-neogenesis necessary for treating AGA/FPHL?

Honestly, except for a small fraction of patients with severe scarring alopecias or congenital hair follicle aplasia (less than 1–3% of all alopecias), stem cell therapy may not offer significant therapeutic benefits with an acceptable cost/benefit ratio for the majority of cases (representing 97–99% of alopecias) (Fig. 11.7).

Over the past decade, preclinical investigations suggest that therapeutic approaches avoiding the direct use of live stem cells may offer a

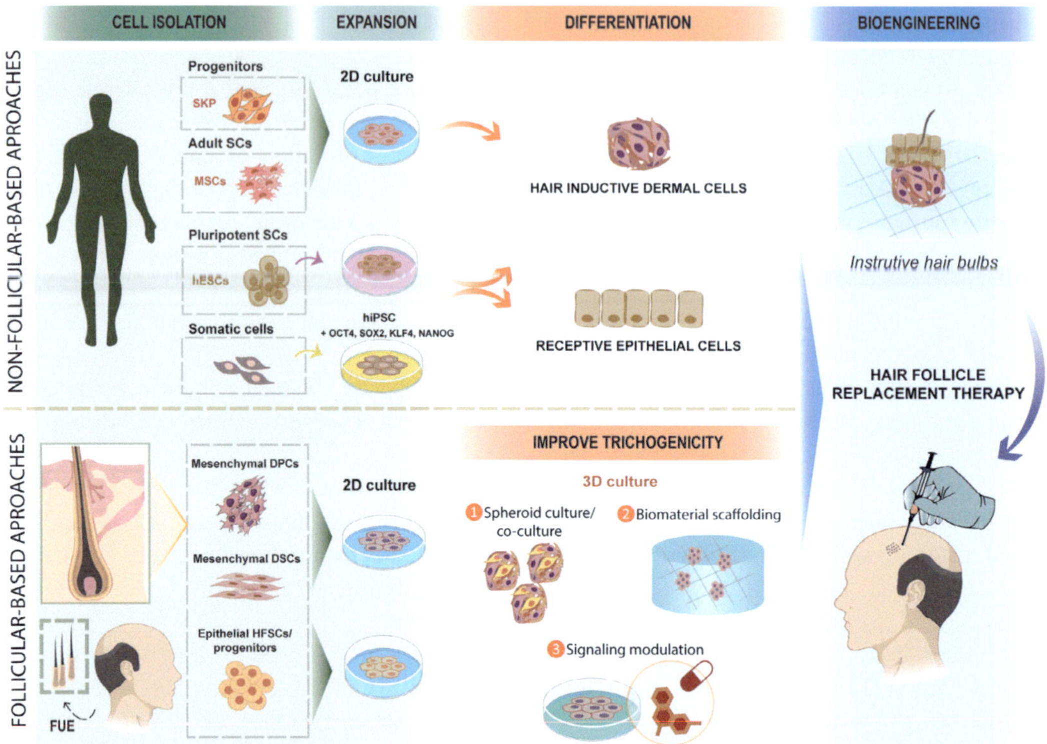

Fig. 11.7 Potential cell-based strategies for regenerating hair follicles (HFs) are being actively investigated, with various cell sources under exploration for HF tissue engineering. Non-follicular cell sources include skin-derived progenitors (SKPs) from human skin, akin to dermal papilla cells (DPCs); adult stem cells (e.g., isolated from bone marrow, MSCs); and pluripotent stem cells (embryonic/ESCs or induced/iPSCs with Yamanaka factors), which can differentiate into either a mesenchymal inductive population resembling follicular DP or a receptive epithelial population. Follicular cell sources encompass DPCs and DSCs as mesenchymal inductive components, along with bulge hair follicle stem cells (HFSCs) as epithelial receptive elements. Considering the potential drawbacks of in vitro follicular cell culture expansion, strategies such as signaling modulation, 3D culture, biomaterial-based culture, or a combination thereof may be employed to preserve cell trichogenicity. Through the integration of epithelial and mesenchymal components, engineered instructive mini-bulbs can be cultivated in vitro, offering a promising tissue engineering solution capable of generating mature and functional HFs on bald scalps (adapted from Castro et al. [139])

safer route to prevent disease progression and initiate regeneration [140]. Consequently, the paracrine action of stem cell secretome is being explored as a potentially safer alternative to the direct use of live stem cells.

Synopsis

Hair follicle neogenesis through post-follicular stem cell implantation presents an intriguing concept that captivates scientists and individuals experiencing hair loss. Envisaging scenarios where stem cells are injected into bald areas, leading to robust and naturally looking hair growth, or cultivating an infinite number of hair follicles in vitro for transplantation onto bald scalps, ignite the imagination. Despite its apparent simplicity as an organ, in-depth characterization of the constituent cells comprising the hair follicle reveals an unexpectedly intricate cellular architecture. Since the late 1990s, considerable scientific advancements have been made; however, the experimental systems published to demonstrate hair regeneration completely lack the ability to safely and efficiently implant cultured follicular cells repeatedly to achieve adequate hair restoration in humans. To be clinically viable, engineered hairs necessitate organized follicular architecture, hair differentiation products, appropriate planar arrangement, and the ability to cycle and regenerate. Subsequent endeavors should concentrate on developing more authentic and aesthetically pleasing models with potential clinical translation into therapies. Encouraged by novel findings centered on stem-cell-based therapies, efforts towards more effective treatments for hair loss are underway. The secretome, a plethora of substances secreted by stem cells, garners increasing attention for its pivotal role in regulating various physiological processes. While these initial strides are promising, there remains to be more clinical data to substantiate stem-cell-based therapies fully. Stem-cell transplants, conditioned media, and exosome therapies exhibit preclinical and some clinical success, albeit each carrying its own set of limitations requiring mitigation. It is imperative to note that hair follicle neogenesis is superfluous for managing common alopecias (>97%) and would primarily find relevance in rare follicular diseases, such as scarring alopecias or other conditions affecting the stem cell populations of the hair follicle (<3%).

References

1. Cotsarelis G. Epithelial stem cells: a folliculocentric view. J Invest Dermatol. 2006;126(7):1459–68.
2. Stenn KS, Cotsarelis G. Bioengineering the hair follicle: fringe benefits of stem cell technology. Curr Opin Biotechnol. 2005;16(5):493–7.
3. Strong AL, Neumeister MW, Levi B. Stem Cells and Tissue Engineering: Regeneration of the Skin and Its Contents. Clin Plast Surg. 2017;44(3):635–50.
4. Toma JG, Akhavan M, Fernandes KJ, Barnabé-Heider F, Sadikot A, Kaplan DR, Miller FD. Isolation of multipotent adult stem cells from the dermis of mammalian skin. Nat Cell Biol. 2001;3(9):778–84V.
5. Anastassakis K. Stem cells and hair follicle cloning/engineering. In: Androgenetic alopecia from A to Z. Cham: Springer; 2023. https://doi.org/10.1007/978-3-031-10613-2_40.
6. Reed M. Hair transplantation. In: Thorne CH, Beasley RW, Aston SJ, Bartlett SP, Gurtner GC, Spear SL, editors. Grabb and Smith's plastic surgery. 6th ed. Philadelphia, PA: Lippincott Williams & Wilkins; 2006. p. 562–72.
7. Cooley J. Follicular cell implantation: an update on "hair follicle cloning". Facial Plast Surg Clin North Am. 2004;12(2):219–24.
8. Stenn KS, Paus R. Controls of hair follicle cycling. Physiol Rev. 2001;81(1):449–94.
9. Anastassakis K. Embryogenesis of pilosebaceous unit. In: Androgenetic alopecia from A to Z. Cham: Springer; 2022. https://doi.org/10.1007/978-3-030-76111-0_3.
10. Zheng Y, Nace A, Chen W, Watkins K, Sergott L, Homan Y, Vandeberg JL, Breen M, Stenn K. Mature hair follicles generated from dissociated cells: a universal mechanism of folliculoneogenesis. Dev Dyn. 2010;239(10):2619–26.
11. Rose K. The beginning of the age of mammals. Baltimore: Johns Hopkins University Press; 2006.
12. Ji S, Zhu Z, Sun X, Fu X. Functional hair follicle regeneration: an updated review. Signal Transduct Target Ther. 2021;6(1):66.
13. Sato T, Vries RG, Snippert HJ, van de Wetering M, Barker N, Stange DE, van Es JH, Abo A, Kujala P, Peters PJ, Clevers H. Single Lgr5 stem cells build crypt-villus structures in vitro without a mesenchymal niche. Nature. 2009;459(7244):262–5.
14. Shackleton M, Vaillant F, Simpson KJ, Stingl J, Smyth GK, Asselin-Labat ML, Wu L, Lindeman GJ, Visvader JE. Generation of a functional mammary gland from a single stem cell. Nature. 2006;439(7072):84–8.
15. Ikeda E, Morita R, Nakao K, et al. Fully functional bioengineered tooth replacement as an organ replacement therapy. Proc Natl Acad Sci U S A. 2009;106(32):13475–80.
16. Garza LA, Yang CC, Zhao T, Cotsarelis G, et al. Bald scalp in men with androgenetic alopecia retains hair follicle stem cells but lacks CD200-rich and CD34-positive hair follicle progenitor cells. J Clin Invest. 2011;121(2):613–22.
17. Benitah SA, Frye M, Glogauer M, Watt FM. Stem cell depletion through epidermal deletion of Rac1. Science. 2005;309(5736):933–5.
18. Dlugosz AA, Hutchin ME. From hair to eternity: hedgehog signaling in skin biology and cancer. Progr in Dermatol Dec. 2005;39:1–12.
19. Yi R, O'Carroll D, Pasolli HA, Zhang Z, Dietrich FS, Tarakhovsky A, Fuchs E. Morphogenesis in skin is governed by discrete sets of differentially expressed microRNAs. Nat Genet. 2006;38(3):356–62.
20. Chuong CM, Cotsarelis G, Stenn K. Defining hair follicles in the age of stem cell bioengineering. J Invest Dermatol. 2007;127(9):2098–100.
21. Ohyama M, Zheng Y, Paus R, Stenn KS. The mesenchymal component of hair follicle neogenesis: background, methods and molecular characterization. Exp Dermatol. 2010;19(2):89–99.
22. Cohen J. The transplantation of individual rat and guineapig whisker papillae. J Embryol Exp Morphol. 1961;9:117–27.
23. Oliver RF. The experimental induction of whisker growth in the hooded rat by implantation of dermal papillae. J Embryol Exp Morphol. 1967;18(1):43–51.

24. Oliver RF. The induction of hair follicle formation in the adult hooded rat by vibrissa dermal papillae. J Embryol Exp Morphol. 1970;23(1):219–36.
25. Jahoda CA. Induction of follicle formation and hair growth by vibrissa dermal papillae implanted into rat ear wounds: vibrissa-type fibres are specified. Development. 1992;115(4):1103–9.
26. Aoi N, Inoue K, Kato H, et al. Clinically applicable transplantation procedure of dermal papilla cells for hair follicle regeneration. J Tissue Eng Regen Med. 2012;6(2):85–95.
27. Jahoda CA, Horne KA, Oliver RF. Induction of hair growth by implantation of cultured dermal papilla cells. Nature. 1984;311(5986):560–2.
28. Lichti U, Weinberg WC, Goodman L, Ledbetter S, Dooley T, Morgan D, Yuspa SH. In vivo regulation of murine hair growth: insights from grafting defined cell populations onto nude mice. J Invest Dermatol. 1993;101(1 Suppl):124S–9S.
29. Weinberg WC, Goodman LV, George C, et al. Reconstitution of hair follicle development in vivo: determination of follicle formation, hair growth, and hair quality by dermal cells. J Invest Dermatol. 1993;100(3):229–36.
30. Kamimura J, Lee D, Baden HP, Brissette J, Dotto GP. Primary mouse keratinocyte cultures contain hair follicle progenitor cells with multiple differentiation potential. J Invest Dermatol. 1997;109(4):534–40.
31. Kishimoto J, Ehama R, Wu L, Jiang S, Jiang N, Burgeson RE. Selective activation of the versican promoter by epithelial- mesenchymal interactions during hair follicle development. Proc Natl Acad Sci U S A. 1999;96(13):7336–41.
32. Ehama R, Ishimatsu-Tsuji Y, Iriyama S, Ideta R, Soma T, Yano K, Kawasaki C, Suzuki S, Shirakata Y, Hashimoto K, Kishimoto J. Hair follicle regeneration using grafted rodent and human cells. J Invest Dermatol. 2007;127(9):2106–15.
33. Reynolds AJ, Jahoda CA. Cultured dermal papilla cells induce follicle formation and hair growth by transdifferentiation of an adult epidermis. Development. 1992;115(2):587–93.
34. Inoue K, Kato H, Sato T, Osada A, Aoi N, Suga H, Eto H, Gonda K, Yoshimura K. Evaluation of animal models for the hair-inducing capacity of cultured human dermal papilla cells. Cells Tissues Organs. 2009;190(2):102–10.
35. Inamatsu M, Matsuzaki T, Iwanari H, Yoshizato K. Establishment of rat dermal papilla cell lines that sustain the potency to induce hair follicles from afollicular skin. J Invest Dermatol. 1998;111(5):767–75.
36. Osada A, Iwabuchi T, Kishimoto J, Hamazaki TS, Okochi H. Long-term culture of mouse vibrissal dermal papilla cells and de novo hair follicle induction. Tissue Eng. 2007;13(5):975–82.
37. Qiao J, Philips E, Teumer J. A graft model for hair development. Exp Dermatol. 2008;17(6):512–8.
38. Qiao J, Zawadzka A, Philips E, Turetsky A, Batchelor S, Peacock J, Durrant S, Garlick D, Kemp P, Teumer J. Hair follicle neogenesis induced by cultured human scalp dermal papilla cells. Regen Med. 2009;4(5):667–76.
39. Ito Y, Hamazaki TS, Ohnuma K, Tamaki K, Asashima M, Okochi H. Isolation of murine hair-inducing cells using the cell surface marker prominin-1/CD133. J Invest Dermatol. 2007;127(5):1052–60.
40. Zheng Y, Du X, Wang W, Boucher M, Parimoo S, Stenn K. Organogenesis from dissociated cells: generation of mature cycling hair follicles from skin-derived cells. J Invest Dermatol. 2005;124(5):867–76.
41. Blanpain C, Lowry WE, Geoghegan A, Polak L, Fuchs E. Self-renewal, multipotency, and the existence of two cell populations within an epithelial stem cell niche. Cell. 2004;118(5):635–48.
42. Morris RJ, Liu Y, Marles L, Yang Z, Trempus C, Li S, Lin JS, Sawicki JA, Cotsarelis G. Capturing and profiling adult hair follicle stem cells. Nat Biotechnol. 2004;22(4):411–7.
43. Oliver RF. Whisker growth after removal of the dermal papilla and lengths of follicle in the hooded rat. J Embryol Exp Morphol. 1966;15(3):331–47.
44. Oliver RF. Histological studies of whisker regeneration in the hooded rat. J Embryol Exp Morphol. 1966;16(2):231–44.
45. Horne KA, Jahoda CA. Restoration of hair growth by surgical implantation of follicular dermal sheath. Development. 1992;116(3):563–71.
46. Reynolds AJ, Lawrence C, Cserhalmi-Friedman PB, Christiano AM, Jahoda CA. Trans-gender induction of hair follicles. Nature. 1999;402(6757):33–4.
47. Paus R, Nickoloff BJ, Ito T. A 'hairy' privilege. Trends Immunol. 2005;26(1):32–40.
48. Itami S, Kurata S, Takayasu S. Androgen induction of follicular epithelial cell growth is mediated via insulin-like growth factor-I from dermal papilla cells. Biochem Biophys Res Commun. 1995;212(3):988–94.
49. Rosenquist TA, Martin GR. Fibroblast growth factor signalling in the hair growth cycle: expression of the fibroblast growth factor receptor and ligand genes in the murine hair follicle. Dev Dyn. 1996;205(4):379–86.
50. Kishimoto J, Burgeson RE, Morgan BA. Wnt signaling maintains the hair-inducing activity of the dermal papilla. Genes Dev. 2000;14(10):1181–5.
51. Chiu HC, Chang CH, Chen JS, Jee SH. Human hair follicle dermal papilla cell, dermal sheath cell and interstitial dermal fibroblast characteristics. J Formos Med Assoc. 1996;95(9):667–74.
52. Jahoda CA, Reynolds AJ, Oliver RF. Induction of hair growth in ear wounds by cultured dermal papilla cells. J Invest Dermatol. 1993;101(4):584–90.
53. Rendl M, Polak L, Fuchs E. BMP signaling in dermal papilla cells is required for their hair follicle-inductive properties. Genes Dev. 2008;22(4):543–57.
54. Inoue K, Aoi N, Yamauchi Y, Sato T, Suga H, Eto H, Kato H, Tabata Y, Yoshimura K. TGF-beta is spe-

cifically expressed in human dermal papilla cells and modulates hair folliculogenesis. J Cell Mol Med. 2009;13(11–12):4643–56.
55. Randall VA, Sundberg JP, Philpott MP. Animal and in vitro models for the study of hair follicles. J Investig Dermatol Symp Proc. 2003;8(1):39–45.
56. Midorikawa T, Chikazawa T, Yoshino T, Takada K, Arase S. Different gene expression profile observed in dermal papilla cells related to androgenic alopecia by DNA macroarray analysis. J Dermatol Sci. 2004;36(1):25–32.
57. Rutberg SE, Kolpak ML, Gourley JA, Tan G, Henry JP, Shander D. Differences in expression of specific biomarkers distinguish human beard from scalp dermal papilla cells. J Invest Dermatol. 2006;126(12):2583–95.
58. Martinez-Lopez A, Montero-Vilchez T, Sierra-Sánchez Á, Molina-Leyva A, Arias-Santiago S. Advanced medical therapies in the management of non-scarring alopecia: areata and androgenic alopecia. Int J Mol Sci. 2020;21(21):8390.
59. Maxson S, Lopez EA, Yoo D, Danilkovitch-Miagkova A, Leroux MA. Concise review: role of mesenchymal stem cells in wound repair. Stem Cells Transl Med. 2012;1(2):142–9.
60. Egger A, Tomic-Canic M, Tosti A. Advances in stem cell-based therapy for hair loss. CellR4 Repair Replace Regen Reprogram. 2020;8:e2894.
61. Chang CL, Sung PH, Chen KH, et al. Adipose-derived mesenchymal stem cell-derived exosomes alleviate overwhelming systemic inflammatory reaction and organ damage and improve outcome in rat sepsis syndrome. Am J Transl Res. 2018;10(4):1053–70.
62. Mizuno H, Tobita M, Uysal AC. Concise review: adipose-derived stem cells as a novel tool for future regenerative medicine. Stem Cells. 2012;30(5):804–10.
63. Cai L, Johnstone BH, Cook TG, Liang Z, Traktuev D, Cornetta K, Ingram DA, Rosen ED, March KL. Suppression of hepatocyte growth factor production impairs the ability of adipose-derived stem cells to promote ischemic tissue revascularization. Stem Cells. 2007;25(12):3234–43.
64. Gnecchi M, He H, Liang OD, Melo LG, Morello F, Mu H, Noiseux N, Zhang L, Pratt RE, Ingwall JS, Dzau VJ. Paracrine action accounts for marked protection of ischemic heart by Akt-modified mesenchymal stem cells. Nat Med. 2005;11(4):367–8.
65. Kinnaird T, Stabile E, Burnett MS, Lee CW, Barr S, Fuchs S, Epstein SE. Marrow-derived stromal cells express genes encoding a broad spectrum of arteriogenic cytokines and promote in vitro and in vivo arteriogenesis through paracrine mechanisms. Circ Res. 2004;94(5):678–85.
66. Maguire G. Stem cell therapy without the cells. Commun Integr Biol. 2013;6(6):e26631.
67. Beer L, Mildner M, Ankersmit HJ. Cell secretome based drug substances in regenerative medicine: when regulatory affairs meet basic science. Ann Transl Med. 2017;5(7):170.
68. Danilenko DM, Ring BD, Pierce GF. Growth factors and cytokines in hair follicle development and cycling: recent insights from animal models and the potentials for clinical therapy. Mol Med Today. 1996;2(11):460–7.
69. Limat A, Hunziker T, Waelti ER, Inaebnit SP, Wiesmann U, Braathen LR. Soluble factors from human hair papilla cells and dermal fibroblasts dramatically increase the clonal growth of outer root sheath cells. Arch Dermatol Res. 1993;285(4):205–10.
70. Won CH, Yoo HG, Kwon OS, Sung MY, Kang YJ, Chung JH, Park BS, Sung JH, Kim S, Kim KH. Hair growth promoting effects of adipose tissue-derived stem cells. J Dermatol Sci. 2010;57(2):134–7.
71. Yuan AR, Bian Q, Gao JQ. Current advances in stem cell-based therapies for hair regeneration. Eur J Pharmacol. 2020;881:173197.
72. Won CH, Park GH, Wu X, Tran TN, Park KY, Park BS, Kim DY, Kwon O, Kim KH. The basic mechanism of hair growth stimulation by adipose-derived stem cells and their secretory factors. Curr Stem Cell Res Ther. 2017;12(7):535–543V.
73. Kim WS, Park BS, Kim HK, Park JS, Kim KJ, Choi JS, Chung SJ, Kim DD, Sung JH. Evidence supporting antioxidant action of adipose-derived stem cells: protection of human dermal fibroblasts from oxidative stress. J Dermatol Sci. 2008;49(2):133–42.
74. Park BS, Jang KA, Sung JH, Park JS, Kwon YH, Kim KJ, Kim WS. Adipose-derived stem cells and their secretory factors as a promising therapy for skin aging. Dermatol Surg. 2008;34(10):1323–6V.
75. Park BS, Kim WS, Choi JS, Kim HK, Won JH, Ohkubo F, Fukuoka H. Hair growth stimulated by conditioned medium of adipose-derived stem cells is enhanced by hypoxia: evidence of increased growth factor secretion. Biomed Res. 2010;31(1):27–34.
76. Lee RH, Kim B, Choi I, Kim H, Choi HS, Suh K, Bae YC, Jung JS. Characterization and expression analysis of mesenchymal stem cells from human bone marrow and adipose tissue. Cell Physiol Biochem. 2004;14(4–6):311–24.
77. Fukuoka H, Tadayuki S, Ohkubo F. Hair regenerated therapy with growth factors in adipose-derived stem cells secreted protein. Jpn J Plast Surg. 2010;53:1095–104.
78. Fukuoka H, Suga H. Hair regeneration treatment using stem cell conditioned medium. Jpn J Plast Surg. 2012;55:1083–9.
79. Fukuoka H, Suga H, Narita, Watanabe R, Shintani S. The latest advance in hair regeneration therapy using proteins secreted by adipose-derived stem cells. Am J Cosmet Surg. 2012;29:273–82.
80. Fukuoka H, Suga H. Hair regeneration treatment using adipose-derived stem cell conditioned medium: follow-up with trichograms. Eplasty. 2015;15:e10.

81. Shin H, Ryu HH, Kwon O, Park BS, Jo SJ. Clinical use of conditioned media of adipose tissue-derived stem cells in female pattern hair loss: a retrospective case series study. Int J Dermatol. 2015;54(6):730–5V.
82. Perez-Meza D, Ziering C, Sforza M, Krishnan G, Ball E, Daniels E. Hair follicle growth by stromal vascular fraction-enhanced adipose transplantation in baldness. Stem Cells Cloning. 2017;10:1–10V.
83. Fukuoka H, Narita K, Suga H. Hair regeneration therapy: application of adipose-derived stem cells. Curr Stem Cell Res Ther. 2017;12(7):531–4.
84. Tsuboi R, Niiyama S, Irisawa R, Harada K, Nakazawa Y, Kishimoto J. Autologous cell-based therapy for male and female pattern hair loss using dermal sheath cup cells: a randomized placebo-controlled double-blinded dose-finding clinical study. J Am Acad Dermatol. 2020;83(1):109–16.
85. Owczarczyk-Saczonek A, Krajewska-Włodarczyk M, Kruszewska A, Banasiak Ł, Placek W, Maksymowicz W, Wojtkiewicz J. Therapeutic potential of stem cells in follicle regeneration. Stem Cells Int. 2018;2018:1049641.
86. Gentile P, Garcovich S. Advances in regenerative stem cell therapy in androgenic alopecia and hair loss: Wnt pathway, growth-factor, and mesenchymal stem cell signaling impact analysis on cell growth and hair follicle development. Cells. 2019;8(5):E466.
87. Alvarez X, Valenzuela M, Tuffet J. Clinical and histological evaluation of the Regenera® method for thetreatment of androgenetic alopecia. IEASRJ. 2018;3:2456–5040.
88. Alvarez X, Valenzuela M, Tuffet J. Microscopic and histologic evaluation of the Regenera® method forthe treatment of androgenetic alopecia in a small number of cases. IJRSMHS. 2017;2:19–22.
89. Gentile P. Autologous cellular method using micrografts of human adipose tissue derived follicle stem cells in androgenic alopecia. Int J Mol Sci. 2019;20(14):E3446.
90. Elmaadawi IH, Mohamed BM, Ibrahim ZAS, et al. Stem cell therapy as a novel therapeutic intervention for resistant cases of alopecia areata and androgenetic alopecia. J Dermatolog Treat. 2018;29(5):431–40.
91. Tak YJ, Lee SY, Cho AR, Kim YS. A randomized, double-blind, vehicle-controlled clinical study of hair regeneration using adipose-derived stem cell constituent extract in androgenetic alopecia. Stem Cells Transl Med. 2020;9(8):839–49.
92. https://clinicaltrials.gov/ct2/show/NCT01673789.
93. https://clinicaltrials.gov/ct2/show/NCT02865421.
94. https://clinicaltrials.gov/ct2/show/NCT03078686.
95. https://clinicaltrials.gov/ct2/show/NCT02849470.
96. https://clinicaltrials.gov/ct2/show/NCT03676400.
97. https://clinicaltrials.gov/ct2/show/NCT01501617.
98. Balañá ME, Charreau HE, Leirós GJ. Epidermal stem cells and skin tissue engineering in hair follicle regeneration. World J Stem Cells. 2015;7(4):711–27.
99. Abaci HE, Coffman A, Doucet Y, Chen J, Jacków J, Wang E, Guo Z, Shin JU, Jahoda CA, Christiano AM. Tissue engineering of human hair follicles using a biomimetic developmental approach. Nat Commun. 2018;9(1):5301.
100. Lee LF, Jiang TX, Garner W, Chuong CM. A simplified procedure to reconstitute hair-producing skin. Tissue Eng Part C Methods. 2011;17(4):391–400.
101. Asakawa K, Toyoshima KE, Ishibashi N, Tobe H, Iwadate A, Kanayama T, Hasegawa T, Nakao K, Toki H, Noguchi S, Ogawa M, Sato A, Tsuji T. Hair organ regeneration via the bioengineered hair follicular unit transplantation. Sci Rep. 2012;2:424.
102. Toyoshima KE, Asakawa K, Ishibashi N, Toki H, Ogawa M, Hasegawa T, Irié T, Tachikawa T, Sato A, Takeda A, Tsuji T. Fully functional hair follicle regeneration through the rearrangement of stem cells and their niches. Nat Commun. 2012;3:784.
103. Nakao K, Morita R, Saji Y, Ishida K, Tomita Y, Ogawa M, Saitoh M, Tomooka Y, Tsuji T. The development of a bioengineered organ germ method. Nat Methods. 2007;4(3):227–30.
104. Qiao J, Turetsky A, Kemp P, Teumer J. Hair morphogenesis in vitro: formation of hair structures suitable for implantation. Regen Med. 2008;3(5):683–92.
105. Fan Z, Miao Y, Qu Q, Xiao S, Wang J, Du L, Liu B, Hu Z. Unlocking the vital role of host cells in hair follicle reconstruction by semi-permeable capsules. PLoS One. 2017;12(6):e0179279.
106. McElwee KJ, Kissling S, Wenzel E, Huth A, Hoffmann R. Cultured peribulbar dermal sheath cells can induce hair follicle development and contribute to the dermal sheath and dermal papilla. J Invest Dermatol. 2003;121(6):1267–75V.
107. Stenn KS, et al. Future directions: bioengineering the hair follicle. In: Trüeb Ralph M, Desmond T, editors. Aging hair. 1st ed. Heidelberg: Springer; 2010. p. 239–48.
108. Jahoda CA, Oliver RF, Reynolds AJ, Forrester JC, Horne KA. Human hair follicle regeneration following amputation and grafting into the nude mouse. J Invest Dermatol. 1996;107(6):804–7.
109. Pisansarakit P, Moore GP. Induction of hair follicles in mouse skin by rat vibrissa dermal papillae. J Embryol Exp Morphol. 1986;94:113–9.
110. Ferraris C, Bernard BA, Dhouailly D. Adult epidermal keratinocytes are endowed with pilosebaceous forming abilities. Int J Dev Biol. 1997;41(3):491–8.
111. Jahoda CA, Oliver RF. Vibrissa dermal papilla cell aggregative behaviour in vivo and in vitro. J Embryol Exp Morphol. 1984;79:211–24.
112. Triel C, Vestergaard ME, Bolund L, Jensen TG, Jensen UB. Side population cells in human and mouse epidermis lack stem cell characteristics. Exp Cell Res. 2004;295(1):79–90. Erratum in: Exp Cell Res. 2007 Nov 1;313(18):3943.
113. Rochat A, Kobayashi K, Barrandon Y. Location of stem cells of human hair follicles by clonal analysis. Cell. 1994;76(6):1063–73.
114. Matsuzaki T, Inamatsu M, Yoshizato K. The upper dermal sheath has a potential to regenerate the hair in the rat follicular epidermis. Differentiation. 1996;60(5):287–97.

115. Paus R, Eichmüller S, Hofmann U, Czarnetzki BM, Robinson P. Expression of classical and non-classical MHC class I antigens in murine hair follicles. Br J Dermatol. 1994;131(2):177–83.
116. Inoue K, Aoi N, Yamauchi Y, et al. TGF-beta is specifically expressed in human dermal papilla cells and modulates hair folliculogenesis. J Cell Mol Med. 2009;13(11–12):4643–56.
117. Jahoda CA. Cell movement in the hair follicle dermis—more than a two-way street? J Invest Dermatol. 2003;121(6):ix–xi.
118. Yamao M, Inamatsu M, Ogawa Y, Toki H, Okada T, Toyoshima KE, Yoshizato K. Contact between dermal papilla cells and dermal sheath cells enhances the ability of DPCs to induce hair growth. J Invest Dermatol. 2010;130(12):2707–18.
119. Kwack MH, Yang JM, Won GH, Kim MK, Kim JC, Sung YK. Establishment and characterization of five immortalized human scalp dermal papilla cell lines. Biochem Biophys Res Commun. 2018;496(2):346–51.
120. Lin CM, Li Y, Ji YC, Huang K, Cai XN, Li GQ. Induction of hair follicle regeneration in rat ear by microencapsulated human hair dermal papilla cells. Chin J Traumatol. 2009;12(1):49–54.
121. Perez-Losada J, Balmain A. Stem-cell hierarchy in skin cancer. Nat Rev Cancer. 2003;3(6):434–43.
122. Stenbäck F. Adnexal participation in formation of cutaneous tumors following topical application of 9,10-dimethyl-benzanthracene. J Cutan Pathol. 1980;7(5):277–94.
123. Morris RJ, Fischer SM, Slaga TJ. Evidence that a slowly cycling subpopulation of adult murine epidermal cells retains carcinogen. Cancer Res. 1986;46(6):3061–6.
124. Morris RJ. Keratinocyte stem cells: targets for cutaneous carcinogens. J Clin Invest. 2000;106(1):3–8.
125. Hutchin ME, Kariapper MS, Grachtchouk M, et al. Sustained Hedgehog signaling is required for basal cell carcinoma proliferation and survival: conditional skin tumorigenesis recapitulates the hair growth cycle. Genes Dev. 2005;19(2):214–23.
126. Verhaegh ME, Arends JW, Majoie IM, Hoekzema R, Neumann HA. Transforming growth factor-beta and bcl-2 distribution patterns distinguish trichoepithelioma from basal cell carcinoma. Dermatol Surg. 1997;23(8):695–700V.
127. Stenn KS, Lawrence L, Veis D, Korsmeyer S, Seiberg M. Expression of the bcl-2 protooncogene in the cycling adult mouse hair follicle. J Invest Dermatol. 1994;103(1):107–11.
128. Oro AE, Higgins KM, Hu Z, Bonifas JM, Epstein EH Jr, Scott MP. Basal cell carcinomas in mice overexpressing sonic hedgehog. Science. 1997;276(5313):817–21.
129. Adolphe C, Narang M, Ellis T, Wicking C, Kaur P, Wainwright B. An in vivo comparative study of sonic, desert and Indian hedgehog reveals that hedgehog pathway activity regulates epidermal stem cell homeostasis. Development. 2004;131(20):5009–19.
130. Headington JT. Tumors of the hair follicle. A review. Am J Pathol. 1976;85(2):479–514.
131. Gailani MR, Sthle-Bäckdahl M, Leffell DJ, Glynn M, Zaphiropoulos PG, Pressman C, Undén AB, Dean M, Brash DE, Bale AE, Toftgrd R. The role of the human homologue of Drosophila patched in sporadic basal cell carcinomas. Nat Genet. 1996;14(1):78–81.
132. Johnson RL, Rothman AL, Xie J, Goodrich LV, Bare JW, Bonifas JM, Quinn G, Myers RM, Cox DR, Epstein EH Jr, Scott MP. Human homolog of patched, a candidate gene for the basal cell nevus syndrome. Science. 1996;272(5268):1668–71.
133. Tan JJY, Kang L. Engineering the future of hair follicle regeneration and delivery. Ther Deliv. 2018;9(5):321–4.
134. Lee LF, Chuong CM. Building complex tissues: high-throughput screening for molecules required in hair engineering. J Invest Dermatol. 2009;129(4):815–7.
135. Adenuga P, Summers P, Bergfeld W. Hair regrowth in a male patient with extensive androgenetic alopecia on estrogen therapy. J Am Acad Dermatol. 2012;67(3):e121–3.
136. https://www.fda.gov/consumers/consumer-updates/fda-warns-about-stem-cell-therapies.
137. https://www.engage.hoganlovells.com/knowledgeservices/news/times-up-new-enforcement-era-for-regenerative-medicines-begins-june-1.
138. Marks PW, Hahn S. Identifying the risks of unproven regenerative medicine therapies. JAMA. 2020;324(3):241–2.
139. Castro AR, Logarinho E. Tissue engineering strategies for human hair follicle regeneration: how far from a hairy goal? Stem Cells Transl Med. 2020;9(3):342–50.
140. Han C, Sun X, Liu L, Jiang H, Shen Y, Xu X, Li J, Zhang G, Huang J, Lin Z, Xiong N, Wang T. Exosomes and their therapeutic potentials of stem cells. Stem Cells Int. 2016;2016:7653489.

Index

P. J. Panagotacos, H. Maibach (eds.), *Hair Loss*, Updates in Clinical Dermatology,
https://doi.org/10.1007/978-3-031-74314-6

MIX
Papier aus verantwortungsvollen Quellen
Paper from responsible sources
FSC® C105338

If you have any concerns about our products,
you can contact us on
ProductSafety@springernature.com

In case Publisher is established outside the EU,
the EU authorized representative is:
Springer Nature Customer Service Center GmbH
Europaplatz 3, 69115 Heidelberg, Germany

Printed by Libri Plureos GmbH
in Hamburg, Germany